TRANSFERENCE-FOCUSED PSYCHOTHERAPY FOR BORDERLINE PERSONALITY DISORDER

A Clinical Guide

TRANSFERENCE-FOCUSED PSYCHOTHERAPY FOR BORDERLINE PERSONALITY DISORDER

A Clinical Guide

Frank E. Yeomans, M.D., Ph.D.

John F. Clarkin, Ph.D.

Otto F. Kernberg, M.D.

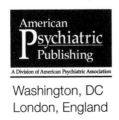

American Psychiatric Publishing

A Division of American Psychiatric Association

Washington, DC
London, England

If you would like to buy between 25 and 99 copies of this or any other American Psychiatric Publishing title, you are eligible for a 20% discount; please contact Customer Service at appi@psych.org or 800-368-5777. If you wish to buy 100 or more copies of the same title, please e-mail us at bulksales@psych.org for a price quote.

Manufactured in the United States of America on acid-free paper
18 17 16 15 14   5 4 3 2 1
First Edition

Typeset in Janson and HelveticNeueLt.

American Psychiatric Publishing

A Division of American Psychiatric Association
1000 Wilson Boulevard
Arlington, VA 22209-3901
www.appi.org

Library of Congress Cataloging-in-Publication Data
Yeomans, Frank E., 1949– , author.
  Transference-focused psychotherapy for borderline personality disorder : a clinical guide / Frank E. Yeomans, John F. Clarkin, Otto F. Kernberg. — First edition.
    p. ; cm.
  Includes bibliographical references and index.
  ISBN 978-1-58562-437-9 (pb : alk. paper)
  I. Clarkin, John F., author. II. Kernberg, Otto F., 1928– , author. III. American Psychiatric Association, issuing body. IV. Title.
  [DNLM: 1. Borderline Personality Disorder—therapy. 2. Psychotherapy—methods. 3. Transference (Psychology) WM 190.5.B5]
  RC569.5.B67
  616.85'8520651—dc23

                                                                    2014035770

British Library Cataloguing in Publication Data
A CIP record is available from the British Library.

CONTENTS

ABOUT THE AUTHORS

John F. Clarkin, Ph.D., is Codirector, Personality Disorders Institute, Weill Cornell Medical College; Clinical Professor of Psychology in Psychiatry, Weill Cornell Medical College, New York, New York

Otto F. Kernberg, M.D., is Director of the Personality Disorders Institute, Weill Cornell Medical College; Professor Emeritus, Weill Cornell Medical College; Training and Supervising Analyst, Columbia University Center for Psychoanalytic Training and Research, New York, New York

Frank E. Yeomans, M.D., Ph.D., is Clinical Associate Professor of Psychiatry, Weill Cornell Medical College; Director of Training, Personality Disorders Institute, Weill Cornell Medical College; Adjunct Associate Professor of Psychiatry, Columbia University Center for Psychoanalytic Training and Research, New York, New York

DISCLOSURE OF INTERESTS

The authors have indicated that they have no financial interests or other affiliations that represent or could appear to represent a competing interest with their contributions to this book.

PREFACE

TREATMENT DEVELOPMENT is a lengthy and highly technical process involving sequential steps from examination of the patient pathology to generating treatment principles and guidelines to the empirical investigation of the effectiveness of the treatment under various conditions. Under our leadership (Director Otto Kernberg, Codirector John Clarkin, and Director of Training Frank Yeomans), the Personality Disorders Institute (PDI) of the New York–Presbyterian Hospital/Weill Cornell Medical Center has pursued the examination and treatment of severe personality disorders since 1980. When we began this effort, we were joined by expert clinicians including Drs. Ann Appelbaum, Steven Bauer, Arthur Carr, Paulina Kernberg, Harold Koenigsberg, John Oldham, and Michael Selzer. Over the years, we have enhanced our group effort with expert clinicians (Monica Carsky, Jill Delaney, and Kay Haran) and expert clinician/researchers in psychopathology and psychotherapy (Nicole Cain, Eve Caligor, Diana Diamond, Karin Ensink, Mark Lenzenweger, Kenneth Levy, Kevin Meehan, Lina Normandin, Mallay Occhiogrosso, and Barry Stern). We have enjoyed the collaboration of neuroscientists BJ Casey, Michael Posner, and David Silbersweig.

Our first treatment manual for patients with borderline personality organization appeared in 1999 (Clarkin et al. 1999). However, the treatment approach that we describe, transference-focused psychotherapy (TFP), is not a static approach. As we have accumulated treatment experience with a wide range of patients with borderline pathology and as our understanding of the pathology has been enriched by theoretical advances and data from developmental and neurocognitive studies, the treatment itself has been amplified and further defined. Our specific goal continues to be one of organizing a treatment for the personality disorder itself, not only for symptoms derived from the pathological personality structure. Our long-range, ambitious goal is to modify the basic personality organization and structure of the person in treatment. In addition, technological advances also enable us to combine the written page with video demonstrations of various aspects of the treatment (available online at www.appi.org/Yeomans) in order to enhance the pedagogical usefulness of this volume. We thank Fatih Ozbay and Alexander Lau for their help in producing the videos and Victor Yalom and Psychotherapy.net for permission to reproduce sections of Video 1, Dr. Kernberg's structural interview. We are grateful to Michele Athena Morgen and Hendrik Grashuis for their skillful acting in our demonstration videos. We are also grateful to Liam Ó Broin for permission to use his drawing of a young girl on our cover. Mr. Ó Broin, who has painted a portrait of Dr. Kernberg, now has also illustrated a book that is central to his work.

The development and advancement of treatment for borderline personality disorders over the last 25 years has been nothing short of phenomenal. We at the PDI have been fortunate to have special contact with two other groups of scholars and researchers investigating this area. In the early years of our work, we were fortunate to have contact with Dr. Marsha Linehan and to profit from her consultation on our first treatment development grant funded by the National Institute of Mental Health. We also enjoyed her presence on our campus during a portion of her sabbatical year, and we had the opportunity to compare our approach with her developing ideas of dialectical behavior therapy.

We have also been most fortunate to enjoy collegial contact with Dr. Peter Fonagy and Dr. Anthony Bateman, the designers and developers of the mentalization-based approach to the treatment of borderline patients. As president of the International Psychoanalytical Association (IPA), Dr. Kernberg was instrumental in fostering an empirical approach to the psychoanalytic orientation to patient treatment. He was instrumental in fostering the Research Training Program (RTP) that is offered for developing scholars and researchers by the IPA and University College London. Since the inception of the RTP, Drs. Fonagy and Clarkin have worked together over 18 years and shared ideas, data, PowerPoint presentations, and many enjoyable hours in collaboration concerning the pathology and treatment of borderline patients.

At its most optimal, clinical and research progress is a collaborative venture. While we were developing and testing the effects of TFP on U.S. soil, we also fostered collegial contacts with clinical and scholarly groups in (roughly in this order) Germany, Austria, Canada, the Netherlands, Italy, Spain, Switzerland, Chile, the United Kingdom, Mexico, Brazil, Denmark, Turkey, Poland, Sweden, Argentina, and Australia. Through the vision and special efforts of Dr. Peter Buchheim, we were able to encourage and support a randomized clinical trial of TFP in Munich, Germany, and Vienna, Austria (Doering et al. 2010), the results of which enhanced our conviction that TFP could be effective in other Western cultures.

Through our work with TFP for adult patients with borderline personality organization, we have also written a treatment guide to apply TFP to patients with higher-level personality organization. This work was done with our colleague Dr. Eve Caligor (Caligor et al. 2007). In order to reach adolescents with borderline personality organization, we have developed TFP for this age group with colleagues Dr. Lina Normandin and Dr. Karin Ensink.

In New York, TFP has been introduced as a popular elective and postgraduate training program at the Columbia University Center for Psychoanalytic Training and Research. Online seminars and supervision groups have extended the training possibilities. A TFP module is being introduced in an increasing number of psychiatry residency training programs, including at Weill Cornell Medical College, NYU Langone Medical Center, and Mount Sinai Hospital. In addition, TFP is taught in graduate programs in clinical psychology, including the doctoral programs at City University of New York, Pennsylvania State University, and Université Laval.

This latest version of our treatment approach is, therefore, a collaborative product based on work done at the PDI in New York, by our colleagues in the United States, and by our international colleagues who are dedicated to the improvement of the treatment of patients with severe personality disorders. This collaborative effort not only is enjoyable but also enhances the applicability of the principles of TFP to different cultural contexts. For this, we are grateful.

This book is intended for all mental health professionals who work with individuals presenting with moderate to severe forms of personality disorder. Our research has been with patients having the DSM-IV diagnosis of borderline personality disorder (BPD; American Psychiatric Association 1994), but in this book we focus on the broader group of patients with borderline personality organization (BPO). In this book, the terms *borderline* and *borderline pathology* refer to BPO, a category that includes the more narrowly defined BPD. We discuss the basics of borderline pathology (Chapters 1 and 2) and describe the initial assessment and the strategies, tactics, and techniques of TFP (Chapters 3–7). In Chapters 8–10 we focus on the early, middle, and late phases of long-term treatment, with the goal of symptom and personality change. In Chapter 11 we review the various ways of understanding the trajectories of change in borderline patients in TFP.

In the early stages of our work, Dr. Gerald Klerman counseled us that a treatment manual should combine principles of intervention with clinical cases that illustrate the principles as applied in somewhat varied situations. We took that advice to heart, and throughout the book we combine in-depth discussion of individual cases with the principles of treatment. Given the diversity of severe personality disorder, every patient and his or her treatment are unique, and therefore we combine the principles of treatment as they are applied to the individual situation. The danger of any treatment manual is that it might be used as one would use numbered dots to construct a painting. A literal application of this manual would produce a lifeless product. Instead, we attempt to describe the preparation of the canvas, followed by the unfolding of the patient's internal world, in the lively, and often intense, interaction with the therapist over time. In this respect, we would like to acknowledge the patients we have had the opportunity to treat and thank them for all they have taught us. It is unfortunately still true that borderline personality disorder and those who have it are subject to continued misunderstanding, stigma, and a lack of adequate treatment resources. We would like to thank Bea and Michael Tusiani, Paul Tusiani-Eng, Dr. Winifred Christ, and the Borderline Personality Disorders Resource Center for their tireless work in addressing these problems.

This book is intended to inform the reader of the strategies, tactics, and techniques of TFP as applied over time in the treatment of patients with borderline personality disorder and borderline personality organization. To achieve this end, the book contains both the principles of the treatment and explication of the principles as applied to individual patients and their unique situations. This is the process that any practitioner will need to replicate: application of the principles of TFP to the specifics of the individual patient. This method does justice both to the long-term dynamic treatment that cannot be delivered effectively in a predetermined, lock-step fashion and to the individuality of the patient.

We owe a special note of gratitude to the two chairs of psychiatry at the Weill Cornell Medical College under whose guidance and support we have been privileged to work. Dr. Robert Michels and Dr. Jack Barchas have appreciated our efforts, encouraged persistence, and tolerated our mistakes.

Frank E. Yeomans
John F. Clarkin
Otto F. Kernberg

VIDEO GUIDE

A MAJOR ADDITION to this latest description of our treatment is the inclusion of video demonstrations of the treatment. The individualized nature of psychotherapy—specific to each patient-therapist dyad—necessitates some discussion of how to use the video examples that accompany this book. Like any real therapy session, they demonstrate a unique interaction that will not exactly resemble any other session. However, we have put together examples that provide relatively clear illustrations of the principles and techniques of the therapy in action. Each session is accompanied by a commentary that links the dialogue and interaction in the session to the material presented in the chapters on strategies, tactics, and techniques. Because therapy sessions are the intersection between a set of ideas and a shared experience, in the videos we try to demonstrate the therapist's need to "think on his feet" about what is going on between him and the patient and how the interaction relates to the patient's themes and to the therapist's own internal experience.

Video 1–1, "Description of Self and Description of Other," should be viewed after Chapter 4, "Assessment Phase." This video provides a brief window into the part of the structural interview when the therapist asks the patient to describe himself and to describe another person. The segment demonstrates how challenging these apparently simple questions are and shows the type of responses that might be given by someone whose internal structure is marked by identity diffusion. The other video segments demonstrate the use of the tactics and techniques of TFP. Videos 1–2 and 1–3 ("Technical Neutrality and Tactful Confrontation"), like Video 1–1, are excerpted from a demonstration video that is available in its entirety in *Psychoanalytic Psychotherapy* and can be found at http://www.psychotherapy.net/video/psychoanalytic-psychotherapy-otto-kernberg. These segments demonstrate the moment in therapy when the therapist has obtained enough information from the process of clarification to move on to tactful confrontations and early interpretations. They should be viewed after Chapter 6, "Techniques of Treatment."

Videos 2–1 and 2–2, "Prevacation Session," with Betty and Dr. Em, should also be viewed after Chapter 6. The commentary provided at the end of that chapter explicates how that first part of a session illustrates the interplay between elaborating the active dyad, attending to the treatment frame, and offering an interpretation. The session fragment also shows how containment and interpretation of an affect can help the patient move from acting it out to reflecting on it.

Videos 3–1, 3–2, and 3–3, "Affect Storm," should be viewed after Chapter 7, "Tactics of Treatment and Clinical Challenges." Although, as with the other videos, the elements of therapy are intertwined, this session illustrates how the therapist, Dr. Hamilton, deals with both a risk of the patient ending the treatment and an affect storm. Dr. Hamilton helps the patient, Carolyn, elaborate the experience of self and other that is underlying the problems and helps her gain awareness of other parts of her internal world that are split off and communicated by other channels of communication.

It should be noted that the videos are based on real therapy cases, but these cases have been 1) highly disguised and 2) combined into composite sessions to maintain the confidentiality of the patients. All of the patients who appear in the videos are actors, not actual patients, and any resemblance to real persons is purely coincidental. The reader should note that although the actors (Michele Athena Morgen and Frank Yeomans) are the same in "Prevacation Session" and "Affect Storm," the sessions represent two different therapies.

 Video Illustration: Video cues provided in the text identify the vignettes by title and run time.

The videos can be viewed online by navigating to www.appi.org/ Yeomans and using the embedded video player. The videos are optimized for most current operating systems, including mobile operating systems iOS 5.1 and Android 4.1 and higher.

VIDEO VIGNETTES

The reader should be aware that Videos 1-2 and 1-3 ("Technical Neutrality and Tactful Confrontation"); Videos 2-1 and 2-2 ("Prevacation Session"); and Videos 3-1, 3-2, and 3-3 ("Affect Storm") each represent a session that, for technical reasons, did not have the interruption that was required. The reader should consider each as a continuous session.

THE NATURE OF NORMAL AND ABNORMAL PERSONALITY ORGANIZATION

THE MODEL OF personality disorder and its treatment described in this book is based on contemporary psychoanalytic object relations theory as developed by Kernberg (1984, 1992) and amplified with current phenomenological and neurobiological research (Clarkin and De Panfilis 2013; Clarkin and Posner 2005; Depue and Lenzenweger 2001). A fundamental premise of a psychodynamic conceptualization and treatment of patients with personality disorders is that the observable behaviors and subjective disturbances of these patients reflect pathological features of underlying psychological structures and the way in which those structures enhance a satisfactory balance between the internal and external challenges that impinge on every individual. Consistent with this conceptualization, we first review the observable behaviors and symptoms of patients with borderline personality disorder (BPD). Following the review of the observable behaviors examined in the empirical literature, we then describe the nature of personality from an object relations point of view in terms of the underlying psychological structures that are hypothesized to guide the observable behaviors. Both the observable behaviors and the underlying structures inform our approach to a diagnostic nosology for personality pathology, assessment issues, and targets for therapeutic intervention.

In this chapter, we do not provide an extensive review of borderline pathology because that has been done elsewhere (Clarkin et al., in press). Our main goal in this chapter is to provide the clinician with a model of borderline pathology that is essential for expert assessment and treatment planning. It is helpful for the clinician to have both a general picture of borderline pathology as it is observed phenomenologically and a model of the mental representations of self and others that these patients have internalized from their developmental experiences. Despite the incomplete models of borderline pathology that exist in the field today (Lenzenweger and Clarkin 2005), the clinician needs an experience-near working model of the disorder to guide his or her moment-to-moment interventions in the interaction with the patient. Therefore, we describe borderline pathology in this chapter first from a phenomenological view and then from a structural view.

TWO APPROACHES TO BORDERLINE PATHOLOGY

Otto Kernberg and John Gunderson were instrumental in the description of borderline pathology and the articulation of the syndrome now called *borderline personality disorder,* as first defined in DSM-III (American Psychiatric Association 1980). The concept of preschizophrenic personality structure, borderline states, psychotic characters, and borderline personality grew out of clinical treatment experience with patients who were severely disturbed and multisymptomatic (Kernberg 1975). Knight (1954), for instance, described the ego weakness that led to severe regression in the transference and the need for modification of psychotherapeutic approaches. On the basis of his experiences with patients with severe personality disorder who were studied as part of the Psychotherapy Research Project of the Menninger Foundation, Kernberg (1975) described these patients as having a specific and stable pathological psychological structure differing from that in neurotic patients and from that in patients in the psychotic range, and he termed this group as having *borderline personality organization* (BPO). When in classical analytic treatment, these patients were prone to developing loss of reality testing and delusional ideas restricted to the transference. Using concepts of defensive splitting (Fairbairn 1943; Jacobson

1954, 1957, 1964; Klein 1946), Kernberg described these patients in terms of both descriptive pathology and the level of structural organization, involving lack of anxiety tolerance, poor impulse control, lack of developed sublimatory channels (ego weakness), and pathological internalized object relations.

When Kernberg (1975, 1984) was describing these patients in terms of descriptive pathology and structural characteristics, other researchers (Grinker et al. 1968; Gunderson and Kolb 1978) were using a purely descriptive approach to identify patients with intense affect, particularly anger and depression, and to indicate subgroups of these patients. Many of the descriptive characteristics of these patients were used to formulate the diagnosis of BPD for the first time in the diagnostic system (American Psychiatric Association 1980).

In the remainder of this chapter, we describe borderline pathology from a structural, object relations view. In Chapter 2, "Empirical Development of Transference-Focused Psychotherapy," we combine the structural understanding with the growing body of research on the behavioral and neurocognitive functioning of patients with borderline pathology.

BORDERLINE PATHOLOGY: STRUCTURAL ORGANIZATION

A fundamental premise of psychodynamic conceptualization and treatment of patients with personality disorders is that the observable behaviors and subjective disturbances of these patients reflect pathological features of underlying psychological structures. A *psychological structure* is a stable and enduring pattern of mental functions that organize the individual's behavior, perceptions, and subjective experience. A central characteristic of the psychological structure of patients with severe personality disorders is the nature and degree of integration of the sense of self and others. The level of personality organization as it relates to the severity of personality disorders—from normal to neurotic to borderline to psychotic—is largely dependent on this degree of integration.

Object relations theory (Jacobson 1964; Kernberg 1980; Klein 1957; Mahler 1971) emphasizes that the drives described by Sigmund Freud—libido and aggression—are always experienced in relation to a specific other, an object of the drive. *Internalized object relations* are the building blocks of psychological structures and serve as the organizers of motivation and behavior. These building blocks are units composed of a representation of the self and a representation of an other, linked by an affect related to or representing a drive (Figure 1–1). These units of self, other, and the affect linking them are *object relations dyads.* It is important to note that the self and the object in the dyad are neither accurate internal representations of the entirety of the self or the other nor accurate representations of real interactions in the past but rather are representations of the self and other as they were experienced and internalized at specific, affectively charged moments in time in the course of early development and then processed by internal forces such as primary affects and fantasies.

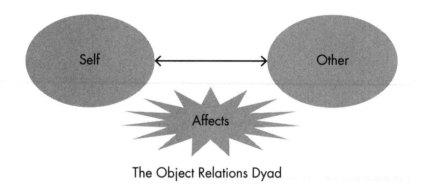

The Object Relations Dyad

FIGURE 1–1.   Theoretical underpinnings of transference-focused psychotherapy: object relations theory.

NORMAL PERSONALITY DEVELOPMENT AND ITS DEVIATIONS

Personality pathology is brought into sharp relief when contrasted with a clear conception of the functioning of the normal personality. In both assessment (Chapter 4, "Assessment Phase") and treatment, the therapist using transference-focused psychotherapy (TFP) constantly compares the functioning of the patient to that of an individual with a normal level of personality organization. Treatment goals are captured in the successive steps of helping a patient advance from abnormal personality functioning toward normal functioning (Table 1–1).

Personality represents the integration of behavior patterns with their roots in temperament, cognitive capacities, character, and internalized value systems (Kernberg and Caligor 2005). *Temperament* refers to the constitutionally based disposition to a pattern of reactions to internal and en-

TABLE 1–1.	Aspects of levels of personality organization		
	Borderline organization	**Neurotic organization**	**Normal organization**
Identity	Incoherent sense of self and others; poor investments in work, relations, leisure	Coherent sense of self and others but one element of psychic life not fully integrated; investments in work, relations, leisure	Integrated sense of self and others; investment in work, relations, leisure
Defenses	Use of primitive defenses	Use of more advanced defenses; rigidity	Use of more advanced defenses; flexibility
Reality testing	Variable empathy with social criteria of reality; some confusion and distortion of self versus nonself, internal versus external	Accurate perception of self versus nonself, internal versus external; empathy with social criteria of reality	Accurate perception of self versus nonself, internal versus external; empathy with social criteria of reality

vironmental stimuli; this includes the intensity, rhythm, and thresholds of affective responses. Constitutionally based thresholds for the activation of positive, pleasurable, rewarding affects and of negative and painful affects represent the most important link between biological and psychological aspects of personality (Kernberg 1994). The intensity, type, and range of affect exhibited by children in a developmental sequence are important in understanding BPO. Not surprisingly, affect is related to the caregiving context (Kochanska 2001). Attachment patterns between a mother and a child as young as 14 months are related to affect display in laboratory settings. In these settings, over time secure children become less angry, whereas insecure children demonstrate more negative affect.

Cognitive processes play a crucial role in the perception of reality and the organization of behavior toward articulated goals. Cognitive processes also play a crucial role in the development and modulation of affective responses. Cognitive representations of affect influence affect activation thresholds. These cognitive processes are crucial in the transformation of primitive affective states into complex emotional experiences. Through an integration of learning from models provided by caregivers and temperamental dispositions, cognitive capacities for attention regulation and effortful control are developed.

Character—the behavioral manifestation of identity—is the dynamic organization of behavior patterns that are characteristic of the particular individual. Character includes the level and degree of organization of behavior patterns and the degree of flexibility or rigidity of behaviors across environmental situations. Character reflects the effects of the integration of myriad internalized relations between self and others that contribute to internal models of behavior. The subjective consequence of character is the structure of identity, that is, the integration of all the self representations of these dyadic units into a stable and complex self concept, related to the complementary integration of object representations into integrated concepts of significant others. Character and identity are mutually complementary aspects. It is identity, composed of the concept, or concepts, of self and of significant others, that provides the psychological structure that determines the dynamic organization of character.

The internalization of significant object relations gives rise to one more crucial subjective structure of an integrated system of ethical values, which in psychoanalytic theory is designated as the *superego*. In the development of borderline pathology, disturbances of this structure have significant clinical, therapeutic, and prognostic implications.

NORMAL PERSONALITY ORGANIZATION

The individual with a normal personality organization has, first of all, an
1. integrated and coherent concept of self and of significant others that is captured in the concept of identity. This concept includes both an internal coherent sense of self and behavior that reflects self-coherence. This coherent
sense of self is basic to self-esteem, enjoyment, a capacity to derive pleasure
from relationships with others and from commitments to work, and a sense
of continuity through time. A coherent and integrated sense of self contributes to the realization of one's capacities, desires, and long-range goals.
Likewise, a coherent and integrated conception of others contributes to a
realistic evaluation of others, involving empathy and social tact, and thus
the ability to interact and relate successfully. An integrated sense of self and
of others contributes to the capacity for mature interdependence with others, which involves a capacity to make emotional commitments to others
while simultaneously maintaining self-coherence and autonomy. The capacity to establish intimate and stable love relations, and to integrate eroticism and tenderness in such relationships, is another consequence of a
coherent identity.

A second structural characteristic of normal personality organization is
2. the presence of a broad spectrum of affective experience. The individual
with normal personality organization has the capacity to experience a range
of complex and well-modulated affects without the loss of impulse control.
This capacity is related to both identity and an individual's level of defense
mechanisms. Defense mechanisms are those aspects of the psychological
apparatus that help an individual negotiate the anxiety related to conflicts
within the self (e.g., between loving feelings and hating feelings or between
urges and internal prohibitions against the urges) or between internal urges
and the exigencies of external reality. A coherent identity associated with
well-functioning psychological defenses allows the individual to experience
intense affects in the context of a consistent and solid foundation of internalized experience that helps the individual both understand and absorb the
affect. For individuals with personality disorders, a basic initial element of
therapy is to create a setting in which the therapist is able to contain the
intense affects that the patient has difficulty containing and therefore metabolizing symbolically through language.

A third characteristic of normal personality organization is the presence
3. of an integrated system of internalized values. With its developmental roots
in parental values and prohibitions, the mature system of internalized values is not rigidly tied to parental prohibitions but is stable, individualized,
and independent of external relations with others. This internal structure

of values is reflected in a sense of personal responsibility, a capacity for realistic self-appraisal and self-criticism, and decision making that is flexible and infused with a commitment to standards, values, and ideals.

DEVELOPMENTAL FACTORS

Internalized object relations dyads are the building blocks of psychological structure. In the course of infant development, multiple internal dyads are created on the basis of affectively intense experiences. These dyads become the prototypes of an individual's experience of self and other. Figure 1–2 illustrates several of the most prominent dyads, among many possible others, that are generally internalized in the course of development.

Object relations theory posits that the combination of an infant's temperament and experiences in affectively intense interactions with caretakers in the environment is crucial to development. The early interactions between infant and caregiver are the operative elements in the gradual internalization by the infant of a representation of the external world. These interactions are internalized in ways that are influenced by the infant's temperament. They involve both affective arousal and cognitive-perceptual elements. An optimal infant-caregiver interaction provides the infant with a nurturing and caring atmosphere in which he or she perceives the caregiver as loving and as accurately understanding the infant's needs, which are met in a satisfying rhythmic interchange (see Gergely and Watson 1996). In this context, the infant develops a secure attachment to the caregiver and begins to create a coherent internal narrative about self and other, with positive and joyful expectations that he or she is safe and cared for. This secure attachment helps the infant deal with the negative experiences—moments of discomfort and pain—that are inevitably part of the developmental path.

During relatively quiescent periods of low affective intensity, the infant takes in the surrounding environment with a general sort of cognitive learning depending on age and neuropsychological development. In contrast, the infant also experiences periods of high affective intensity. These periods are usually related to needs or wishes for pleasure ("I need help," "I want more") or to fears or wishes to get away from pain ("Get me away from that!"). The infant's affects are intense because affects have the biological function of helping immature mammals survive through pleasure/nurturance seeking and harm avoidance and through signaling needs via affect expression to the caregiver. A typical experience of pleasure or satisfaction occurs when the infant is acutely hungry and the mother is present and responds, whereas a typical experience of pain or frustration occurs when the caretaker, for whatever reason, does not respond to the infant's felt needs.

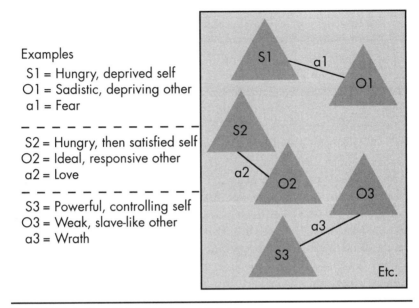

Examples

S1 = Hungry, deprived self
O1 = Sadistic, depriving other
a1 = Fear

- - - - - - - - - -

S2 = Hungry, then satisfied self
O2 = Ideal, responsive other
a2 = Love

- - - - - - - - - -

S3 = Powerful, controlling self
O3 = Weak, slave-like other
a3 = Wrath

FIGURE 1–2.   Infant's internal world.

Note.   a=affect; O=object representation; S=self representation.

During a child's early life, the intensity of these moments is not yet cushioned by a broad internalized context of experience.

These periods of peak affective intensity involve the self in relation to the other and are involved in the *laying down of affect-laden memory structures* in the developing psyche (see Figure 1–2). As stated by Kernberg (1992), "Peak-affect experiences may facilitate the internalization of primitive object relations organized along the axis of rewarding, or all-good, or aversive, or all-bad, ones. In other words, the experience of self and object when the infant is in a peak-affect state acquires an intensity that facilitates the laying down of affective memory structures" (p. 13). These affect-laden memory structures influence the developing individual's motivational system because under peak affect states an infant is likely to internalize what seems important for survival—that is, obtaining what is needed and avoiding what is painful or threatening.

With regard to the object relations dyads, the infant's satisfying experiences involve an ideal image of a perfect nurturing other and a content, satisfied self, whereas the frustrating experiences involve a totally negative image of a depriving or even sadistic other and a needy, helpless, anxious self. Although these images are representative of specific moments in time, rather than of the totality or continuity of the object, they are encoded in memory structures as a partial representation of a larger reality. This system is such that an infant whose caregiver is generally attentive and nurturing may nevertheless internalize images of a sadistic, depriving object because of experiences of temporary frustration or deprivation. In a similar fashion, an infant whose caregiver is generally neglectful or abusive may have rare satisfying experiences that, in combination with a longing for gratification, lead to an internalized image of a loving, nurturing object.

Disruptions in the infant-caregiver interaction lead to deviations in this optimal developmental path that may cause negative experiences to take on a more dominant role in the developing mind. The conception of self and others develops from an early age and depends on the emergence of language and the encoding of semantic (objective information about the world) and episodic (reexperiencing of past events) memories. Autobiographical memory is referred to as that form of episodic memory that forms personal and long-lasting conceptions of one's own story over time (Nelson and Fivush 2004). There is a sequence in the development of self representations, progressing from unrealistically positive or negative evaluations with all-or-none thinking in childhood to the presence of positive and negative evaluations with the ability to integrate opposing attributes in middle to late childhood (Harter 1999).

Disruptions in the relationship between the child and caregivers and/or the presence of trauma have a profound effect on the developing conception of self and others (Harter 1999). Early sexual abuse occurs in the history of some borderline patients, and caregiver neglect, indifference, and empathic failures have been identified as additional factors with profound deleterious effects (Cicchetti et al. 1990; Westen 1993). Children reared in these disturbed environments form insecure attachments with their primary caregivers (Cicchetti et al. 1990; Westen 1993) that interfere with the development of capacities for effortful control and self-regulation, and the internalization of conceptions of self and other are compromised by intense negative affect and defensive operations that distort the information system in an attempt to avoid pain.

MOTIVATIONAL ASPECTS: AFFECTS AND INTERNAL OBJECT RELATIONS

Affects are the inborn dispositions that emerge in the early stages of human development. Constitutionally and genetically determined experiences of positive and negative affect are gradually organized into broader drives, involving motivation, as the affects associated with specific relationship dyads sort out into broader positive and negative segments. Gratifying, pleasurable affects are organized as libido, whereas painful, aversive, negative affects are organized as aggression. It is the affectively driven development of an individual's set of internal object relations, based on interactions that were experienced and then elaborated by unconscious fantasy processes, that is laid down in memory and becomes the individual's inner world of object relations—that is, images of self and object representations with their affective charge. Affects, then, are the building blocks of the drives, and they signal the activation of drives in the context of particular internalized object relations.

In the course of the infant's development, multiple affectively charged experiences are internalized in such a way that a segment of the psyche is built up with these idealized images on the basis of satisfying experiences on one side, and a segment is built up with negative, aversive, hostile images on the other. In early development, an active separation of these segments develops within the psyche (Figure 1–3).

In the normally developing child, there is a gradual integration, over the first few years of life, of these extreme good and bad representations of self and others that results in internal representations of self and objects[1] that are more complex and realistic—acknowledging the reality that every person is a mix of good and bad attributes and is capable of being satisfying at some times and frustrating at others (Figure 1–4).

In patients who will develop borderline pathology, this process of integration does not evolve, and a more permanent division between the idealized and persecutory sectors of peak affect experiences remains as a stable, pathological intrapsychic structure (see Figure 1–3). Dyads such as those seen in Figure 1–2 play a prominent role in this split internal structure: the "hungry, deprived self" may be experienced as the "victim" in relation to the "sadistic, depriving other," and the "hungry, then satisfied self" may be experienced as the "perfectly loved object" of the "ideal, responsive other." This separation "protects" the idealized representations, imbued with warm, loving feelings toward the object perceived as satisfying, from the negative representations that are associated with the affects of anxiety, rage, and hatred. One aspect of object relations theory that distinguishes it from a more purely cognitive psychology is the emphasis that these representa-

---

[1]The term *other* refers to people in the individual's life. The term *object representation* refers to the representation in the mind of the object of affects and drives. The object representation derives from experiences with others but does not correspond exactly to their objective reality.

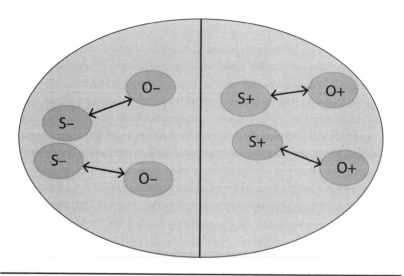

FIGURE 1-3. Split organization: consciousness of all-bad or all-good internal representations.

O=object representation; S=self representation.

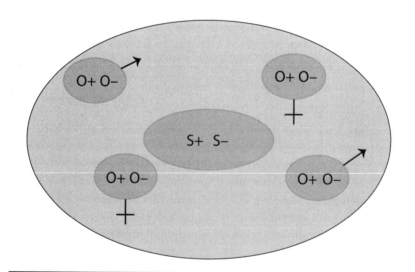

FIGURE 1-4. Normal organization: integration with awareness of complexity.

O=object representation; S=self representation.

tions are not merely cognitive images but also are connected to intense primitive affects, including hatred of the depriving object. Because hatred is defined by the wish to destroy, a separation of the good and bad segments is necessary in this primitive psychic organization to protect the "ideal" representations of self and object from the danger of destruction by the hatred associated with the "bad" ones. This separation is the internal mechanism of splitting, which is the paradigm of primitive defense mechanisms and is central to borderline pathology. Although this radical splitting of affects into extreme opposite camps does not help an individual adapt well to the complexity of external reality, it nonetheless provides a modicum of relief from anxiety in that it provides a first attempt at organizing the confusing mix of affects an individual experiences in response to the world and therefore may be hard for an individual to abandon as the process of change puts that system into question.

Melanie Klein (1946) referred to this split internal world as the *paranoid-schizoid position*, characterized by all-good and all-bad internal representations. The schizoid quality of this position comes from its split nature. The paranoid quality comes from the tendency to project the "bad" persecutory object onto external objects and therefore to live in fear of aggression from the outside. This psychological structure is thus an obstacle to intimacy because getting close to someone means getting close to a likely source of aggression. In the course of normal development, individuals evolve beyond the split paranoid-schizoid position to achieve an integrated and more nuanced psychological structure that acknowledges the blend of loving and aggressive affects in the self and in others; the individual moves from the realm of extremes, which includes only the possibilities of either the perfect other or self or the totally negative self or other, to the realm of more realistic and complex representations that can still be "good enough." Klein labeled this latter psychological structure the *depressive position* for two reasons. First, it entails the loss of and need to mourn the unrealistic ideal image of provider and of self, a difficult step that might involve the shift of the quest for the ideal to more symbolic realms such as art or spirituality. Second, it involves accepting one's own aggression that had previously been experienced as existing solely in others, leading to the experience of guilt and remorse that accompanies the conscious awareness of aggression that might have been acted out toward others with no awareness or guilt when those others were perceived through the lens of the internal all-bad object. A goal of TFP is to help the patient advance from the paranoid-schizoid position to the depressive position, with further work to then resolve issues of the depressive position and achieve a harmonious psychological balance.

If the infant cannot avoid what is bad and obtain what is good, he or she signals the caregiver for help. The caregiver with a capacity to read those signals knows how to respond, in terms of both behavior and expression of affect (Fonagy et al. 2007). However, if the interactional system between infant and caregiver is distorted by abnormal attachment, characterized by a mismatch between signal and response, the infant suffers from overwhelming negative affect. A result of this process is that normal integration of affectively opposite experiences does not take place: the child does not internalize the fact that frustration can be tolerated in the context of knowing that a generally reliable system is in place. As these negative experiences accumulate, there develops an entire motivational system, a dissociated motivational system that functions independently from the positive rewarding one, which engenders a series of mental mechanisms to deal with the intensity of negative affects. Projective defense mechanisms attempt to get rid of negative affect and perceive it as coming from the outside. Other primitive defense mechanisms idealize some relationships as protection against danger from activation of negative affects. Unrealistic idealized distortions alternate with unrealistic paranoid distortions.

This alternation of distortions has an impact on relational systems in that an individual experiencing internal conflict may feel well ("I am safe") but then suddenly experience aggression as threatening from the outside. With the development of an exaggerated, hypertrophied negative segment of affective experience, the individual becomes both hyperalert to any potentially negative stimulus and hyperreactive to negative and threatening experiences. The way to survive is to withdraw or to counterattack, leading to difficulty identifying with others and deficits in the internalized morality that is based on identification with a consistent system of shared values. This process creates an interruption to the developing mental social system.

Eventually, in the course of normal development, patterns of behavior are established by which the intense motivational system of splitting off and projecting negative affects is modulated and integrated into the individual's adaptive mechanisms and general aspirations, improving adaptation to the complexity of the real world. However, in borderline individuals the split between the extreme negative and idealized segments of the psyche remains intact, impeding the development of an integrated sense of who they are and leaving relationships with others seriously distorted. These individuals cannot acquire an integrated sense of self that would permit them to accurately evaluate their specific mental state and that of others in the light of a generally balanced view of self and human interactions. These concepts have more recently been taken up and studied in the theory of mentalization (Bateman and Fonagy 2004).

Finally, important to the organization and guidance of patterns of behavior is the system of internalized values. This moral compass is derived developmentally from the internalization of parental and cultural demands and prohibitions in the first phase of moral development and coherent realistic values as the system matures. From a psychoanalytic object relations view, the development of a coherent system of moral values is related to the successful integration of internal representations of self and others. Moral development proceeds from harsh internalized punitive voices to identification with a harmonious system of consistent values (Jacobson 1964). In a series of studies, Kochanska and colleagues have traced the development of effortful control with the emergence of conscience. During early childhood, effortful control emerges by age 45 months as a traitlike attribute. Children with higher effortful control have greater conscience development and fewer externalizing problems (Kochanska and Knaack 2003).

In summary, healthy and adaptive self-reflection depends on a series of mechanisms: the internalization of dyadic relationships with the integration of concept of self and integration of concept of significant others. The latter also enables one to acquire a view of the other person in depth and judge the concrete behavior of another in the context of the overall pattern of that person's behavior. Interpretation of the self concept enables one to differentiate and circumscribe a momentary affect state within the context of one's more complex affective dispositions. If evaluation of the other in total is distorted by the projection of narrow internal images, one cannot reflect realistically about the other—one cannot see beyond the internal object representation that he or she triggers in the immediate interaction. This leads to thinking that how the other person is right now defines him or her, in contrast to being able to judge another person beyond that person's emotional state and actions in the moment.

A picture emerges of a developmental pathway characterized by the confluence of effortful control and other self-regulatory skills emerging in the context of a nurturing and securely rhythmic and predictable relationship between child and caregiver. The interaction of the benevolent, empathic, and attentive caregiver and the child yields growing self-regulation, the predominance of positive over negative affect, the beginnings of conscience, and increasingly smooth interactions with peers. This path of normal development may be disrupted by a genetic constitution characterized by abnormally intense levels of affect activation (temperament) and/or an environment characterized by physical or emotional neglect or by physical or sexual abuse. The result is a child who demonstrates predominantly negative affect, poor self-regulation, disruptions in conceptions of self and others, and disturbed relations with peers. Although no developmental studies of borderline patients yet exist, this emerging picture resembles the adult presentation of BPO with its identity diffusion, preponderance of negative affect, poor self-regulation, and compromised relations with others.

AN OBJECT RELATIONS MODEL OF NOSOLOGY

Consistent with our fundamental premise that one can understand personality and its pathology only by examining observable behavior with reference to subjective experience and the underlying psychological structures, we have constructed a psychoanalytic model of nosology based on these elements. Figure 1–5 illustrates a theoretical classification of personality disorders that combines categorical (i.e., DSM-5 disorders [American Psychiatric Association 2013] and other personality disorders) and dimensional constructs (i.e., relative severity of pathology, relative degree of infusion of mental life with aggression, and introversion vs. extroversion) for understanding the entire realm of personality disorder.

At the behavioral level, personality pathology is manifest in inhibition of normal behaviors and/or exaggeration of certain behaviors (e.g., sexual inhibition or sexual promiscuity) and also the presence of oscillation between contradictory behaviors. At the structural level, the personality can be organized either with a coherent and integrated sense of self and others or without this coherent sense of identity (identity diffusion). By considering the concept of identity along with related concepts of defense mechanisms, reality testing, object relations, aggression, and moral values, one can conceptualize levels or degrees of pathology of personality organization, ranging from healthy to increasingly dysfunctional organization as one progresses from normal to neurotic to borderline to psychotic personality organization (see Table 1–1).

NEUROTIC PERSONALITY ORGANIZATION

In contrast to patients with BPO, patients with neurotic personality organization (NPO) have an integrated identity (i.e., integrated sense of self and others). These patients generally use mature defensive operations that are organized around repression rather than splitting; that is, they more successfully keep their disturbing thoughts and affects at bay. These defensive operations do not lead to abrupt changes in affect states or manifest behavioral characteristics that acutely distort the patient's life experience and interpersonal interactions. Neurotic defenses, in contrast to splitting, involve integrated, ego-syntonic representations of self and objects that have combined into a complex whole that defines a consistent self concept and a re-

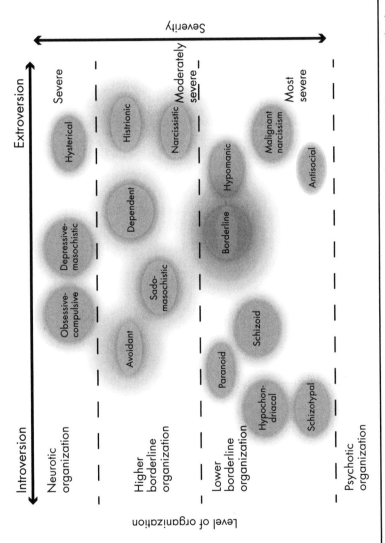

FIGURE 1–5. Structured diagnoses: classification of personality disorders combining categorical and dimensional constructs.

Severity reflects 1) identity diffusion, 2) predominance of primitive defenses, and 3) intensity of aggression.

alistic repertoire of representations of others that provide a stability lacking in BPO. A typical example of this is reaction formation. A neurotic individual with a conflict around aggression might function in accordance with a predominant sense of self as a polite but subservient individual in relation to a powerful authority while consistently repressing from consciousness a single isolated dyad, not integrated with the otherwise coherent sense of self, that involves a rebellious self aggressively challenging a sadistic authority. This latter dyad is consistently repressed and has no access to consciousness in the neurotic individual except in the case of regression, such as an explosive angry outburst, dreams, or neurotic symptoms such as anxiety when a rebellious urge comes close to consciousness. In most circumstances, this individual would demonstrate an even level of functioning, albeit limited in the fulfillment of competitive strivings. Neurotic level personality disorders, including hysterical personality disorder, obsessive-compulsive personality disorder, and depressive-masochistic personality disorder (diagnoses not found in DSM-5), are the least severe personality disorders (see Figure 1–5).

BORDERLINE PERSONALITY ORGANIZATION

Patients with BPO experience primitive intense emotions that are not linked to each other internally; therefore, whatever emotion is experienced in the moment overwhelms the patient's subjective experience, becomes his or her entire sense of reality, and impairs his or her ability to cognitively assess situations accurately. Although aware of the cognition associated in his or her mind with the intense affect, the patient is not effective in appraising the external situation. This is not simply affect dysregulation but rather dysregulation of cognition and affect.

The borderline level of personality organization includes both specific personality disorders described in DSM-5 and other personality disorders not mentioned in DSM-5 (hypomanic personality disorder, sadomasochistic personality disorder, hypochondriacal personality disorder, and the syndrome of malignant narcissism) (Kernberg and Caligor 2005).

Constituent Elements of Borderline Personality Organization

Patients with BPO are characterized by the fragmented nature of their identity, the use of primitive defenses, generally intact but fragile reality testing, impaired affect regulation and sexual and aggressive expression, inconsistent internalized values, and poor quality of relations with others (see Table 1–1).

The pathological structure of BPO consists of a lack of integration of the primitive positive (idealized) and negative (persecutory) segments of early object relations that were laid down as memory traces in the course of early intense affective experiences. This lack of internal integration—of a coherent sense of self and coherent representation of significant others—constitutes the syndrome of identity diffusion, the opposite of a normal identity and sense of self. Clinically, the lack of integration of these internal representations of self and others becomes evident in the patient's nonreflective, contradictory, or chaotic experience of self and others and in the inability to integrate or even to become aware of these contradictions.

Behavioral correlates of this borderline psychic structure include emotional lability, anger, interpersonal chaos, impulsive self-destructive behaviors, and proneness to lapses in reality testing (i.e., the types of symptoms described in DSM-5). A typical specific manifestation of this diffuse and fragmented identity is the abrupt shift from a calm moment in a relationship to rage because of a perceived slight.

Primitive Defenses

The predominant use of primitive defensive operations is manifest in behaviors that interfere with the patient's functioning and, in the context of therapy, distort the patient-therapist interaction in ways that become material to work on. The purpose of defense mechanisms in general is to negotiate conflicts among the competing pressures exerted by affect states and drives, internalized prohibitions against drives, and external reality. Successful mature defenses minimize the anxiety stemming from these conflicts and maximize the individual's ability to act flexibly and succeed in love and work. In the course of normal psychological development, individuals proceed from the primitive defenses, such as splitting, that predominate in infancy and childhood as a first attempt to establish some order among the internal forces in conflict to the mature defenses that predominate in the psychological life of the healthy individual, such as rationalization, intellectualization, humor, and sublimation.

Primitive defenses are a first attempt to deal with anxiety, but they are rigid and inflexible and do not allow for successful adaptation in life. They emerge in the first years when the developing child is attempting to cope with the interface of intense affects and their related drives in relation to each other and in relation to external reality. The first effort at protecting from the anxiety of colliding libidinal and aggressive affects is to strictly separate these affects, as well as to separate the objects of these affects. Primitive defenses are organized around *splitting*, the radical separation of good and bad affect, of good and bad object. These defense mechanisms are an attempt to protect an idealized segment of the individual's psyche, or internal world, from an aggressive segment (see Figure 1–3). This separation,

[handwritten margin note: Defense Mech's in general]

which provides a certain sense of order (i.e., of distinguishing good from bad and attempting to distinguish self from other), is maintained at the expense of the integration of the images in the psyche. Because these defenses can impede successful cognitive processing of the external world or of internal affects, they often lead to behavioral manifestations of distress rather than internal mastery of it.

This split internal organization of the psyche imposes itself on the individual's perception of the world, which is experienced in categorical terms. Opinions are strong, but they are not stable. Things are good or bad in such an extreme way that there is a poor fit with reality. The good must be so completely good that any failing or shortcoming catapults it into the bad category. Consequently, what is good and what is bad can quickly shift according to the immediate circumstances. These sudden changes contribute to the chaotic nature of the borderline individual's experience. If the individual feels a friend has disappointed her, that person may be abruptly relegated to a "blacklist"; later, a positive experience may shift things back as the wish to find the totally good object comes back into play. The good versus bad responses to the world influence the individual's moods: a single frustration may make everything seem bleak, resulting in a depressed mood. A happy surprise may shift everything temporarily to euphoria. The rigid good versus bad categories provide little flexibility for dealing with the complexity of the world and, in particular, of interpersonal interactions. The individual is not able to appreciate the subtle shadings of a situation or to tolerate ambiguity. The individual is predisposed to distortions in perceptions because external reality is filtered through the rigid and primitive internal structure of self and object representations. Splitting does not provide for successful adaptation to life and can explain much of the emotional and interpersonal chaos and symptoms of patients with BPO.

In the borderline individual in whom splitting predominates, each part of the split has access to consciousness and to expression, although in a discontinuous, abrupt, and dissociated form. This individual experiences, in a chaotic way, contradictory thinking, affects, and behaviors. When split-off material enters consciousness, it does so with the full accompanying affect, resulting in the experience of intense emotional chaos.

Splitting, or primitive dissociation, can be manifested by projective identification, an unconscious tendency to induce in another person affect states that are difficult to tolerate; the other individual is made the repository of the dissociated affect that the self cannot tolerate. This concept will be very important in the therapist's interactions with the patient as the therapist's awareness of what he or she is "made to feel" in the interaction provides valuable information about what the patient has difficulty integrating within himself or herself. Projective identification is intimately linked with the defense of omnipotent control (Kernberg 1995). The patient who has deposited unwanted parts of the self into another feels the need to control the other person because the projection of that part of the self makes the other seem dangerous and threatening (e.g., a source of anger, aggression, abandonment). Primitive idealization, devaluation, and denial are other dominant primitive mechanisms that complement or reinforce splitting, projective identification, and omnipotent control. Primitive denial involves the conscious cognitive awareness of an affective state or behavior that the individual experiences at another time but without any capacity for emotional connection with that experience at the present time.

Reality Testing

Individuals with both borderline and neurotic personality organization can experience intact reality testing—that is, the capacity to identify with ordinary social criteria of reality. However, the borderline patient's reality testing is subject to fluctuation not found in neurotic patients. Borderline patients typically lack subtle tactfulness in social interactions, particularly under stress, and may regress to paranoid thinking related to lack of clarity about whether an affect "in the room" stems from the patient or from the other person in the interaction. There can be confusion as to which elements of an interaction come from the self and which come from the other. In contrast, neurotic personality organization presents with a more fine-tuned sense of tactfulness, empathy, discretion, and self-reflection.

Object Relations

In normal development, the internal object relations dyads become linked and develop into the larger organizing structures making up the mature psychic apparatus: the id, the ego, and the superego (Kernberg 1980). Relatively stable conflicts among these psychic structures underlie neurotic symptoms. Borderline individuals remain at the level of more fragmented, and not necessarily accurate, internal representations of self and others that correspond to a psychological landscape of more isolated impulses and prohibitions, in contrast to an organized system of them. This results, first, in a view of the world in which loving nurturing objects and punitive depriving objects alternate with no realistic middle ground and, second, in a poorly developed sense of self with shifts from experiencing oneself (more or less consciously) as needy and helpless to experiencing oneself as omnipotent. Disturbed object relations are manifested in a lack of capacity for empathy with others and a lack of mature evaluation of others. Because others are perceived alternately as idealized or persecutory and/or devalued, the borderline individual has difficulty establishing and maintaining relationships in depth and, in particular, intimate relationships. Corresponding to this, sexual pathology takes the form of either inhibition of sexual experience or chaotic sexuality.

A particular variant of BPO that is common in clinical practice is narcissistic personality disorder (NPD). Individuals with NPD share the identity diffusion characteristic of all personality disorders organized at the borderline level. However, their defensive structure differs in that, in an attempt to escape the distress and sense of emptiness associated with identity diffusion, individuals with NPD retreat into an imaged grandiose self that can appear integrated but is fragile and brittle in that it does not correspond to objective reality. Patients with NPD constitute an increasing challenge in clinical practice. Although the methods of TFP outlined in this book apply to therapy for patients with NPD, practical constraints have kept us from including a full discussion of narcissistic pathology and modifications of TFP to address the particular challenges of NPD. A fuller discussion of these topics is available elsewhere (Diamond et al. 2011; Stern et al. 2013; D. Diamond, F.E. Yeomans, and B.L. Stem, A Clinical Guide for Treating Narcissistic Pathology: A Transference Focused Psychotherapy, in preparation).

Moral Values

The mature superego is constituted developmentally by successive layers of value systems related to internalized self and object representations (Jacobson 1964; Kernberg 1984). The first developmental layer reflects the demanding and primitive morality experienced by the child as caregivers make demands that prohibit the expression of aggressive, sexual, and dependent impulses. The second layer is constituted by the ideal representations of self and object a reflection of early childhood ideals. The third layer of the superego evolves as the earliest persecutory level and the later idealizing level of superego functions are integrated, toned down, and made more realistic, facilitating the internalization of more realistic parental and cultural demands and prohibitions. This third layer of integrated superego operating as an internalized value system allows the individual to be less dependent on external confirmation and behavior control and capable of deeper commitments to values and to others. It undergoes processes of abstraction, generalization, and individualization that usually are completed by late adolescence.

The extent of superego pathology, which at its most extreme involves antisocial traits, is particularly important in terms of its negative prognostic implications for all psychotherapeutic approaches to the personality disorders. This overriding prognostic indicator is matched in importance only by the presence (or absence) of intense relationships with significant others, chaotic or disturbed as they may be. The more severe the antisocial traits are and the more isolated the patient is over an extended period of time, the worse the prognosis is. Conversely, severe personality disorders with maintained interpersonal behavior and absence of antisocial features can present a positive prognosis for psychotherapy.

Aggression

We previously discussed the central role of the constitutionally derived affects that are the earliest powerful motivators of human behavior (see section "Borderline Pathology: Structural Organization"). These affects emerge in the earliest stages of development, and through interaction with the environment and especially the major caregivers, the pleasurable, gratifying affects are organized as libido and the painful, negative affects are organized as aggression. Sexual excitement constitutes the core affect of libido, which evolves out of the early experiences of elation and body surface sensual pleasures. The erotic system gradually acquires a central role in the integration of positive affective systems—that is, libido. Aggression is related to the origins of the more differentiated affects of irritability, anger, rage, envy, and hatred.

Affects are the primary psychological motivators in the sense that one seeks what is desirable and tries to flee from what is undesirable, painful, or harmful. A complex variant is an abnormal development of the generally normal integration of positive and negative affective systems—namely, the recruitment of sexual pleasure at the service of aggression through inordinate sadism or pleasure in self-harming. Under these circumstances, the experience of aggression becomes a source of pleasure. Regardless of the cause of the negative affect—either constitutional negative affect and/or environmentally mediated experiences of trauma, disturbed relationships with caregivers, or overwhelming pain—its internalized representations and related distortions have an important impact on what the individual feels and how he or she perceives things.

Patients with low-level BPO (toward the bottom of Figure 1–5) suffer from more overt aggression that invades their object relations and thus have more serious lacunae in superego development than do patients with high-level BPO. In terms of DSM diagnoses, patients with low-level BPO are likely to have BPD with comorbid narcissistic, paranoid, and antisocial personality disorder or traits. Patients with low-level BPO are more difficult to treat than are patients with high-level BPO and at times approach the limits of treatability (Koenigsberg et al. 2000a; Stone 2006). Patients in the less severe group (upper part of Figure 1–5) demonstrate a greater proportion of libidinal affect (albeit frustrated) in relation to aggressive affect, a greater capacity for dependent relationships with significant others, more capacity for investing in work and social relations, and fewer nonspecific manifestations of ego weakness.

Object Relations Nosology and DSM-5

The DSM system has the tendency to anchor the diagnostic criteria to observable behaviors. The limitation in this approach is that the same behaviors can have very different functions and meaning (Horowitz 2004) depending on the underlying personality organization (Kernberg and Caligor 2005). Behaviors related to social timidity or inhibition, for example, may contribute to a diagnosis of schizoid or avoidant personality disorder, yet these same surface behaviors may, in fact, reflect the cautiousness of a paranoid individual or the reticence of a narcissistically grandiose individual to expose his or her deep yearnings.

In light of the history noted earlier in this chapter of the concepts of BPD and BPO that predated DSM-III (see section "Two Approaches to Borderline Pathology"), it is interesting to consider the two views of the personality disorders presented in DSM-5. After fierce debate and disagreement, the personality disorder categories from DSM-IV (American Psychiatric Association 1994) have been retained in DSM-5, but the deliberations of the Personality Disorders Work Group are presented in DSM-5 Section III, "Emerging Measures and Models," as the "Alternative DSM-5 Model for Personality Disorders." The core of personality disorder is defined in the alternative model as disturbances in self and interpersonal functioning. *Self-functioning* is described by the domains of identity and self-direction, and *interpersonal functioning* is described by the domains of empathy and intimacy. This definition, adapted by the Personality Disorders Work Group, is in line with a growing consensus in the field that self and other functioning is at the center of personality and personality disorder (Bender and Skodol 2007; Gunderson and Lyons-Ruth 2008; Horowitz 2004; Livesley 2001; Meyer and Pilkonis 2005; Pincus 2005). This is a view that has long been espoused in object relations theory (Kernberg 1984). These difficulties in self and interpersonal functioning are intertwined and lead to the final common pathway of subjective experience and interpersonal behavior.

The revised and improved definition of personality disorder in DSM-5 Section III may lead to a more refined assessment of the core aspects of personality disorder and to advancements in the assessment of outcome of treatment for individuals with these disorders. To date, the treatments for personality disorder have concentrated on the reduction of symptom behaviors and feelings. Although various treatments have resulted in significant changes in symptoms, the core issues of self-functioning and interpersonal functioning have received less attention. The alternative DSM-5 model balances attention to personality disorder diagnoses or types with dimensional traits that capture important domains of dysfunction with estimates of severity. The alternative model includes five broad domains of personality trait variation: negative affectivity, detachment, antagonism, disinhibition, and psychoticism. The object relations concept of identity includes investment in relations with others, which would relate to traits of antagonism and detachment. The object relations concept of reality testing includes but is broader than the trait of psychoticism. The traits of negative affect and antagonism are similar to the dimension of aggression in the object relations model. The object relations concept of moral values is not covered in the traits of the alternative DSM-5 model.

Traits are chosen to describe individuals in terms of their stable patterns across environmental situations. Because this is basically a descriptive process, trait theory fails to explain how or why the behaviors occur. Only with the study of personality processes can one begin to understand how and in what way personality traits have their impact (Hampson 2012). By understanding both personality traits and personality processes (e.g., emotion regulation) (Cervone 2005; Mischel and Shoda 2008), one can achieve a fuller picture of personality functioning. This fuller picture has implications for the clinical assessment of the individual with suspected personality pathology. The rating of salient traits and their severity is only the first step in treatment planning and must be followed with interview assessment of the situations in which the troublesome trait is manifested and with details about the specific context.

Key Clinical Concepts

- Object relations theory postulates that human drives are always experienced in a relation between self and others and focuses on an individual's internal mental representations of self and others (objects of the drives) linked by affects.

- Through the interaction of temperamental predispositions and experience in the infant-caregiver context, symbolic cognitive-affective representations of self and others are internalized by the developing individual. These *object relations dyads* can be considered the building blocks of psychological structure, especially with regard to identity.

- A clinically useful nosology of personality pathology combines dimensional variables (level of identity integration, defenses, reality testing, quality of object relations, aggression, moral values) and categorical zones of organization.

* Key to structural diagnosis is the concept of the split internal structure within which "bad" aggressive and persecutory affects are radically separated from "ideal" loving and libidinal affects. The former are projected and experienced as coming from outside. Growth and integration involve an individual's gaining awareness of and taking responsibility for the full range of his or her affect states.

SELECTED READINGS

Akhtar S: Broken Structures: Severe Personality Disorders and Their Treatment. Northvale, NJ, Jason Aronson, 1992 [A sophisticated discussion of the nature of the personality disorders.]

Auchincloss EL, Samberg E. Psychoanalytic Terms and Concepts. New Haven, CT, Yale University Press, 2012

Jacobson E: The Self and the Object World. New York, International Universities Press, 1964

Kernberg OF: Psychoanalysis: Freud's theories and their contemporary development, in New Oxford Textbook of Psychiatry, 2nd Edition, Vol 1. Edited by Gelder MG, Andreasen NC, Lopez-Ibor Jr JJ, et al. Oxford, UK, Oxford University Press, 2009 [For those relatively unconversant with basic psychodynamic concepts, this is a chapter that relates basic concepts of pathology and treatment with current trends.]

Klein M: Notes on some schizoid mechanisms. Int J Psychoanal 27:99–110, 1946

Lenzenweger MF, Clarkin JF (eds): Major Theories of Personality Disorder. New York, Guilford, 2005 [This text can help one place the object relations theory of personality disorder (see Chapter 3 by Kernberg and Caligor) within the context of other (i.e., neurobiological, attachment, schema) theories of personality pathology.]

2

EMPIRICAL DEVELOPMENT OF TRANSFERENCE- FOCUSED PSYCHOTHERAPY

A Clinical Research Process

IN THIS CHAPTER we describe the steps in the empirical development of transference-focused psychotherapy (TFP), proceeding from a conceptualization of borderline pathology to an articulation of the treatment focus and process and to empirical assessment of TFP. We relate the emerging core pathological processes to treatment foci, with special attention to the real-time functioning of patients with borderline pathology as identified by empirical methodological advances. Because TFP and other major empirically supported treatments for borderline personality disorder

---

Dr. Chiara De Panfilis was a significant contributor to the articulation of neurocognitive functioning and borderline pathology in this chapter.

(BPD) focus on current functioning of the patient, this refinement of understanding of real-time functioning is crucial for treatment development.

STEPS IN THE EMPIRICAL DEVELOPMENT OF TFP

The empirical development of a psychotherapeutic intervention has been described as involving six essential steps: 1) theory and research on the nature of the particular clinical dysfunction; 2) specification of the treatment, preferably in written manual form; 3) preliminary tests of treatment outcome; 4) theory and research on the change processes or mechanisms of change; 5) tests of the influence of moderators (such as pretreatment patient characteristics) on which the outcome depends; and 6) assessment of how the treatment generalizes to ordinary clinical conditions (Kazdin 2004).

Our path of treatment development for BPD and organization has progressed from articulations of borderline pathology in our clinical work to examination of treatment of patients with borderline pathology by experienced therapists to generation of treatment principles and articulation of a treatment manual. We proceeded from an examination of the effects of this treatment in a small study without a comparison group to a randomized controlled trial (RCT) with attention to outcome and to an approach highlighting the mechanisms of change. Each of the steps along our path calls for some elucidation.

THE EVOLVING UNDERSTANDING OF BORDERLINE PATHOLOGY

The history of research and clinical exploration into the nature of borderline pathology has been described as progressing from clinical descriptions to the emergence of diagnostic criteria to empirical validation of the criteria with behavioral correlates and finally to examination of the core psychological and neurocognitive processes in borderline functioning (Lenzenweger and Cicchetti 2005). In Chapter 1, "The Nature of Normal and Abnormal Personality Organization," we discussed how Kernberg (1975) identified borderline organization on the basis of difficult treatment experiences with patients now described as having severe personality disorder. Gunderson and Kolb (1978) developed a phenomenological description of these same patients that heavily influenced articulation of the DSM-III (American Psychiatric Association 1980) description of BPD. This introduction of specific criteria for the diagnosis was extremely productive in initiating a tremendous wave of research on both the pathology and treatment of these patients. The emphasis was on reliability, and issues of validity were not equally addressed. The diagnostic criteria have been very effective in identifying borderline samples and stimulating treatment research, but problems with the system have become more apparent with time. Exclusive reliance on criteria in the DSM descriptions has a number of limitations.

One legacy of the polythetic criteria sets for BPD (i.e., meeting any combination of five or more of the total of nine criteria) used in DSM-III to DSM-5 (American Psychiatric Association 2013) is the heterogeneity of the patients selected with these criteria (Lenzenweger 2010). These patients manifest rampant comorbidity with other personality disorders, as well as a range of symptom disorders.

Heterogeneity at the phenotypic level is problematic in many ways. It confounds any attempt to search for related endophenotypes and the genetic factors in BPD. This heterogeneity has also confounded the empirical investigation of treatment of borderline patients. The existing RCTs on the treatment of borderline patients neither identify subgroups of patients in their examination of treatment effects nor select for a specific type of borderline patient.

The group of patients captured by the DSM BPD criteria is an extremely heterogeneous group of individuals. The dismantling of this heterogeneity is a major task facing the field at this time. Understanding the heterogeneity of BPD is necessary to describe domains of the pathology that are likely to have different etiological roots and to describe treatments with refined approaches to the various domains of pathology currently nested under the wide borderline construct.

SYMPTOM FACTOR STRUCTURE

Since the introduction of personality disorders in 1980, the eight, and subsequently nine, criteria defining BPD have been examined in terms of their frequency, co-occurrence, factor structure, and predictive validity. Factor analytic studies of the criteria in DSM-III (Clarkin et al. 1993; Sanislow et al. 2000) and DSM-IV (American Psychiatric Association 1994; Johansen et al. 2004) resulted in two to four factors, depending on the sample and instruments used. The main components of BPD are commonly described as identity problems, negative relationships, affective instability, and self-harm (Distel et al. 2010).

Because factor analysis is not the most effective statistical approach to identifying clinically relevant subgroups of individuals, we have used a sophisticated statistical procedure called finite mixture modeling. This effort has identified three subgroups of patients with BPD (Lenzenweger et al.

2008), which are characterized by different combinations of paranoid and suspicious orientation to others, aggressive attitudes and behavior, and antisocial behaviors and traits. Group 1 is relatively low on paranoia, aggression, and antisocial traits; group 2 is characterized by paranoia but is relatively low on the other two variables; and group 3 is high on aggression and antisocial traits. These results have been replicated (Hallquist and Pilkonis 2012; Yun et al. 2013), suggesting that these subtypes may be important for guiding further efforts to understand underlying endophenotypes and genotypes. These identifiable subtypes also have clinical implications, as we explore more fully in Chapter 11, "Trajectories of Change in Transference-Focused Psychotherapy."

TRAIT DESCRIPTIONS

Some researchers (e.g., Widiger and Simonsen 2006) advocate the trait description of individuals in order to capture both the individuality of the patient and the dimensional similarities among groups of patients with personality disorders. This is a useful but limited approach. We and our colleagues have examined borderline pathology at the trait level (Sanderson and Clarkin 2013) and in terms of the psychodynamic constructs of identity, defenses, and reality testing (Lenzenweger et al. 2001, 2012b). Patients with BPD are high on measures of trait alienation, aggression, and absorption, and these traits represent important linkages to psychodynamic processes such as primitive defenses and reality-testing impairments.

Traits describe individuals in terms of their stable behavior patterns across different environmental situations but fail to explain how or why these behaviors occur. Only through the study of personality processes can one begin to understand how and why the personality traits have their impact (Hampson 2012). Combined understanding of personality traits and personality processes (Caspi et al. 2005; Cervone 2005; Mischel and Shoda 2008) can provide a fuller picture of personality functioning. We have attempted to combine information on borderline patients from traits to real-time processes.

REAL-TIME PROCESSES IN BPD

There are compelling reasons to focus on real-time processes within patients with BPD and other severe personality disorders. Successful therapy must focus on patients' current reality and help them change their current functioning because their behavior is destructive and impedes their movement toward a more normal existence. Many treatments help these patients to reduce symptoms, but relatively little information is available about how these treatments have their effects—that is, about the mechanisms of change. Which therapist interventions coupled with patient responses in a progression through the treatment lead to successful treatment outcome? It will become clear to the reader that our view of the necessary mechanisms of change in the treatment of these patients must involve attention to behavioral control combined with significant change in the patients' active and current representations of themselves and others that guide their behavior.

Two notable advances in scientific methodology—ecological momentary assessment (EMA) and the methods of social neurocognitive science—have contributed to understanding real-time dysfunctional processes in borderline individuals. Experience sampling methods and EMA are advances over self-report methods that are highly subject to memory bias. These newer methods use self-reports or indicators of behavior, cognition, and emotions using recall close in time to the actual events (Trull and Ebner-Priemer 2009). Functional magnetic resonance imaging (fMRI) provides advanced knowledge of the underlying neurocircuitry that is involved in the real-time functioning of borderline individuals, especially in their perception of and reactions to social challenge (for a review, see Frith and Frith 2012). These two approaches have facilitated a more detailed description and perception of the borderline patient in action, especially in the perception of self and others in social interactions.

Both EMA and social neurocognitive science enable the field to progress beyond a trait description of the personality disorders and provide important details on borderline real-time functioning from the processing of incoming stimuli to behavioral response. These methods describe how personality is organized in action. EMA provides data on the individual across time, with a focus on how the individual's behavior is organized and repeated across certain kinds of situations. EMA also begins to reveal how the individual perceives the other across interactions. In both approaches, there is increasing recognition of the emotional and cognitive systems of functioning by borderline patients as compared with those by normal individuals in real time.

Emotion Regulation

Functional imaging studies of borderline patients suggest some specific areas of difficulty these patients experience in the processing of emotional stimuli and serve to further the early speculations by Kernberg (1984) about the defense mechanisms used by borderline patients. Empirical work on emotion regulation began with studies of defense mechanisms as postulated by psychodynamic thinkers in the 1960s, and contemporary models of cognitive emotion regulation built on that background by use of fMRI studies of appraisal and reappraisal (Ochsner and Gross 2008).

Emotions arise from brain systems that appraise the significance of stimuli given the goals and needs of the individual, and reappraisal can be used to rethink the stimuli and modulate the affective response. Reappraisal depends on interactions between the prefrontal and cingulated regions, which are implicated in control, and the amygdala and insula, which are implicated in emotional responding.

Borderline patients have particular difficulty processing negative stimuli efficiently and effectively (Silbersweig et al. 2007). These patients rely on reflexive, automatically responding networks, whereas psychiatrically healthy controls make more use of networks with access to higher-level conscious cortical processing (Koenigsberg et al. 2009a). Furthermore, borderline patients are deficient in their ability to reduce negative affect through reappraisal (Koenigsberg et al. 2009a); this finding is quite important to borderline pathology and to potential treatment implications. In individuals without personality disorders, affect regulation by reappraisal in contrast to suppression is associated with greater positive emotion, reduced negative emotion, and better interpersonal functioning (Gross and John 2003). Both TFP and mentalization-based treatment encourage reappraisal, especially in the interpersonal perception of self and others, by the use of clarification, mentalizing, and interpretation.

Self-Regulation and Its Failures

Effortful control has been described as the ability to inhibit a dominant response in order to perform a subdominant response (Posner and Rothbart 2000; Posner et al. 2002; Rothbart and Bates 1998). Impulsivity in behavior is inversely related to the capacity for effortful control, a self-regulation dimension of temperament (Ahadi and Rothbart 1994).The individual with effortful control is able to voluntarily inhibit, activate, or change attention and thus potentially modify and modulate subsequent affect. There is growing evidence that the development of effortful control in infants and toddlers is central in the regulation of affect and in the development of mature social relations and conscience (Eisenberg et al. 2004).

Effortful self-regulation involves a variety of processes through which individuals pursue their long-term goals regardless of transient distractors, temptations, or biases. This is an intrinsically interactive process between the individual and the environment. All individuals are confronted with stressful situations requiring them to simultaneously regulate their emotions, thoughts, and behaviors. Under the usual circumstances of daily life, multiple stimuli compete for attention, and this competition is greatly influenced by bottom-up stimulus salience. Importantly, negatively charged affective stimuli (e.g., negative affects, threat-related cues) are of high salience and require increased cognitive control to maintain emotion regulation. Cognitive resources are limited in everyone, and for patients with BPD the struggle to regulate the emotional domain may result in a decreased availability of cognitive control skills necessary for regulating other domains. If the intensity of negative stimuli is not counterbalanced by top-down cognitive control processes that enable emotion regulation, negative affect could "sensitize" the individual toward subsequent self-regulatory failures in other domains (Heatherton and Wagner 2011), impeding the effective self-regulation in perception, behavior, and processing of social stimuli. Negative affect may well contribute to borderline patients' reflexive (rather than reflective) pattern of social cognition, inability to process rejection-related stimuli, and misperception of others' perspective.

Patients with BPD manifest difficulties with both aspects of emotion regulation, demonstrating a relative inability for top-down control and reappraisal of negative emotions (Koenigsberg et al. 2009b). Under conditions of negative affect, patients with BPD show a bottom-up impairment in conflict resolution and cognitive control (Silbersweig et al. 2007). In terms of neurocognitive functioning, patients with BPD have been found to have difficulties in attentional tasks even when the tasks do not involve affective arousal (Posner et al. 2002) and in processing emotional stimuli (Silbersweig et al. 2007).

Interpersonal Functioning

A core feature of BPD is severe disruptions in interpersonal behavior (American Psychiatric Association 2013; Clarkin et al. 1983) that endure even after other symptoms have declined (Skodol et al. 2005). There is a growing consensus that personality disorder involves most centrally difficulties with self definition and chronic interpersonal dysfunction (Bender and Skodol 2007; Livesley 2001), a view that has been long espoused by an object relations approach (Kernberg 1975, 1984). Disturbed and disturbing interpersonal behavior is the final common pathway of a number of dysfunctional processes in individuals with personality disorder, including those with BPD. The central issue in the field of personality disorders is which functions of the human organism are essential to adaptation and, therefore, which functions are disordered in those with personality disorders (Livesley 2001). These dysfunctional processes lead to disturbed interpersonal behaviors that have been conceptualized as a sequence of situation selection, situation modification, attentional deployment, cognitive change, and response modulation (Gross and Thompson 2007).

The intense idealized positive affect states and devaluing negative states that borderline patients experience are often stimulated by aspects of interpersonal relations such as interpersonal disruptions (Jovev and Jackson 2006) and perception of rejection (Herpertz 1995; Stiglmayr et al. 2005). Using an event-contingent EMA procedure, Russell et al. (2007) found that borderline patients experienced more unpleasant affect, were less dominant and more submissive, and were more quarrelsome in their interpersonal behavior than were nonclinical controls. Patients with BPD showed greater variability in the use of these behaviors. In contrast to patients with other personality disorders and psychiatric disorders without personality disorder, patients with BPD showed more disagreements, confusion, hostility, emptiness, and ambivalence in their social interactions (Stepp et al. 2009). These findings are consistent with the clinical hypothesis that borderline patients lack a stable sense of self to help guide them smoothly and efficiently through various interpersonal situations (Kernberg 1975). Indeed, information processing biases may be linked to internal beliefs, assumptions, and working models of self and others, which, in turn, guide interpersonal behavior. Beliefs about the social world, such as that one is powerless and vulnerable in the face of a malevolent social environment (Beck et al. 2004), may bias appraisal of the environment. Individuals with BPD selectively remember negative information (Korfine and Hooley 2000) while having an increased awareness of others' emotions (Fertuck et al. 2006).

Interpersonal Trust

The centrality of disturbed self-other representations is reflected in the inability of borderline individuals to deal with two interrelated challenges of human interactions: 1) the need to trust and cooperate with others and 2) the need to obtain social acceptance and avoid rejection. As will become evident from the clinical cases illustrated in this book, these issues of mistrust and perception of rejection occur over and over again between borderline patient and therapist.

Deciding whether to trust others depends in part on the ability to accurately infer the intentions of the other in a social exchange that leads to reciprocal cooperation. The development of expectations of others as trustworthy is a multistage process. First, it requires the recruitment of brain regions involved in representing others' mental states. Second, it activates brain areas implicated in the modulation of various aspects of social functioning, such as social memory, learning, and attachment behavior. By developing positive mental models, partners accumulate sufficient mutual trust to become socially attached to each other and to cooperate in advantageous ways. Healthy individuals build a trust relationship by learning that they can safely depend on each other (Krueger et al. 2007), but this is a dysfunctional process in patients with BPD. Borderline patients show atypical social norms in perception of social exchanges, which are consistent with fixed and pervasive social expectations of untrustworthiness that are not modified by the actual social experience. These biased perceptions of others eventually lead to the inability to benefit from cooperative exchange (King-Casas et al. 2008).

Rejection Sensitivity

The tendency to trust or mistrust others can be logically related to the concept of rejection sensitivity (RS), a concept that has grown out of the cognitive-affective processing model of personality functioning (Mischel and Shoda 2008). *Rejection sensitivity* is defined as "the processing disposition to anxiously expect, readily perceive and intensively (negatively) react to rejection cues" (Downey and Feldman 1996, p. 1327). Individuals with high RS focus extensively on anxious expectations of rejection, which can result in the perception of rejection even in the ambiguous and/or innocuous behavior of others. These individuals have a tendency to automatically interpret any social situation as confirming their rejection fears. Such an "automatic" ascription of negative dispositions to others accounts for increasing interpersonal conflicts by eliciting a self-fulfilling prophecy of rejection. The bias of expecting rejection results in a variety of adverse personal and interpersonal outcomes (Ayduk et al. 2000). RS can be conceptualized as a particular object relations dyad, one in which the other is seen as rejecting, the self is seen as vulnerable, and both are united with affects of anxiety and fear.

RS features seem central to the interpersonal difficulties of people with BPD (Ayduk et al. 2008; Staebler et al. 2011b) and can account for the association between BPD features and the increased tendency to interpret neutral social faces as untrustworthy (Miano et al. 2013). These results suggest that disturbed representation of others (as malevolent and rejecting) and self (as rejected or abandoned) may underlie the impairment in trust appraisal among patients with BPD, thus contributing to their extensive difficulties in depending on and cooperating with others. Given a history of physical and emotional neglect, and, in some cases, outright physical and sexual abuse, it is not surprising that patients with BPD might approach social situations with a bias toward rejection or worse. Yet because only a minority of individuals with a history of abuse go on to develop a psychiatric illness (Paris 1994) it is likely that aspects of the BPD patient's mind combine with the history of abuse to result in the disorders. Converging findings suggest that the nature of RS in BPD involves a relative inability to process social interactions in a reflective, emotionally regulated way. Borderline patients react in a defensive manner and feel rejected regardless of actual interpersonal acceptance or rejection (Renneberg et al. 2012; Staebler et al. 2011a).

RS alone may not account for the interpersonal behaviors distinguishing normal individuals from those with borderline pathology. In nonclinical individuals, social rejection and threats to acceptance signal the need to increase cognitive control in order to help interpret rejection-related stimuli in ways that minimize personal distress and promote adjustment by responding to the immediate moment with emotional balance (Eisenberger et al. 2003). This mechanism can explain why the deployment of effortful attentional strategies accounts for a successful adjustment following interpersonal conflicts (Hooker et al. 2010). However, such a function seems to be lost or missing in individuals with BPD. Importantly, having low executive control abilities increases the risk of developing borderline features in individuals high in RS (Ayduk et al. 2008), indicating that the capacity to effortfully control rejection cues may play a major role in the pathogenesis and maintenance of the disorder. Interestingly, effortful cognitive abilities are required for inhibiting one's own self-experience (e.g., perceived distress or rejection) to foster an unbiased consideration of another's state of mind (e.g., neutral intention, context-dependent evaluation rather than hostile attributions) (Lieberman 2007). Patients with BPD, however, show a reflexive hypersensitivity to negative social cues (Koenigsberg et al. 2009a) as well as reduced perspective taking and increased personal distress (Dziòbek et al. 2011).

These data suggest that patients with BPD find it difficult to represent alternative explanations for others' behaviors independently from their own internal and predetermined perspective. Their disturbed self-other representations combined with poor emotion regulation are manifest as a reflexive processing of human actions and assessment of intentions when facing social stimuli. Such automatic ascription of social attributions may depend on a relative inability to deploy the effortful self-regulatory skills necessary to process rejection-trust dilemmas in a reflective way. Recent insights on the social neuroscience of self-regulation failures may help in clarifying these mechanisms.

Social Exclusion

Stimuli that signal social exclusion are associated with an increase in negative affect (Sadikaj et al. 2010), negative other-focused emotions (Renneberg et al. 2012; Staebler et al. 2011a), emotion dysregulation, and problem behaviors (Selby et al. 2010) in individuals with BPD. Borderline patients show impaired social problem solving when experiencing negative affect induced by social rejection cues (Dixon-Gordon et al. 2011). In contexts perceived as abandoning or rejecting, patients with BPD, in contrast to nonclinical controls, showed an increased polarity in representations of others, which in turn predicted subsequent impulsive behaviors (Coifman et al. 2012). These empirical findings are consistent with the object relations understanding of defensive splitting that results in extreme and polarized perceptions and affective shifts.

These considerations suggest that BPD psychopathology may be viewed as a dysregulated, reflexive response to managing perceptions of self and others, especially in situations involving rejection and trust issues. The polarized and distorted self-other representations, as captured by the dynamics of RS, are not buffered by the adoption of "controlled" emotion and social regulation strategies, which could lead to interpersonal maladaptive responses.

The object relations perspective adds importantly to this view of personality functioning and personality pathology. The cognitive-affective units referred to in object relations theory as dyads are not static but rather are in constant activation, depending on the interpersonal context as the patient with BPD perceives it. Defensive mechanisms such as splitting that are more obvious in those with severe personality pathology complicate the functioning of the cognitive-affective units that are activated. The representation of self and other with related affect are prone to reversal—that is, the individual may perceive self as victim and later treat the other as victim at the hands of the self as persecutor.

This conceptualization of BPD pathology may contribute to illuminating the phenotypic heterogeneity of the disorder. It is quite plausible that patients with BPD may exhibit different types of maladaptive "solutions" to deal with rejection-trust dilemmas. For instance, patients with BPD may react to threats of rejection with increased anger, rage, and hostility (Berenson et al. 2011), or they may avoid social threats in an effort to defensively downregulate the experience of threat and rejection-related distress (Berenson et al. 2009). A reflexive (rather than reflective), poorly regulated vulnerability to social rejection in borderline individuals may be a central feature of the disorder that results in subgroups of different phenotypic responses in these individuals, thus resulting in identifiable phenotypes (e.g., Lenzenweger et al. 2008). Perceived rejection in patients with BPD could trigger different maladaptive defensive behaviors, depending on the interpersonal context and each patient's individual dispositional cognitive-affective processing.

Focus on self-other representation as cognitive representations of self and others and related affects, as described by the RS dynamics, represents a promising venue for exploring the phenomenology of BPD. Specifically, emerging evidence suggests that failures in reflective social and emotional regulation may underlie and perpetuate such distorted self (as rejected) and other (as untrustworthy) representations, in this way accounting for the extensive dysfunction in interpersonal adjustment of borderline patients. Finally, the diverse behavioral and defensive strategies that patients adopt to deal with expected or perceived interpersonal rejection from significant others may shape BPD phenomenology and severity.

REPRESENTATIONS OF SELF AND OTHERS

Attachment and developmental research suggests that disturbed self-other representations and related deficits and distortions in mentalizing processes play a major role in shaping the risk for BPD. Barone (2003) reported that individuals with BPD invariably suffer from insecure attachment as measured by the Adult Attachment Interview, which assesses the coherence of one's view of significant others. In a study of the attachment styles of patients with BPD, Levy et al. (2006) found almost universal anxious attachment, with a dominance of dismissive and preoccupied styles. With the vulnerability of insecure attachment, patients with BPD are prone to instability in their perception of self in relation to others. Not only are their perceptions of others unstable, but borderline individuals show more "malevolent" representations of their caregivers than do patients with major depressive disorder, especially in the context of a history of sexual abuse (Baker et al. 1992). Among individuals with a history of abuse, the successful development of reflective function, or the ability to correctly infer others' mental states and intentions, seems to protect against the risk of a BPD diagnosis (Fonagy et al. 1996). Therefore, the formation of malevolent representations of others may confer risk of developing BPD, at least among individuals with a history of abuse. Measures of disturbed self representations in childhood and adolescence mediate the link between attachment disorganization in infancy and BPD symptoms in adulthood (Carlson et al. 2009). Taken together, these findings suggest that disturbed self-other representations may act as carriers of (adverse) experience into later life and may account for the developmental process by which early adverse experience is linked to BPD.

LONGITUDINAL COURSE

Our clinical and personal experience confirms that personality is a consistent and enduring aspect of the individual, and this assumption has been built into the DSM definition of personality disorder. However, a number of studies have revealed that personality disorder, as defined and identified by the DSM criteria, tends to decline categorically and dimensionally over time in both community samples and clinical samples. The Collaborative Longitudinal Personality Disorders Study found a significant decrease in personality disorder diagnoses over a 2-year time period (Shea et al. 2002) among patients with Axis II diagnoses residing in the community, and a similar decline was found in a sample of university students followed for 12 years (Lenzenweger et al. 2004).

A major limitation in these studies is the exclusive reliance on DSM Axis II criteria, which often do not reflect long-standing aspects of the person but instead reflect transient behavioral manifestations (e.g., suicidal acts). The DSM criteria sets contain a mixture of feelings, symptomatic behaviors, more traitlike patterns of interacting with others, and internal constructs relating to social behavior such as identity diffusion. One would expect different degrees of stability and change among the individual criteria over time. It is important to note in this regard that this differential is an indication of what is ephemeral (e.g., symptoms) and what is more consistent (e.g., interpersonal and work functioning).

The general finding of a decrease in personality disorder criteria over time has resulted in speculation about what precisely is changing over time and what remains relatively stable, an issue that has been of central concern in personality theory. Zanarini et al. (2003) proposed that among borderline patients, the remission of acute symptoms such as suicidal behavior has a different time course than remission of more stable temperamental features such as chronic anger. Likewise, Clark (2007) suggested that basic temperamental dimensions are responsible for the enduring aspects of the personality disorders.

A unique effort to understand change in personality disorder has been reported in a three-wave study over 12 years that hypothesized that change in personality disorder features would be related to change in underlying neurobiological systems (Lenzenweger et al. 2004). Elevated levels of the agentic positive emotion system predicted more rapid decline in Cluster B personality disorder features over time. The authors suggest that individuals with personality disorder features who are nonetheless able to engage with the world and to use rewards and incentives for self-regulation find themselves less susceptible to continuing personality dysfunction over time.

Most relevant to this book on the treatment of adults with BPD and borderline personality organization (BPO) is the progression of symptoms and functioning of these individuals through their adult years. In a prospective follow-up study over a 16-year period of a large group of patients with BPD between ages 18 and 35 treated at McLean Hospital, Zanarini et al. (2012) made comparisons between the patients with BPD and subjects treated at the same hospital with personality disorders other than BPD. Whereas patients with BPD were slower than the comparison patients to achieve symptomatic reductions, both groups had achieved high rates of remission at the 16-year follow-up. It is more sobering to consider that only 40% of the patients with BPD attained symptom recovery of 8 years or longer, in contrast to 75% of the patients with other personality disorders. The authors noted that vocational impairment was the main reason that the patients with BPD failed to attain or maintain both symptom remission and good social and vocational functioning. Contemporary specialized treatments for BPD are not effective in significantly enhancing social and work functioning (McMain et al. 2012).

OUR CURRENT UNDERSTANDING OF BPD

Personality disorder is an emergent end product of interacting processes, with neurobehavioral systems underpinning the psychological organization and observable behavior as the individual interacts with the environment (Lenzenweger 2010). The resulting configured personality disorder phenotypes are not reducible to the underlying components, and, furthermore, the match between emerging phenotypes and existing descriptions of the personality disorders has yet to be determined.

For a full appreciation of personality pathology, including severe personality pathology in the form of BPD and BPO, one must consider three relevant levels of the organism: 1) observable behavior, 2) subjective experience, and 3) neurocognitive functioning. The basic assumption of the object relations model is that the individual with BPO suffers from a chronic lack of integration of both the negative and the positive aspects of experience. Lacking integration, the borderline individual is dominated by intensely felt negative aspects of experience. This is manifested clinically by the proclivity of these individuals to perceive neutral and sometimes even positive stimuli as negative; to distort the intentions of others in a negative direction; to project and attribute aggression to others; and to behave toward others as if the others are negatively motivated. With a focus on the subjective experience of these patients, object relations theory predicts that these individuals will have impulse dysregulation, project their own aggression onto others, misperceive the immediate motivation of others, and have difficulty placing the momentary response of the other into a larger context of the other's usual behavior. This theoretical formulation based on years of clinical experience with patients is consistent with the findings of empirical studies, especially those that capture the real-time functioning of these patients as reviewed previously in this chapter (see subsection "Real-Time Processes in BPD").

Psychoanalytic treatment with borderline patients has provided information about the patients' subjective experience, including their perceptions of self and others infused with intense and often negative affect, and their defensive attempts to organize their experience. Psychological research investigating the observable behaviors of BPD pathology and psychological trait research are informative at the descriptive and phenomenological levels. Finally, neurocognitive science is furthering understanding of how the brain functions while executing crucial tasks, including memory, working memory, perceptions of self and others in interpersonal interactions, and emotion regulation.

Because of the greater precision in detecting the interpersonal behavior of individuals with BPD in real time, the field is approaching an integration of the phenomenological approach of Gunderson (Gunderson and Kolb 1978) and the structural approach of Kernberg (1975). Patients with BPD are constantly faced with an approach-avoidance dilemma in which they desperately want to connect to others while being intensely threatened by the prospect of rejection. However, patients may show different types of maladaptive "solutions" to deal with this dilemma, resulting in different phenomenological subtypes.

TREATMENT OF PATIENTS WITH BPD IN A CLINICAL STUDY GROUP

Our psychodynamically informed treatment for borderline patients was developed by a group of senior clinicians who had experience in treating these patients and who used video recordings to examine clinical sessions in detail. Group review and discussions of these sessions led to the generation of principles of intervention that could be articulated and agreed on, which are represented in this treatment manual as the strategies of this treatment. This development took place in the early 1980s at a time when analytically oriented therapists were reticent to audio or video record sessions from fear that such procedures would interfere with their transference work. It became clear to us through experience that the video recording was well accepted by the patients who readily gave their written consent to the procedure. In contrast, the therapists were not accustomed to having their work viewed by others. This issue was discussed, and an atmosphere of support and mutual positive suggestions without criticism led to the continued use of the process.

THE TFP TREATMENT MODEL

The treatment of BPO is informed by the nature of the pathology, in terms of both the observable dysfunctional behaviors and the internal representations of self and other. TFP combines attention to the specific need of borderline patients for structure in the form of a clear treatment frame with core psychodynamic concerns, such as a concern with helping each individual find a balance among the forces that have an impact on his or her feelings, thoughts, and behaviors: biological urges, internal constraints against these urges, and the values and constraints of the individual's social reality. The goal is a balance allowing adequate satisfaction of urges while maintaining adequate control to successfully adapt to the external world. TFP helps the patient understand unconscious irrational patterns of thinking and feeling—and the conflicts between different sets of them—that often underlie behavioral symptoms. We believe that as these unconscious thoughts and feelings come into awareness, the understanding will allow the patient to master aspects of self, as well as internal conflicts among different aspects of self, that had previously exerted unconscious control over the patient's feelings and behaviors.

GOAL OF TFP

The goal of TFP is to help patients integrate all aspects of their internal world (rather than defensively split off shameful, painful, or "unacceptable" thoughts, feelings, and motivations) in order to experience themselves and others in a coherent, balanced way. The TFP therapist helps integrate these disparate psychological states using the transference relationship as a vehicle for understanding internal relational patterns that underlie feeling states and behaviors but are outside of the patient's awareness.

Given that a number of structured treatments for BPD significantly reduce symptoms and that no single treatment is superior to others in this regard (Levy et al. 2012), it is important for us to discuss how TFP is unique. The contribution of TFP begins with its ambitious treatment goals. TFP is structured and organized with the goal of changing the personality organization of the patient. That goal of treatment can be identified and measured at several levels of observation. The proximate goal is to have a significant impact and change in the borderline patient's perceptions of self and others. A normalization in the representations of self and others will guide interpersonal behavior and lead to significant changes in the domains of interpersonal functioning. Measurement of the representations of self and others can use standardized techniques such as the Adult Attachment Interview (C. George, N. Kaplan, and M. Main: Adult Attachment Interview protocol, 3rd Edition, unpublished manuscript, University of California, Berkeley, 1996) and material scored with the reflective functioning scale (Fonagy P, Steele M, Steele H, et al: Reflective-function manual: version 5.0, unpublished manuscript, University College London, 1998). At another level of measurement and observation, the success of the patient in friendship and intimate relations and in work relations is a major goal of TFP. Symptom reduction is important as a step toward engaging in normal satisfactions of friendships, intimate relations, and work investment and success.

TFP is unique in its ambitious goals of symptom change; change in representations of self and others; and success in friendships, intimate relations, and work functioning. These extensive goals of TFP influence the entire process, including the techniques of intervention, the focus of individual sessions, and the duration of treatment. It should be noted in this regard that although borderline patients share many common symptoms, the level of severity varies greatly, including their adjustment in love and work. The implication is that the process and duration of TFP will vary according to each patient's level of severity of dysfunction at the beginning of treatment. We return to this theme in Chapter 11 when we consider the multitude of trajectories of treatment after explicating the main concepts and tools of treatment in the central chapters of this book.

ACTIVATION OF OBJECT RELATIONS IN SAFE CONTEXT

In contrast to other treatment models, TFP provides a setting that encourages the full activation of the patient's internal representations of self and other in the developing relationship between therapist and patient. It is to be expected that primitive object relations—intense internalized experiences of self and other—are activated in the treatment setting because they are activated in all domains of the patient's life and underlie the patient's dominant motivational systems. Patients can use the treatment opportunity to let the primitive object relations unfold in a setting where TFP therapists analyze and clarify what the patient perceives and experiences at the most profound level. These scenarios are not simply a literal reproduction of what has happened in the past but instead a combination of what happened, what the patient imagined happened, and what the patient defensively set up to avoid painful awareness.

In TFP the patient's relationship with the therapist is structured under controlled conditions to prevent intense affects from totally exploding and overwhelming the communication. We create a treatment frame, described in Chapter 5, "Establishing the Treatment Frame," which makes it safe to reactivate those past pathogenic experiences. The safety and stability of the therapeutic environment allows the patient to begin to reflect about what he or she is experiencing and to relate that experience to internal representations that may not correspond to the objective reality and eventually to what went on in the past because current perceptions are at times based more on internal representations than on what is realistically going on now. *Technical neutrality* on the part of the therapist assists in the activation of internal representations and in establishing an observing stance toward them. Neutrality consists of observing all the parts of the patient's experience and helping the patient join the therapist in that observation without the therapist favoring one aspect of the patient's experience in a way that would inhibit full expression or consideration of the full set of factors having an impact on the patient's thoughts, emotions, and behaviors.

TFP fosters change by reactivation of primitive object relations under controlled circumstances without creating the vicious circle of the reaction of the normal environment when the patient behaves with emotion dysregulation. In this way TFP suspends the ordinary reaction of a normal environment to a disturbed patient and allows the patient to live out the internal pathological relationships in controlled conditions. This is the essence of transference. Instead of attempting to deter these perceptions and behaviors by educative means, we allow their activation in order to observe, reflect on, and understand them.

This process has limitations, however. Because of the condensation of what happened in memory and at different times in the past, we can never assume this reactivation is an exact reproduction of what factually happened in the past because transformational processes, progression, regression, and fixation occur.[1] The treatment does not reproduce a specific experience in time but rather produces an internal construction, the ultimate origin of which cannot be identified precisely. We are not concerned about what is actually fantasy and what is a precise description of the past. It is a current psychic reality that is a fundamental motivational factor in the patient's life because it reflects a psychic structure, and this structure is the focus of modification in the treatment (Table 2–1). A fundamental mechanism of change is the facilitation of reactivation of dissociated, repressed, or projected internalized object relations under controlled circumstances. This is the facilitation of a regressive process—regression in terms of time, mode of functioning, and experience in the service of the development of introspection or self-reflection.[2] The patient's increase in reflection is an essential mechanism of change.

The reactivation of internal object relations in relation to the therapist

---

[1]This is one case of what the French call *après coup*. The concept in the German literature is *Nachträglichkeit*, retrospective modification of the trauma.

[2]We prefer the term *introspection* to the term *reflective functioning*.

is called *transference*, which is the unconscious activation of dominant pathogenic internalized object relations in the present relationship established by the patient. The therapist's initial instructions to the patient (encouraging free association in relation to the problems that brought the patient to therapy) and listening attitude (with evenly suspended attention) signal the setting up of a specific object relationship—that of one who needs help combined with realistic trust that the facilitator (therapist) wishes to help with authentic interest and knowledge but not omnipotence. Transference emergence is signaled by any evidence of distortion of a "normal" (friendly) relationship by the emergence of the patient's primitive, split-off, persecutory, and idealized internal object relationship dyads in the interaction with the therapist.

The unconscious conflicts related to the core of identity diffusion will emerge in the therapeutic interaction, and analysis of this emergence is a core aspect of the technical approach of TFP. The therapist's cognitive formulation of this experience is called *interpretation*, which involves the formulation of a hypothesis of unconscious meaning of the transference or other aspects of the patient's experiences or behavior. The protective treatment frame (spelled out in the treatment contract) contributes fundamentally to containment or holding of the strong affects that accompany and contribute to the internal conflicts. *Holding* refers to the affective containment, or to the affective framing, and does not refer to the therapist's being overtly warm and sympathetic (although the therapist treats the patient with civility and courtesy rather than the cold "neutrality" that is the caricature of a psychoanalytic therapist).

Containment refers more to the cognitive structuring of what at first seems cognitively chaotic. In working with highly disturbed patients, the therapist may have to accept periods in which his or her primary role is to be exposed to and accept the patient's most unbearable and intense affective states—states the patient may find intolerable and tend to discharge through acting-out behaviors. The therapist's capacity to sit with these affects without denying them or reacting to them may be essential in helping the patient experience what was previously intolerable long enough to begin to reflect on it. At that point the process of interpretation can begin.

DESTRUCTION OF THINKING

The disorganization of the patient involves not only concepts of self and others, relationships with self and others, and predominance of primitive affects but also the defensive processes that prevent full awareness. These processes erase and distort awareness and thinking. Healthier, neurotic patients attempt

TABLE 2–1.   Mechanisms of change in transference-focused psychotherapy

Therapist interventions	Patient behavior and responses
Negotiation of treatment frame; position of technical neutrality; containment of affect in countertransference	The result is less impulsive action in the patient's daily life and activation of pathological object relations in reference to the therapist.
Identification and exploration of pathological object relations activated in the treatment, involving the following steps:	
1. Clarification: identification, description, and elaboration of the cognitive contents of intense affective states in terms of object relations	Highly charged affect states and acting-out are transformed and contained by cognitive elaboration. This leads to some degree of affective modulation and containment.
2. Confrontation: the tactful exploration of discrepancies and contradictions in a patient's communication, behaviors, or states of mind	This invites the patient to reflect. The patient begins to become aware of contradictory nature of experience, of oscillation between idealized and persecutory experiences. The patient becomes better able to observe own mental experience. There are moments of increasing capacity for the triangulation of thought and the capacity to appreciate the symbolic nature of thought; this leads to further containment of affect and reduction of the overwhelming nature of affective experience.
3. Interpretation of defensive motivations for splitting and other primitive defense mechanisms	This leads to a deepening observation of mental experience as symbolic—with increasing awareness of how thought processes and behaviors have concealed aspects of the self.

TABLE 2–1. Mechanisms of change in transference-focused psychotherapy *(continued)*

Therapist interventions	Patient behavior and responses
Identification and exploration of pathological object relations activated in the treatment, involving the following steps: *(continued)*	
4. Interpretation of splitting	This leads to further owning and containment of negative affect and appreciation of symbolic nature of thought with an increase in the capacity to reflect and appreciate the triangular nature of thought. There is a gradual and initially transient integration of idealized and persecutory experiences with a toning down of primitive affective experience. Cycles of decreased anxiety and decreased splitting may alternate with regressions to paranoid anxiety in the midphase of therapy as there is a gradual movement toward the "depressive position" with its more integrated and realistic views of self and others.

to eliminate unacceptable thoughts, affects, and memories by the process of repression, which creates a relatively steady and even system, albeit one that may involve symptoms such as anxiety. More primitive patients manifest a fragmentation and a disconnection of thinking with attacks on the linking of thoughts (Bion 1967), so the person's very thought processes are affected. These processes can be so powerfully affected that affects, particularly the most negative ones, are expressed in action without the patient's cognitive awareness of their existence in the self. In other words, these patients may behave extremely aggressively but with no conscious awareness of the aggression. The affect is only in the action, as in the case of Amy, which we discuss in Chapters 8, 9, and 10, the chapters on the phases of treatment. An example from her case is when Amy cut herself while a guard was watching over her, although she had no awareness of the aggression involved in the action.

TFP works to understand the patient's action and any related affect in terms of the object relations—the experience of self and other—that underlie the action. Another mechanism of change in TFP is the transformation of action (of "acting out") into emotional cognition—that is, the transformation of behavioral actions into an understanding of the internalized representations of self and other that constitute their motivating system. The treatment seeks to activate in the transference and then explicate the internalized object relations that constitute character structure and underlie acting out. Mechanized, automatized behavior is retransformed into the internal relationship(s) that gave origin to it—what the attachment theorists call the "internal working models." The concept of an internalized relational scenario that encompasses an image of self in interaction with another and that involves expectations of interpersonal transactions is common to both object relations dyads and to the internal working model of attachment elaborated in attachment theory. Given the primitive disorganization of affects and of their connection with cognitive processes, the therapist facilitates the patient's development of the cognitive capacity to represent affect. The therapist assists the patient in bringing together cognition and affect that was abnormally dissociated and disorganized.

PROGRESSION OF TFP

There is an orderly progression to the delivery of TFP. The therapeutic frame contributes to containment by providing an atmosphere of safety, allowing safe reactivation of internalized dyads in the transference. The patient will naturally resist the developing relationship within the frame because of anxieties about attachment and paranoid aspects of the transference and may act out in ways to escape from or diffuse the affective intensity. Analyzing the patient's efforts to resist the relationship will help in understanding the underlying assumptions and expectations regarding relationships. By encouraging free communication in the context of a treatment frame, the therapist allows the reactivation of relationship tangles that characterize the patient's life.

In TFP, first we analyze the patient's defenses. This may sound risky, but the containment provided by the treatment frame serves as an anchor and supports control in a space where the patient can regress. This analysis is followed by the steps of interpretation and the development of self-reflection. TFP is a repetitive process; nothing is resolved neatly the first time around. There are repetitive cycles in which modification and change are a gradual process. For example, affect storms may at first seem uncontrollable and un-available to reflection, but they eventually become modulated and then dis-appear as the patient progresses through cycles of modulating affects through increased reflection and further increasing reflection in the context of more modulated affects. An example of working with an affect storm is seen in Videos 3–1, 3–2, and 3–3 (see Chapter 7, "Tactics of Treatment and Clinical Challenges").

In borderline patients negative affects become hierarchically organized as a general tendency to protect oneself against pain and suffering by at-tacking and potentially destroying what, or who, is seen as causing it. There is a general destructive urge against others as well as against oneself. Chronic anger and aggression can crystallize into hate experienced in rela-tion to objects perceived as causing suffering. The urge is to eliminate or destroy the source of pain, with a possible concurrent urge to take revenge and to make the other suffer, resulting in a reversal of the situation that the patient may not be aware of. Pleasure and pain can become combined with aggression and lead to prominent sadomasochistic dynamics. At less severe levels of aggression, there is a need to control the other rather than take re-venge. One feels safe as long as one is in control, which is reflected in the active primitive defense of omnipotent control.

The pain-inducing object may be perceived as external or experienced as an internal object. The aggression therefore may be redirected against the self, with frequent confusion and chaos derived from projective iden-tification and reintrojection of the source of the negative affect. There may be strong urges to direct aggression against the self; under the most ex-treme circumstances, the wish to destroy the self becomes the dominant drive.

Directing the aggression against the self (i.e., through suicide and para-suicidal behavior) is an expression in action of different motivations that can emerge in the transference. There is not one type of suicide, but many. Sometimes the thinking and behavior reflect identification with a sadistic caretaker. The following statement of Fairbairn (1952) is relevant: "It is better to be a sinner in a world ruled by God than to live in a world ruled by the Devil" (pp. 66–67). In other words, it is better to hold out for pure goodness than to accept the fundamental presence of aggression. In this way, masochism may become a safety system by which savage attacks are in-ternalized, creating a sense of safety as long as the aggression is directed against the self, sparing the idealized other. At other times the individual is more directly internalizing and identifying with a sadistic object to main-tain the relationship with the aggressive caretaker. The attempt to kill the self is an attempt to identify with and unite with the aggressive other.

In a successful midphase of treatment, when acting out has decreased and affects are contained within the treatment frame, the patient's dominant internal object relations can be recognized and clarified as they repeat themselves. There are several aspects to the gradual change in the patient. The patient becomes able to introspect and, at the same time, to tolerate the gradual bringing together of affects with opposite valence. The increase in introspection and gradual integration of contradictory affects lead to modulation of the affects and, in turn, foster further introspection.

ROLE OF THE HUMAN RELATIONSHIP IN TFP

To what extent the direct, helpful human relationship between therapist and patient is important is an issue that has been discussed extensively in the literature (Mitchell and Aron 1999). Under ordinary circumstances human relationships help individuals. However, the more disturbed the patient, the less he or she is capable of being responsive to ordinary human relationships. That is the tragedy of severe personality pathology: the ordinary channels of mutuality in communication and of redress of grievances with others are distorted and destroyed. In contrast to the assumption that it is the warm, giving human relationship that permits the growth of the patient, it is the exploration of the intense negative affects through analysis of the transference that gradually permits the patient to accept a new relationship as something valuable that he or she can use for growth and gratification. It is the work in therapy that allows the patient to move from being trapped in fixed internal images that determine his or her experience of others to the ability to get to know others as different and unique. The relationship with the therapist is a nonspecific effect that probably takes place in all treatments, but it is particularly instrumental in TFP and other analytic treatments with patients whose internal images and projections destroy the possibility of relating in depth. Initially, the essential quality in the therapist is not warmth, which is often misinterpreted by borderline patients as being insincere or even dangerously seductive, but rather is the therapist's ability to accept and contain the intensity of the patient's affects without defensively withdrawing or retaliating. In the final phase of treatment, the more nonspecific factor of a helping human relationship becomes operative. In contrast to the commonsense assumption that first a therapist has to build up a good relationship with the patient, the therapeutic alliance with borderline patients is a consequence of the treatment, not a precondition; it is a result of the systematic resolution of the negative aspects of the transference and integration of the internal world. The precondition is containment of intense affect.

DURATION OF TFP

As we have described, patients who meet the BPD diagnosis are a hetero-geneous group, varying in degree of severity of both symptoms and deficits in intimate relations and work. For this reason it is impossible to describe a uniform time frame for treatment. Our research, which uses frequent as-sessment and statistics to analyze the trajectory of change, enables us to de-scribe some observed treatment durations as related to some specific changes in these patients. For example, we have seen many cases in which the patient's acting out comes under control within the first 6 months of treatment and in which the use of primitive defense mechanisms is signif-icantly decreased in the second year of treatment. These changes set the stage for focusing more directly on resolving the patient's identity diffu-sion, consolidating a more integrated identity, and refining the under-standing and progress with regard to the patient's problems in love, work, and leisure. (See Chapter 11 for more on what can be accomplished across time.)

GENERATION OF A TREATMENT MANUAL

Through ongoing review of the videotaped therapy sessions, it was an easy step to articulate in writing the principles of intervention that arose from group discussions. We generated a treatment manual by combining the prin-ciples of intervention with the specific clinical examples that arose in our clin-ical work (Clarkin et al. 1999). However, that manual is not a static written product but rather is an evolving document that has been updated to reflect our continuing experience with borderline patients. We subsequently wrote a primer for TFP (Yeomans et al. 2002) and a second manual (Clarkin et al. 2006). In this current manual, we include new developments based on more experience with the midphase and late phase of treatment, more experience with what results can be expected over time, and more differentiation of the treatment as it is applied to the various subgroups of patients with BPO, such as those with high-level BPO, low-level BPO with and without narcissism, or malignant narcissism.

The written treatment manual was introduced into the psychotherapy research tool kit in order to specify the treatment in sufficient detail to al-low others to replicate the treatment for further investigation. This pur-pose and the need for instruction to our students stimulated our writing of the manual. In addition, we have found in teaching TFP that the videotaped sessions of experienced therapists and clinicians in the progress of learning the treatment are excellent tools for instructing others in the treatment. For this reason, this book includes access to online videos of composite cases using actors as the patients (available at www.appi.org/Yeomans).

TEACHING TFP TO ADHERENCE AND COMPETENCE

Our clinical research group at the Personality Disorders Institute has accumulated experience in training clinicians in TFP to acceptable levels of adherence and competence. The typical training involves the initial steps of seminar instruction, followed by watching videotapes of adherent TFP therapists. The therapist then treats two borderline patients using TFP with regular supervision. We have developed an adherence and competence rating form that enables certified TFP therapists to evaluate the performance of those in training (available on request). The regular rating of the adherence and competence of TFP therapists is essential to ensure that quality TFP is being delivered.

PRELIMINARY TESTS OF TREATMENT OUTCOME

During the development of TFP, we received a treatment development grant (R21), with John Clarkin as principal investigator, from the National Institute of Mental Health. With funding from this grant, we treated 17 borderline patients in 1 year of TFP without a control group. This study enabled us to apply the newly generated treatment manual and to further the clinical process of consulting on a regular basis on each other's cases. The focus of these collaborative meetings was not exclusively on what happened in the last session but also on using that information to plan the next sessions and further the intervention. The outcome of this study was encouraging (Clarkin et al. 2001). During the treatment year, compared with the year prior to treatment, the number of patients who made suicide attempts decreased significantly, as did the medical risk and severity of medical condition following self-injurious behavior. Also, study patients had significantly fewer hospitalizations as well as total days of hospitalization during that year compared with the year prior to treatment.

RANDOMIZED CONTROLLED TRIALS

AN RCT IN NEW YORK

The Borderline Research Foundation, a private foundation located in Switzerland, sought us out to explore the possibility of funding our treatment development work. With the encouragement and collaboration of our department chair, Dr. Jack Barchas, we successfully competed for funds, and along with three other sites we were able to mount an RCT comparing TFP with other manualized treatments. We chose to compare TFP with dialectical behavior therapy (DBT), the then recognized empirically tested treatment of borderline patients, and with a manualized supportive psychodynamic treatment, which was similar to TFP with the exception of not using what we considered to be a crucial agent of change in TFP: interpretations in the here and now. The study (Clarkin et al. 2007) found that although TFP, DBT, and supportive psychotherapy all showed significant positive change in patients' depression, anxiety, global functioning, and social adjustment across 1 year of treatment, only TFP was significantly predictive of change in irritability and verbal and direct assault. Both TFP and DBT were significantly associated with improvement in suicidality, and both TFP and supportive psychotherapy were associated with improvement in anger and facets of impulsivity. Most importantly, patients in TFP but not those in DBT or supportive psychotherapy showed significant changes in reflective function (RF), a hypothesized mechanism of change in TFP (Levy et al. 2006).

AN RCT IN EUROPE

With the evidence that TFP was effective in reducing symptoms and was as effective as DBT, it was then important to show that TFP could be delivered with clinical impact at a site other than that of the originator of the treatment. With encouragement and extensive collegial effort with Dr. Peter Buchheim, a psychiatrist in Munich, Germany, we were able to teach clinicians in Munich and other German-speaking cities to use TFP in their clinical work. The TFP manual was translated into and published in German. This development led to the opportunity to design an RCT and compare TFP to the treatment usually delivered by local expert therapists in the German and Austrian health care systems. Doering et al. (2010) completed an RCT comparing 1 year of TFP to treatment by experienced community psychotherapists. Patients improved in both treatments, although patients randomly assigned to TFP evidenced a lower dropout rate; significantly greater reductions in numbers of suicide attempts, inpatient admissions, and BPD symptoms; and significantly greater improvements in personality organization and psychosocial functioning. Both groups improved significantly in depression and anxiety, and the TFP group improved in general psychopathology, all without significant group differences. The results from this study suggest that TFP is an efficacious treatment for BPD.

TREATMENT EFFECTS BEYOND SYMPTOM CHANGE

A number of RCTs have established the efficacy of various manualized cognitive and psychodynamic treatments for patients with BPD (Bateman and Fonagy 1999; Clarkin et al. 2007; Giesen-Bloo et al. 2006; Linehan et al. 1991). The results suggest that common elements across the treatments are helpful with these patients and raise the following question about the mechanisms of change: What are the operative elements in these treatments that lead to change? For example, it is postulated in the respective treatment manuals that key therapeutic strategies and techniques, such as skills training (Linehan 1993), enhancing mentalization (Bateman and Fonagy 1999), and the use of a transference interpretation process in TFP (Clarkin et al. 2006), are pathways to change. Although these treatments have shown success in significantly reducing symptoms, limited data are available to indicate that specific therapist techniques are related to the changes that are found. A second and related question regards the aim of outcomes in the various treatments. In TFP we have always argued that symptom change in borderline patients is essential but that to achieve true personality change, the patient must alter the way he or she mentally represents self and others and achieve success in intimate relations and work functioning. Several aspects of our research have approached these questions.

In the RCT comparing TFP with DBT and a supportive treatment (Clarkin et al. 2007), we used the Adult Attachment Interview (George et al. 1996) prior to and after 1 year of treatment to provide material to rate each patient's level of RF. RF measured in this way has been posited by Fonagy et al. (1998) as an operationalized measure of the ability to mentalize—that is, the ability to represent self and others in terms of attitudes, emotions, and motivations. We hypothesized that TFP, with its emphasis on helping the patient to expand the understanding and articulation of representations of self and others in the interaction with the therapist, would significantly improve the borderline patient's level of RF and that DBT and a supportive treatment that did not include the operative element of transference interpretation would not enhance RF. Indeed, this is precisely what we found (Levy et al. 2006). The fact that TFP significantly reduces symptoms and raises the level of RF is quite consistent with the hypothesized mechanisms of action in the treatment. We interpret the significant rise in RF during TFP as a result of the therapists' inviting patients to clarify their conceptions of self and others, confronting inconsistencies, and helping patients to integrate complex representations of self and others through interpretation in the here and now.

In the European RCT (Doering et al. 2010), the Structured Interview for Personality Organization (STIPO), a semistructured interview based on object relations theory, was used prior to and after 1 year of treatment to assess personality functioning. It was found in that study that TFP significantly improved overall personality functioning as measured on the STIPO, but such progress was not found in the comparison treatment.

CURRENT EMPIRICAL STATUS OF TFP

The clinical research described in the preceding sections has contributed to the current status of TFP. TFP can be learned and utilized with adherence and competence by therapists not only at its site of origin (the Weill Cornell Personality Disorders Institute) but also in other locations. TFP has demonstrated significant symptom change in two RCTs following 1 year of treatment (Clarkin et al. 2007; Doering et al. 2010). TFP is superior to treatment as usual by expert therapists in the community (Doering et al. 2010) and is at least as effective as DBT, a standard in the field (Clarkin et al. 2007). Finally, TFP produces change that goes beyond mere symptom change; that is, TFP results in changes in RF (Levy et al. 2006) and significant improvement in personality functioning (Doering et al. 2010).

THE CLINICAL CASE IN RELATION TO PROCESS AND OUTCOME DATA

Much has been written about the gap between clinical care and empirical research. Clinicians emphasize the individual patient and the individual therapist-patient relationship. Clinicians write case histories that are strong in detail and may leave the reader wondering how this particular story can generalize to other patients and treatments. In contrast, researchers emphasize group data and the need for objective data across multiple individuals, homogeneous in dysfunction, obtained using a clearly defined treatment approach. Researchers complain that clinicians do not use their data, and clinicians assert that the research is not specific enough to inform their work. This seems like an insoluble situation in which both sides are on parallel tracks that will never meet.

Both the clinical and the empirical approaches exert an important point of view because both are partially correct. Our view is that the issue is not clinical orientation versus an empirical orientation but rather how a clinical research group can benefit from both approaches. This treatment manual is an attempt to combine the benefits of both approaches. As the reader will discover, in this treatment manual we emphasize the importance of the clinical case, and we use individual clinical cases extensively as we describe the strategies, tactics, and techniques of TFP as used in the early, middle, and final phases of treatment. Because we have outcome data on all of these cases, which come from our multiple empirical trials of TFP, we are able to combine the power and detail of the individual case with the overall process and outcome data on the groups of patients with BPO whom we have investigated. Because of our knowledge of the individual case and the group statistical outcome scores, we can place the individual case into the context of overall outcome parameters.

The primary goal of this book is to help the clinician treat the individual patient who presents with the symptoms and difficulties of BPO. TFP is a principle-driven treatment approach; that is, we enunciate the principles of treatment (strategies, tactics, and techniques) as applied to the individual patient. Readers must absorb the principles as we describe them and apply them to individual cases we have encountered and treated. Then, as the readers proceed in the clinical process, they must use the principles and apply them to individual cases using their best clinical judgment.

It is useful to provide a guide to the reader concerning the individual cases that are presented in detail in this manual. Although each of these patients is unique, all of them meet the criteria for BPD and BPO. Among the numerous cases cited, we have selected the treatment of two individuals, Amy and Betty, to illustrate the progression of treatment and patient changes (see Chapters 8, 9, and 10). Other shorter vignettes are used throughout to illustrate the application of specific principles of TFP.

Key Clinical Concepts

- TFP has been developed by a clinical research group starting with immersion in the treatment of borderline patients.

- TFP has been empirically developed in a stepwise fashion, progressing from manualization of the therapy model to randomized clinical trials.

- A combination of outcome research and in-depth experience of individual cases supports the principles of TFP.

- The understanding of borderline pathology has been furthered by research focused on real-time functioning, especially in social situations, in borderline individuals.

SELECTED READINGS

Barber JP, Muran C, McCarthy KS, et al: Research on dynamic therapies in Bergin and Garfield's Handbook of Psychotherapy and Behavior Change, 6th Edition. Edited by Lambert MJ, New York, Wiley, 2013, pp 443–494 [A review that puts TFP in the context of the effectiveness of dynamic treatments.]

Kazdin A: Psychotherapy for children and adolescents, in Bergin and Garfield's Handbook of Psychotherapy and Behavior Change, 5th Edition. Edited by Lambert MJ, New York, Wiley, 2004, pp 543–589 [The best description of the stepwise process in the development of a psychotherapeutic treatment.]

Levy KN, Meehan KB, Yeomans FE: An update and overview of the empirical evidence for transference-focused psychotherapy and other psychotherapies for borderline personality disorder, in Psychodynamic Psychotherapy Research. Edited by Levy RA, Ablon JS, Kachele H. New York, Springer, 2012, pp 139–168 [A comparison of the strengths and weaknesses and evidence for the specialized treatments for BPD.]

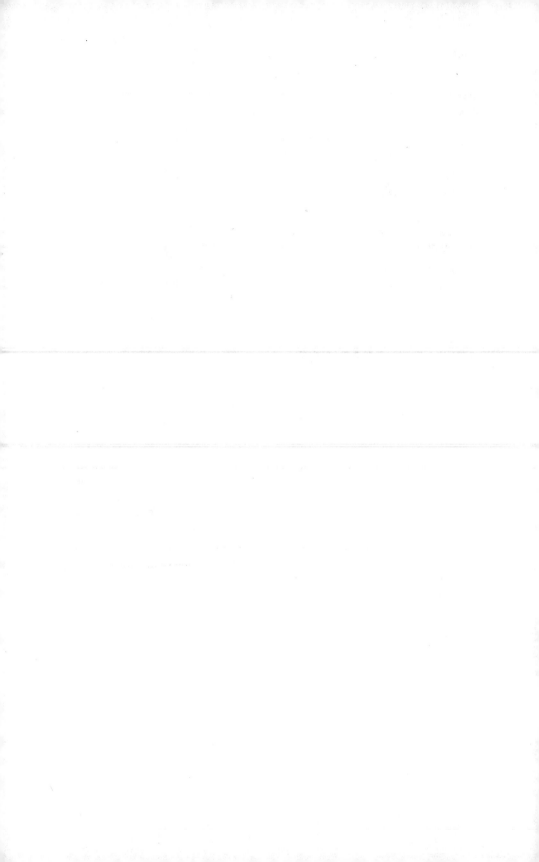

STRATEGIES OF TRANSFERENCE-FOCUSED PSYCHOTHERAPY

THE GOAL OF transference-focused psychotherapy (TFP) is identity consolidation—the integration of mutually split off idealized and persecutory internalized object relations in the transference in order to achieve a coherent, realistic, and stable experience of self and others. This internal state of identity consolidation is congruent with emotion regulation and cooperative, positive relationships with others. This goal is achieved by the therapeutic interventions that can be conceptualized at different levels of abstraction and specificity. The *strategies* of TFP are the overarching approaches defining the sequential steps in the process of interpreting object relations activated in the transference. The *techniques* are the moment-to-moment interventions of the therapist. Finally, the *tactics* of TFP are the maneuvers the therapist uses to lay the groundwork for the proper use of interpretation and other treatment techniques. We describe the strategies of TFP in this chapter; the techniques in Chapter 6, "Techniques of Treatment," and the tactics in Chapter 7, "Tactics of Treatment and Clinical Challenges."

The strategies derive from object relations theory. Part-self and part-object representations are integrated through a process in which underlying representations are identified and labeled by the therapist and then traced as they contribute to the patient's experience of interpersonal relationships. When the patient has begun to recognize characteristic patterns of relating, and when contradictory self and object images begin to re-emerge predictably, the therapist begins to demonstrate the patient's active effort to keep them separated (i.e., the splitting that attempts to avoid the anxiety that would be experienced if these opposing characteristics were perceived simultaneously). The four strategies are listed in Table 3–1 and are described in detail in the following sections.

STRATEGY 1: DEFINING THE DOMINANT OBJECT RELATIONS—TRANSFORMING ACTION INTO OBJECT RELATIONS

The first strategy of TFP calls for the therapist to listen to the patient, observe the patient's ways of relating to the therapist, and gradually define the dominant object relations dyad that the patient is exhibiting or experiencing in the here-and-now interaction. Operationally, this means applying the model depicted in Figure 3–1: perceiving which of the patient's internal object relations dyads is active in the moment and identifying the representation of the self and the representation of the other that is projected onto the therapist. One can delineate a number of steps in the first strategy.

STEP 1: EXPERIENCING AND TOLERATING THE CONFUSION

Often as early as the first session, the therapist working with a borderline patient will become aware of a perplexing, troubling, confusing, and frustrating atmosphere. This experience may be quite distressing, especially because the patient frequently conveys a sense of urgency; the confusion can result in the therapist's feeling impotent. The patient, although apparently intent on seeking professional help, may speak hardly at all, act as if the therapist has a malignant ulterior motive, berate the therapist, or display a storm of affect. The patient may make statements that are mutually contradictory or that contradict his or her current affect or behavior. Such an atmosphere is a hallmark of the early work with borderline patients. The therapist's first task is to sort out his or her own feeling states.

Rather than resisting or denying the experience of confusion or attempting to quash it immediately by reaching a premature "understand-

TABLE 3–1.	Strategies of transference-focused psychotherapy
Strategy 1	Define the dominant object relations dyads
Strategy 2	Observe and interpret role reversals with the dyad
Strategy 3	Observe and interpret linkages between object relations dyads that defend against each other
Strategy 4	Work through the patient's capacity to experience a relationship differently in the transference and review the patient's other significant relationships

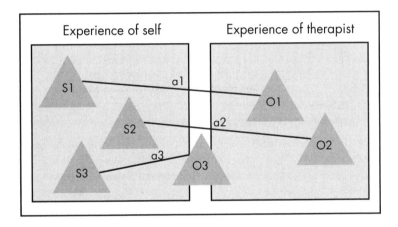

FIGURE 3–1. Transference: the immediate experience of self and other.

The box on the left represents the patient's experience of self and the one on the right represents the experience of the other, the therapist in this case. The three dyads are three different experiences of self and other that could be activated by a "trigger event." When one dyad is active, the others are out of awareness.

The therapist's role is twofold: 1) to initially accept the projected object representation and 2) to "hover above" the situation in a position that observes the interaction, trying to engage the patient in the observation and exploration of the "action" below.

The third dyad shows the kind of movement that corresponds to the patient beginning to understand that what he or she has experienced in the therapist may correspond to something in him or her. The object representation may alternate from being projected to being accepted as part of the self over a period of time in the midphase of therapy.

Note: a=affect; O=other (in this case, the therapist); S=self.

ing," the therapist should experience the confusion freely. The therapist should pay attention to the specific quality of the feelings being evoked in him or her (countertransference) because this may be an important clue to either a similar feeling state or a complementary feeling state active at that moment within the patient. For example, the feeling of impotent rage, mobilized in the therapist by the uncooperative yet urgently demanding patient, may in fact represent the patient's own predominant experience of feeling cornered by a dangerously omnipotent therapist. Alternatively, the therapist's feeling of impotent rage may be the complement to the patient's current state of powerful sadistic control. By not forcing premature closure, the therapist demonstrates the ability to tolerate intense, opposing feeling states. The patient who perceives this quality in the therapist is often reassured, because if the therapist can tolerate the confusion, perhaps he or she can be open to the full range of affects in the patient's internal world. The therapist's accepting the confusion is an initial form of empathy.

STEP 2: IDENTIFYING THE DOMINANT OBJECT RELATIONS

The representations that constitute the patient's internal object world are not directly observable; inferences can be made about the internalized objects by noting recurring patterns in the patient's interactions with others, especially with the therapist. A useful way of making sense of the patient's overt behaviors is to consider the interchanges as scenes in a drama, with different actors playing different roles. The various roles necessary to cast the scene reflect the activated part-self and part-object representations. By imagining the role that the patient is playing at the moment and the role into which the therapist has been cast, the therapist may gain a vivid sense of the patient's internal representational world. For example, the roles might involve first a starved, needy infant in relation to a withholding, disgusted parent, and then a spontaneous, uninhibited child in relation to a loving, tolerant parent. Additional examples of caricatured roles are listed in Table 3–2. This list is far from exhaustive; the therapist should formulate a cast of characters for each patient, choosing words to characterize the actors and the interaction as specifically as possible. In Table 3–2, the roles are arranged in likely pairings, but the pairings could differ with various patients.

To define the cast of object relations dyads that the patient brings to the interpersonal drama, the therapist needs considerable data about the patient's current feeling state, active wishes, and fears, as well as of the patient's expectations and perceptions of the therapist. The therapist gathers these data by encouraging the patient to describe the experience of inter-

TABLE 3-2.   Sample Illustrative role pairs for patient and therapist

Patient	Therapist
Destructive, bad infant	Punitive, sadistic parent
Controlled, enraged child	Controlling parent
Unwanted child	Uncaring, self-involved parent
Defective, worthless child	Contemptuous parent
Abused victim	Sadistic attacker/persecutor
Deprived child	Selfish parent
Out-of-control, angry child	Impotent parent
Attacking child	Fearful, submissive parent
Sexually excited child	Seductive parent
Sexually excited child	Castrating parent
Dependent, gratified child	Perfect provider
Child longing to be loved	Withholding parent
Controlling, omnipotent self	Weak, slavelike other
Friendly, submissive self	Doting, admiring parent
Aggressive, competitive self	Punitive, vengeful other

Note. The left column reflects the common self representations, and the right column the common object relations; however, it must be remembered that the role pairs alternate constantly. The therapist and the patient become, in rapid turns, the depositories of part-self and part-object representations.

acting with the therapist in the here and now. This process, part of the work of clarification, involves actively inquiring about the patient's immediate experience and presenting the therapist's understanding of the patient's experience for the patient to correct and refine. This process of clarification is similar to the approach of mentalization-based therapy (Bateman and Fonagy 2004), which has been developed subsequent to TFP. Thus, the therapist might say to the patient, "Since the session began today, you have been somewhat secretive and evasive, as though you see me as dangerous. Am I right in this?" The patient's response might correct the statement and add important refinements: "Why should I talk to you? You never answer my questions but just rephrase what I have already told you." The therapist might then amend the original hypothesis: "So your secretiveness is a reaction to your perception of me as a withholding person. Would that be more correct?" This process continues until the patient and therapist can either agree on the way in which the therapist is currently caricatured or agree that they cannot agree. The patient's current self representation is elicited in a similar manner. Sometimes patient and therapist do not reach agreement. The patient is then presented with the therapist's best description of the relationship with the understanding that, for the present, they see the interaction differently. An effort to understand the sources of their perceptual differences is often quite productive.

The patient sometimes rejects every suggestion made by the therapist, giving ample evidence in the process that this reaction occurs automatically and unreflectively. Such a devaluation of all that comes from the therapist in itself characterizes a primitive object relation activated in the transference. The patient should be presented with this description, and its meaning should be interpreted.

The therapist's internal feeling state is often a clue to the existence of object representations activated within him or her by the patient. The therapist therefore monitors internal states, noticing alien feeling states, urges to deviate from role, intense affects, intrusive fantasies, or wishes to withdraw.

STEP 3: NAMING THE ACTORS AND THE ACTION

The Level of Individual Dyads

Once the therapist has an opinion about the important self and object representations active at the moment, he or she conveys this impression to the patient. The patient can best hear such communications if they are offered at a moment when the patient displays some spontaneous curiosity about the nature of the interaction with the therapist and has achieved some distance from its immediacy (i.e., interpretations are best offered while the patient is emotionally involved in the session but as the intensity of affect is declining). The therapist, too, requires some distance from the intensity of the interaction in order to compose a succinct, evocative comment. The therapist should try to characterize the process as specifically as is possible at the moment, trying to capture nuances that reflect the individuality of the patient. To demonstrate that the therapist is not omniscient, that the process of therapy is not magic, and that the patient must provide data, the therapist should describe for the patient how the characterization was reached. The therapist might say, for example, "You have spoken in an increasingly low tone of voice despite my repeated statements that I can't hear you. That fits my notion that you're angry with me." It is important to include the linking affect as well as the self and object representations involved.

A metaphor selected from the patient's own language often can serve as a particularly vivid, succinct, and emotionally rich way for patient and therapist to talk about complex self and object images. The following statements illustrate the use of metaphor and the therapist's attempt at specificity in characterizing the active part-self and part-object representations.

- "I have noticed that you have been reacting to me as though I am an adversary with total power over you, as if I am your jailer and you are a cowering, defenseless prisoner."
- "So I am a stingy, depriving adversary, and your only recourse is to act like a word miser, giving me very little in return."
- "Everything would be all right [to you] if I were to obey you, and for this reason I'm like a stubborn child rebelling against a dominant, insistent, rigid mother."
- "You acted as if you had the right to be a child who is not responsible for her actions, where the mother has the responsibility of picking up after her child regardless."

The therapist should enter this process of naming roles as the presentation of a hypothesis to be tested and refined on the basis of the patient's response, not as truth to be accepted. The therapist should attend carefully to the patient's manifest agreement or disagreement as implied by the subsequent associations. If the therapist recognizes that he or she was incorrect, or even somewhat off the mark, he or she should feel free to acknowledge this and provide a revised impression.

Identification of Types of Transference Themes

The transference pattern of a particular patient can be seen as predominantly antisocial (lack of honest communication and receptiveness), paranoid (fearful and suspicious), or depressive (self-blaming and guilt-ridden). Variations on these themes include, among others, narcissistic, erotic, and dependent transference patterns. Although the psyche of the borderline individual is characterized by a fragmented structure made up of a theoretically limitless number of object relations dyads, in practice we find that each patient generally presents with a finite number of dominant dyads. Consequently, although borderline patients are characterized by rapid shifts in the presentation of transference patterns, each patient generally presents with a central, underlying transference disposition when he or she enters treatment. The transference can shift rapidly according to which internalized relationship is being reexperienced at the moment and which role within the relationship is being unconsciously assigned to the patient and which to the therapist. Yet, even in the setting of these rapidly shifting transferences, a borderline patient brings to the therapy a *predominant baseline transference* that, if treatment is effective, will evolve over time. The baseline transference is like a leitmotif among the shifting dyads. The rapid shifts may represent a variation on the baseline predominant transference or may represent an alternative that surfaces temporarily.

From a developmental point of view, the core issues in the early stages of therapy with a borderline patient generally stem from the pre-oedipal level of development, involving experiences of satisfaction and frustration in relation to the caregiver and the interaction of these experiences and constitutional factors on the development of libidinal and aggressive drives.

STEP 4: ATTENDING TO THE PATIENT'S REACTION

Having labeled the active dyad, the therapist should carefully note the patient's response. Manifest agreement or disagreement is less important than the course of the patient's subsequent associations and any changes that emerge in the nature of the interaction with the therapist. A correct characterization of the predominant object relationship may lead to several possible developments. First, the self-object interaction just labeled may become more pronounced. Second, there may be a sudden interchange of roles in which the self image just named is projected onto the therapist and the object image is reintrojected into the patient. Thus, the patient who has just been described as a controlling mother treating the therapist as a naughty but defenseless child may feel defenseless and criticized by an all-powerful therapist-mother. The third possible outcome of a correct characterization would be evidence of insight. The patient might acknowledge with emotional conviction what the therapist is describing and may spontaneously describe other interactions demonstrating a similar pattern. A correct characterization may lead to previously unreported material or to new memories that are linked to the described self-object dyad. A fourth outcome might be the sudden activation of a different object relations dyad. Finally, a correct naming of roles might be met by total denial.

Incorrect naming of roles may lead to overt disagreement, denial, or even acknowledged agreement emerging from an effort to please the therapist. The patient may respond with relief if an inexact characterization organizes a previously chaotic experience—even the incorrect formulation may be taken by the patient as a gift from the therapist, as a token of the therapist's belief that understanding is possible. Alternatively, the patient may react with dismay, realizing that the therapist cannot always understand, is not omniscient, and is separate. Thus, the therapist may not immediately be able to assess the correctness of the intervention. In such situations the therapist should continue to entertain the possibility of being incorrect and should listen patiently as additional material emerges to confirm or refute the hypothesis. At times the therapist will need to tolerate such uncertainty for a long period.

As the treatment progresses, correct interventions will more often lead to shifts away from the described dyad and toward activation of an opposite dyad. Opposing self images and opposing object images thus may emerge within the same session. When this occurs, an interpretation of splitting may be most meaningful to the patient. For example, when the patient has reacted to the therapist as a cold, distant parent at one point in the session and as a warm, loving parent at another point, the therapist may point out how feelings toward the therapist-mother as a hateful, cold witch have been kept separate from feelings of the therapist as a nurturing mother in order to avoid experiencing hate toward one who is loved—a state that would produce intolerable anxiety. Correct interpretations of the object relationships do not often lead to insight the first time they are offered; repeated interpretations as the same pattern recurs are typically required.

STRATEGY 2: OBSERVING AND INTERPRETING PATIENT ROLE REVERSALS

As noted in the discussion of strategy 1, examples of caricature roles as played out by the patient in the interaction with the therapist are multiple but recognizable because they are repetitive and characteristic for the individual patient. An interesting characteristic of the self and object representations that make up a dyad is that in the course of the session (as in real life) they often alternate, or change places, so that what first characterized the self switches to the object, and vice versa (Figure 3–2). This oscillation is especially important for the therapist to be aware of because the change in roles is often in the patient's behavior and not in his or her awareness. Therefore, a first step in enlarging a patient's awareness of his or her internal world is often to point out that the patient is enacting a role that he or she usually experiences as belonging to the other. For example, at one point in a session, a patient's interaction with her therapist appears to be the activation of the patient's self representation as a defenseless victim being controlled by an omnipotent force. However, after the patient notices the therapist look at the clock, she begins to attack the therapist, vigorously berating him for being a "selfish egotist who only cares about getting his next victim into the office." The patient may not be aware of the change but, in effect, she has become the powerful one. The patient is often not conscious of the role she is experiencing and enacting; rather, the patient probably believes she is just reacting reasonably. This is because her behavior may appear reasonable in relation to her internal world. At this point the therapist feels controlled by the patient and unfairly victimized. A reversal has occurred. The same self-object dyad is active, but, by means of projective and introjective mechanisms, the roles played by patient and therapist have been interchanged. This alternation of roles is often what has occurred when the therapist experiences a sudden sense of having lost track of what is going on. When feeling perplexed the therapist should consider the possibility that a reversal of self and object roles has occurred.

STRATEGY 3: OBSERVING AND INTERPRETING LINKAGES BETWEEN OBJECT RELATIONS DYADS THAT DEFEND AGAINST EACH OTHER

After having begun to delineate the patient's set of internal object relations dyads, the therapist seeks to carry his or her understanding of the patient's internal world a step further. The self-object dyads do not exist merely as fragmented, split-off elements of the patient's psyche totally independent of one another. The organization of an individual's internal world includes a level of complexity beyond that described thus far involving the individual's set of object relations dyads. We have emphasized the discrete and discontinuous nature of the internal representations of self and other—representations that are split off internally from each other. This system is not static; there are patterns of interrelation between the self and object representations. A first pattern within this system was described in strategy 2: Any dyad can *oscillate* so that the characteristics attributed to the self abruptly shift to the object and those attributed to the object shift to the self. (In this sense both the "self" representation and the "object" representation are ultimately self representations.) This abrupt oscillation explains some of the confusion in the borderline individual's subjective experience, affect dysregulation, and interpersonal relations, especially because the individual is often not consciously aware of the change.

A second pattern is that the internal representational system includes dyads that are opposite of each other (Figure 3–3), although one of the opposites may be closer to consciousness than the other: this is the crux of splitting. Splitting is *not* the stark contrast between a "good" self representation (victim) and a "bad" object representation (aggressor) within the same dyad: both of those representations are imbued with negative affect. Splitting is more fundamentally the unbridgeable gap between a dyad totally imbued with negative, hateful affect and one imbued with positive, ideal, loving affect. These dyads coexist but are totally dissociated from one another. This dissociation serves the defensive purpose of protecting each dyad from contamination or destruction by the other. The split protects the dyad imbued with love and caring from destruction by the hatred carried in the opposite dyad. In a symmetric way, the split protects the hate-filled dyad from contamination by any positive affect. It may at first be less clear

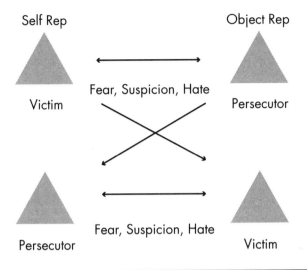

FIGURE 3–2.   Object relationship interactions: oscillation of the roles within a dyad.

The oscillation is usually in behavior, not in consciousness.

Note.   Object Rep=object representation; Self Rep=self representation.

why the hateful dyad should be protected, but in borderline pathology a clear and unadulterated sense of hatred can provide a temporary respite from the confusion of identity diffusion and protect against guilt feelings because of the patient's own aggression to the (at other times) good object.

The hate-laden dyad is usually, but not always, closer to the surface in the beginning stages of therapy with borderline patients. The internal experience of being loved and cared for is more hidden and fragile and is evident only in glimpses of longing, to which the therapist must be very attentive. By helping the patient gain some awareness of this internal possibility of love in the place of hatred, the therapist helps the patient understand the intensity of the hatred as a desperate attempt to keep the fragile longing for love hidden and protected from the risk that it would be destroyed if it were to see the light of day.

The above paragraph describes the most classic example of an object relations dyad defending against the opposite dyad in a borderline patient. However, the system of internal object relations is such that any specific dyad can defend against another dyad, each one representing a part of an intrapsychic conflict. The internal dyads, each with its specific affect, may represent libidinal or aggressive drives in conflict either with internal pro-

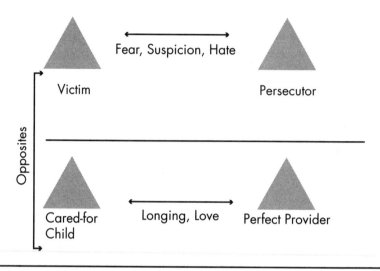

FIGURE 3-3.   Object relationship interactions: a dyad defending against its opposite.

hibitions to them or with each other. Both drives and prohibitions are represented in the individual's internal world by object relations dyads. For example, a libidinally laden dyad involving a representation of the sexually aroused self and a representation of a maternal other may be in conflict with an anxiety-laden dyad involving a representation of the fearful self and a representation of a menacing paternal other.

In another example, a libidinally invested dyad involving a passive, submissive self representation linked by longing with a powerful, distant paternal object representation may be in conflict with an aggressively invested dyad involving a cutthroat, competitive representation of self linked by rage with a threatening, tyrannical paternal object representation. According to the individual's makeup, either one of these dyads could be the more conscious, predominant one defending against the other, generally dissociated, one. A borderline individual has no simultaneous conscious awareness of the more predominant dyad and of the suppressed, split-off one, even though the latter may surface in acting-out behaviors and even in moments of awareness of it. Conflicts that are kept out of consciousness are experienced as either 1) behaviors, through acting out, or 2) physical symptoms, in somatization.

Splitting involves a dyad being unconsciously paired off with another dyad against which it defends, each representing one side of an internal conflict. This is because internal drives and the prohibitions directed against them are represented in the psyche by corresponding affectively charged pairs of self and object representations.

An example is a patient who often experiences herself as a frightened, paralyzed victim and who angrily denounces the therapist as being a sadistic prison guard to whose arbitrary and self-serving rules she is being forced to submit. At other times, the patient experiences the therapist as a perfect, all-giving mother, with the image of being a fully satisfied baby kangaroo ensconced in the mother kangaroo's pouch. In the first dyad, the prison guard represents a bad, frustrating, teasing, and rejecting caretaker-mother, and the victim represents an enraged baby who wants to take revenge but is afraid of being destroyed because of the projection of her own rage onto the mother. This terrible mother–suffering infant relationship is kept completely separate from the idealized one out of fear of contaminating the idealized one with the persecutory one and of destroying all hope that—in spite of the rageful, revengeful attacks on the bad mother—the perfect relationship with the ideal mother might be recovered. In terms of drives, this latter dyad is invested libidinally, whereas the sadistic mother–victim child dyad is invested with aggression. Each dyad, when conscious, defends against concurrent awareness of the other dyad.

Understanding the function of affect-laden dyads in representing drives and the defenses against them adds a new level of complexity to the task of the therapist. Drives stem from primary affect states. From a practical point of view, drives can be defined as the supraordinate common motivational force of all similar affect states. The most basic drives are the libidinal and the aggressive, which represent, respectively, the integration of all the positive, pleasurable affiliative affect states related to attachment, play bonding, and eroticism and the integration of all the negative, aversive affect states related to pain, rage, fight-flight, anxiety, panic, shame, and disgust. In patients with borderline personality organization, the drives generally remain fundamentally split and defend against each other. This is illustrated in the preceding example in which a dyad invested with an overriding aggressive affect defends against a dyad invested with the opposite, libidinal, affect. The system is unstable, with abrupt shifts between the dyad/affect/drive that are conscious and the dyad/affect/drive being defended against.

In summary, the therapist working with borderline patients not only must delineate the different caricatures constituting the dyads and the oscillation between self representation and other representation within the dyad but also must note the function that one dyad may play in relation to another in order to fully understand the fragmentation and conflicts within the patient's internal world. To achieve this level of understanding, the therapist first must be constantly attentive to the different affect-invested roles the patient experiences in the transference or enacts and also to the roles evoked in the countertransference. The therapist must then consider how these role pairs, or dyads, can carry the drives and defenses and organize them in a way that provides a primitive attempt at stability based on an internally fragmented state, maintained by splitting and projection, whose elements cannot be brought together in a complex way that corresponds to mature psychological development.

STRATEGY 4: WORKING THROUGH THE PATIENT'S CAPACITY TO EXPERIENCE A RELATIONSHIP DIFFERENTLY, STARTING WITH THE TRANSFERENCE

INTEGRATING SPLIT-OFF PART OBJECTS

The process of integration of split-off part objects is a repetitive process. Over and over again, the therapist must identify in the here-and-now interaction the contradictory aspects of self that the patient manifests in the sessions. Over a period of months, then within a few weeks, and finally within the same session, the therapist may bring together two opposite pairs of self and object representations, helping the patient to understand the reasons for the defensive splits of these two units. In the process both an integrated concept of self and an integrated concept of significant others will emerge, often initially in a more realistic and in-depth perception of the therapist, in parallel with a corresponding growth of the capacity to relate to others as well as in more realistic and deeper ways.

MARKERS OF GRADUAL INTEGRATION BY THE PATIENT

The shifts that occur in the patient's behavior in the sessions that manifest a progression in the integration of split-off part-self and part-object are subtle but cumulative. We describe the markers of this shift here because these expectable changes, although subtle and only gradual in emerging, are helpful markers for the therapist and help define the overall strategies of the therapy.

1. *Patient statements implying either expansion or further exploration of the therapist's comments.* The issue here is not whether or not the patient agrees with an interpretation or goes along with a suggested topic for exploration but the extent to which the patient does or does not reflect

on what the therapist has said and the extent to which an automatic rejection or denial of the therapist's comments is evident. The issue is not whether the transference is positive or negative but whether there is some degree of cooperation in clarifying what is going on.

2. *Tolerance of the awareness of aggression and hatred and the ability to contain the affect.* Awareness and containment of aggression and hatred, in contrast to the affect's expression by self-destructive actions, somatization, or destruction of the communication with the therapist, are central to patient progress. This is often the most difficult step in treatment.

3. *Tolerance of fantasy and the opening of a transitional space.* The issue is the extent to which the patient may become open to free associations that are not under his or her rigid control, with the implicit "danger" that the therapist may gain understanding about what is going on in the patient's mind before the patient is fully aware of it. For example, the need for omnipotent control in narcissistic patients tends to inhibit free association and reduce the availability of fantasy material.

4. *Tolerance of and capacity to integrate the interpretation of primitive defensive mechanisms, particularly projective identification.* Because of the dominance of projective identification and related primitive defenses in the transferences, the patient's capacity to acknowledge his or her attribution to the therapist of aspects of his or her own unconscious identification with, for example, persecutory or sadistic figures is of central importance to the process of integration.

5. *Working through of the pathological grandiose self in the transference.* This marker is relevant only for patients at the borderline level of organization diagnosed with narcissistic personality disorder, characterized by a pathological, grandiose self structure as the core of their self concept (Stern et al. 2013; D. Diamond, F.E. Yeomans, and B.L. Stem, A Clinical Guide for Treating Narcissistic Pathology: A Transference Focused Psychotherapy, in preparation). Under these circumstances, a grandiose self representation relating to a depreciated object representation is the predominant unit in the transference over extended periods of time. This condition requires systematic elaboration and interpretive resolution before the more typical, underlying, split-off units of self and object representations that are concealed by the apparently monolithic grandiose self emerge in the transference. This transformation—that is, the dissolution of the pathological grandiose self—is an important marker for that particular subgroup of patients. That chronic transference position has to give way to more complex and fragmented acute transference experiences.

6. *Shifts in predominant transference paradigms.* Insofar as the same, mutually split-off units of idealized and persecutory self and object represen-

tations are activated repeatedly in the transference over a period of many months, the development of significant shifts in such dominant units toward other, more integrated transference units not manifest in earlier stages of the treatment is an indication of significant intrapsychic structural change.

7. *Capacity for experiencing guilt and entering the depressive position.* The term *depressive position* refers to the condition in which the patient's aggressively invested, persecutory units of self and object representations and the patient's idealized, all-good self and object representations become integrated. This position is depressive in that the individual must mourn the primitive *ideal* object and accept the reality that no such ideal object exists. A more integrated, realistic, mixed good *and* bad representation of self emerges, evolving into a more mature self concept, while the integration of all-good and all-bad representations of significant others creates more sophisticated, differentiated representations of others with a consequent capacity of understanding others in depth and relating to them more appropriately. This stage of development is characterized by the patient's acknowledgment of his or her own ambivalence toward important, needed, loved objects and the related capacity for experiencing feelings of guilt and concern over dependent and loving relationships that might have been threatened by his or her earlier aggressive reactions. This capacity for guilt and concern also goes hand in hand with efforts to carry out reparative actions toward realistically loved objects and is the basis for more mature dependency, gratitude, and collaborative work with the therapist as well as for the expansion of this capacity into relationships outside the treatment setting.

We present the following case to illustrate both the treatment strategies and some of the markers of integration. We will return to this case in Chapter 9, "Midphase of Treatment," as an illustration of the eroticized transference.

CASE EXAMPLE

Gabby presented with many of the classic features of borderline pathology: a years-long history of cutting herself and taking overdoses, with periods of anorexia and with chronically stormy and chaotic interpersonal relationships. She described her initial attitude toward others to her therapist, Dr. Tam, as follows: "I'm here because I want to get over my crazy behaviors that keep getting me in trouble. I just want to be strong so that I don't have to depend on anyone. You can't depend on anyone. People are rotten and just take advantage of each other. My problem is that I'm not good at that. I'm weak. I'm vulnerable. I get upset and hurt myself. I want to get over that so that I can take care of myself, make a lot of money, leave my husband,

and live all by myself with no connection to anyone else." Dr. Tam understood Gabby as describing the following dyad:

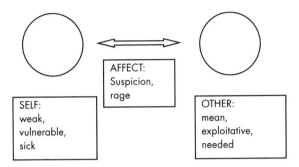

However, Dr. Tam also experienced a different dyad in the patient's attitude toward him and in his countertransference. In this dyad, contempt is a radical devaluation, a complex aggressive affect, typical for envious borderline patients:

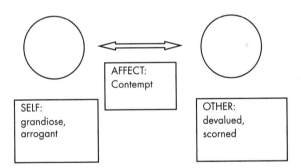

This second dyad was, to a large degree, the reversal of the self and object representations in the first dyad, demonstrating that Dr. Tam is thinking in terms of strategies 1 and 2. His interventions with the patient will reflect this. We should note that this case has been simplified for educational purposes. As with most borderline patients, Gabby presented Dr. Tam with much chaotic material, mixing discussion of her feelings about him with crises in her marriage, problems at work, references to her past, and descriptions of intense, intolerable affect states. Because we believe that an understanding of the internal structure of object relations helps to re-solve this whole spectrum of problems, we teach the therapist to focus on that level, as illustrated in this example. For example, Gabby frequently crit-icized Dr. Tam for the conditions of the treatment contract. Although she had agreed to them, she later stated that she had done so only because she felt it was necessary in order to get treatment and that she experienced these conditions as proof of Dr. Tam's callous disregard for her. According to Gabby, these conditions were just to make his life easy and "cover his ass" if the case did not turn out well. She went so far as to question his medical ethics, to call him a charlatan and mock him. Dr. Tam attempted to bring Gabby's attention to what he observed going on between them. Although he accepted Gabby's description of her subjective experience of herself as weak and vulnerable, he suggested that the nature of her interaction with him revealed aspects of herself that she did not seem to be aware of, such as the kind of callous meanness that she said was all she could expect from oth-ers. Gabby rejected these interventions, saying that she was only doing what she had to do to protect herself.

Attending to the patient's reaction, Dr. Tam reflected on what seemed to be an intensification of her conscious self representation. He wondered, how-ever, from what was she "protecting herself." Suspecting a projective process, he imagined that although Gabby experienced him as the threat, the threat might be hidden deeper in her. He waited for more evidence as to how to un-derstand this threat. He wondered about the possibility of feelings in her that conflicted with her overt suspicion and distrust. He noted that at times she appeared to feel close to her husband and at times appeared to feel that way toward Dr. Tam himself because, for example, she lingered at the end of ses-sions and appeared not to want to leave. Dr. Tam suggested this to Gabby, but she held to her position, stating flatly that he was wrong and that the idea he proposed was just further proof of how incompetent and uncaring he was and that he did not have even the faintest idea of who she was.

The first 2 months of therapy were characterized by this discussion, with other themes also entering into the sessions. Other typical themes were her feelings that she was inadequate as a mother and that she was stu-pid. Gabby linked these themes with her claim that she just needed to be stronger. Dr. Tam related these themes to his idea that there was a cruel part of her and that it was behind these attacks on herself. She rejected these comments. Outside of sessions, she continued to act out at times by cutting herself superficially on her arms and legs.

In the third month of therapy, Dr. Tam notified Gabby that he would be away for a week the following month. She expressed indifference to his going away and even mocked him for making a big deal of it. When he returned, she reported that her week had been routine and, in fact, it was better than usual because she did not have to bother to come to her sessions. Dr. Tam was re-lieved internally that she did not react with the anxiety and aggression many pa-tients expressed when he went away. Another 2 months went by with similar themes to what had preceded. Then Dr. Tam announced that he would be away again for a week. This time Gabby's reaction was different: she exclaimed, "You can't go away!" as if her saying it would control him. Dr. Tam was seeing the breaking through of the split-off side of the patient's internal conflict. This allowed him to work more overtly at the level of strategy 3. Over the months he had worked with Gabby, an intense attachment had developed, but she had succeeded in denying it until now. Then the emergence of this material in such a dramatic way gave Dr. Tam more data to support his interpretation that Gabby was torn internally by a terrible conflict between wanting to be attached and cared for and wanting to be independent and dismissive: "We're now seeing a part of you that is very important but that is very hard for you to tolerate and experience. Your reaction shows that in spite of your general experience of others as threatening and dangerous, you can become attached. And I think you become attached because, deep down inside of you, you have a longing for a goodness and caring you wish for. However, this longing is the scariest thing of all, scary because of your assumption that you will only encounter hurt and deception. Probably, the closer you get to thinking that someone could be caring and kind to you, the more anxious you get. As bad as it is to think of others as mean and exploitative, it is actually less scary than to think that someone could be caring because then you could get hurt in the worst way possible: to have your trust betrayed, to be seduced and then abused, so to speak."

Gabby's longing for love and caring was radically split off from her mistrust and rage, as shown in the following dyads:

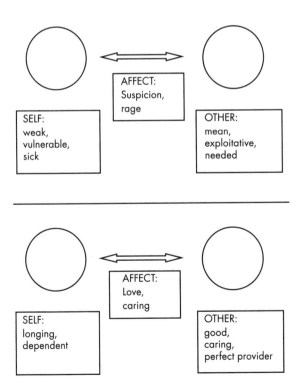

This exchange between Dr. Tam and Gabby represented progress. However, the work on this internal split continued to be intense and challenging. Gabby acknowledged that she might experience some wish to be close but pointed to Dr. Tam's going away as confirmation of her stronger wish to extinguish those feelings and become totally independent: "You see, I'm right. I can't count on anyone. You're going away...just when I was beginning to trust you. How can you do that? You're like everyone else. You wait until I need you and then you disappear."

Dr. Tam attempted to work on Gabby's need for a perfect object in order to feel she could trust any object and included discussion of the role of her aggression in her experience of abandonment: "We can now understand better the difficulty you have letting yourself experience the longing for attachment that you have. If there is any flaw, any deviation from a perfect attention to you, you experience that as proof that the other person doesn't care at all. At that point, I suspect something more happens; you react with anger and rage at the disappointment you feel and you attack the image of the other person in your mind. For instance, it is true that I am going away. But instead of holding on to the image of me that you have in your mind, your rage wipes out that image, leaving you feeling alone and empty. I think, in the end, that it's not my going away for a week that is leaving you feeling totally empty so much as it is you're attacking the image of me you have in your mind."

The kind of discussion encapsulated in the above remarks by the patient and therapist can continue for a long period—months to years—in the therapy. Of course, there are variations and there is evolution, but the struggle between the patient's internal representations and more realistic representations of self and others usually is a slow one. Gabby continued to accuse Dr. Tam of being "just like everyone else" in disappointing and even betraying her, yet she continued to come to therapy diligently, suggesting a side that felt differently. Dr. Tam, rather than trying to convince her that he was genuine and trustworthy, tried to explore her transference in depth: If he did, indeed, want to gain her trust only to trick her and hurt her, what was his motivation for this? Was he dishonest in presenting himself as a therapist who wished to help her? Was he perhaps sadistic, getting pleasure from the suffering he witnessed in her? Gabby sometimes was able to see that some of these ideas seemed extreme and not to correspond to the reality of Dr. Tam's being available to her on a consistent basis, as he had defined in the beginning of the treatment. Yet, at other times, the reality of the situation seemed to matter little, and Gabby experienced an occurrence such as the end of a session as proof of Dr. Tam's indifference to her. This alternation between a distorted perception and a more realistic one can continue for long periods and requires patience and skillful interventions on the part of the therapist.

How does the therapist integrate material from the past into the focus on the transference? As the therapist draws out the patient's internal representations as they emerge in the transference, the therapist can use material from the past to inform his or her understanding of representations of others. However, in doing so, the therapist is careful to remember that the description of the past that he or she is hearing is what the patient has internalized and not an objective representation of a past reality. This is not to say that the patient's descriptions are not connected to the past reality. However, the unintegrated structure of the borderline patient's psyche may result in characterizations that are partial and contradictory. Therefore, the therapist refers, for example, to "a mother who…" rather than "your mother." In the case of Gabby, the therapist knew that the patient's mother had recurrent depression and would drink and take drugs rather than seek treatment when she was depressed. In discussing Gabby's conviction that he was indifferent, Dr. Tam would make reference to this part of the patient's internalized past in describing the object representation that was active in the transference at those times: "You are reacting to me as though I am a doped-up mother who is totally unresponsive to the needy girl in front of me. Your experience of me is of somebody who is inexpressive and expressionless as if he were doped…and who only reacts under extreme circumstances."

These references to the internalized past enlarge the discussion to allow for elaboration of internal images as they relate to the remembered past and also to elements of the past that may have been suppressed or repressed. Some of the past may emerge as it is relived in the transference without conscious memories of it. It may be through the reliving in the transference that the patient gains awareness of some parts of his or her internal world and thus becomes more able to integrate those parts into a more meaningful and complete sense of self. However, linking material in the transference with internalized images from the past does not necessarily, in and of itself, lead to integration or resolve conflicts.

For example, Gabby agreed with Dr. Tam's references to "a doped-up mother," but this did not immediately resolve her intensely negative transference. She responded, "I live 24 hours a day replicating those thousand interchanges; I can't get away from it! Only in church do I feel relief for a minute." Her reference to church provided Dr. Tam with more data with which to address her internal split: "It is as though you can only believe in someone's care and concern for you in a setting defined as pure goodness, and even then the good feeling is very transient. If there is any ambiguity or uncertainty, as in most life situations—including this one—you switch to your 'default' position of experiencing the other as cold and indifferent—'doped.'"

One reason that linking the transference to the internalized past does not necessarily lead to integration is, of course, that the internalized images are partial and split from one another. Gabby, like many patients, could shift from a negative image of her mother to an idealized one: "But she was an invalid…what could you expect from her? I knew she wanted the best for me. There must have been something wrong with me that I couldn't make her happy. I'm just too stupid…I am now and I was as a child." The therapist is again required to follow strategy 2 of following the reversals of self and object representations and the shifts in dyads.

Gabby eventually showed evidence of integration of her internal world. In fact, her own words were like a layman's description of Melanie Klein's (1946) concept of moving from the paranoid-schizoid to the depressive position: "I know now people aren't perfect. Maybe it's that I've had high standards, but you've helped me realize I can't find somebody perfect. But I've wanted that fairy tale love that makes you high. I always believed it could happen… it has a few times, but it never stayed that way. It breaks my heart. I'm the most romantic person…. If I care, it's 500%, but then I can get mad too." This statement communicates a higher level of awareness but also the sadness that accompanies the loss of the ideal object.

REPETITIVE NATURE OF THE WORK

The necessity of repetitive clarification, confrontation, and interpretation of the dominant split-off object representations in the therapy hours can be discouraging to even an experienced therapist. However, the therapist must evaluate the nature and course of the repetitive working-through. There is certainly a diagnostic question of distinguishing between fruitful repetitive working-through that is having therapeutic impact and an endless repetition that is the sign of unchanging defensive operations seen in a therapeutic impasse. A fruitful and productive working-through will be manifested in at least two ways: 1) the patient will show a gradual decrease of acting-out behavior outside the sessions, while at the same time the affective intensity of the object relations being repeated in the transference will increase in the sessions, and 2) there will be a shift from early to advanced stages of treatment as manifested in the therapy hours according to the criteria described above in our discussion of markers of gradual integration.

Key Clinical Concepts

* The object relations model of borderline pathology emphasizes the impact of internal representations of self and others, how these internal representations are organized, and how they influence behavior.

* The strategies of TFP reflect the overarching objective of the therapy: to move from splitting and fragmentation to identity integration or, in other terms, to move from the projection of negative motivations to the capacity to take responsibility for one's thoughts, feelings, and actions as one integrates them.

* The strategies guide the therapist to observe 1) the object relations dyad that is active in the moment, 2) role reversals within dyads, and 3) the defensive splitting of idealized dyads from persecutory ones.

SELECTED READINGS

Britton R: Naming and containing, in Belief and Imagination. London, Routledge, 1998, pp 19–28

Britton R: Subjectivity, objectivity, and triangular space. Psychoanal Q 73:47–61, 2004

Caligor E, Diamond D, Yeomans FE, et al: The interpretive process in the psychoanalytic psychotherapy of borderline personality pathology. J Am Psychoanal Assoc 57:71–301, 2009

Gill M: Analysis of transference. J Am Psychoanal Assoc 27:263–288, 1979

Klein M: Notes on some schizoid mechanisms. Int J Psychoanal 27(Pt 3–4):99–110, 1946

4

ASSESSMENT PHASE

Clinical Evaluation and Treatment Selection

AN OBJECT RELATIONS approach to the nosology of the personality disorders (see Chapter 1, "The Nature of Normal and Abnormal Personality Organization") is based on the patient's subjective experience, observable behavior, and underlying psychological structures. Therefore, clinical assessment, which precedes treatment selection, must examine each of these three areas: 1) subjective experience (e.g., symptoms such as anxiety, depression), 2) observable behaviors (e.g., investments in relationships and work, deficit areas in functioning), and 3) psychological structures (e.g., identity and identity diffusion, defenses, reality testing) (Caligor and Clarkin 2010). This method of evaluation is not purely descriptive, as is sometimes the case in psychiatry, which often focuses primarily on symptoms. Nor is this method of assessment a traditional psychoanalytic one with a focus on history and underlying dynamics related to the past. Rather, we maintain that the nature of the treatment experience will be shaped by the level of personality organization (neurotic personality organization [NPO], high- or low-level borderline personality organization [BPO]), the symptoms the patient experiences, and the areas of functioning that are compromised.

The structure of personality organization is central to the manner in which the patient integrates and organizes all of his or her experiences and behavior. The specific symptom constellations (depression, eating disorders, substance abuse, suicidal behavior) and areas of dysfunction (social relations, work) vary across the levels of personality organization. The primary goal of patient assessment, therefore, is to correctly identify the patient's symptoms, areas of dysfunction, and personality organization because these directly influence the focus, process, and outcome of treatment. After an assessment of these areas and the establishment of an appropriate treatment frame (see Chapter 5, "Establishing the Treatment Frame"), treatment can begin with a focus on the emerging transference themes and underlying psychodynamics.

The patient with BPO often wants to "begin therapy" without attention to the preliminary details of history taking and establishment of the treatment contract. In fact, many patients with BPO come to therapy in self-defined "crisis," asking for immediate attention to such issues as refill of medication, a sudden eruption of suicidal ideation, or a disruption in a previous psychotherapy that has lapsed or gone sour. Our approach is to tactfully acknowledge the patient's situation but at the same time to proceed with adequate assessment prior to committing to engaging in a treatment per se. In response to any request for treatment, the therapist should explain that an assessment is necessary to understand the nature of the problems and make appropriate treatment recommendations. While respecting the felt need for immediate therapy and change, the therapist indicates that effective help depends on an understanding of the problem and a clear agreement between the two participants as to how to proceed. If the patient's situation constitutes a clinical crisis, the patient is referred to emergency services. Careful assessment and treatment contracting can be carried out later, after the emergency has been addressed.

Because patients with BPO suffer from defective internal structure and organization that are manifested in their chaotic behavior, the external structure provided by the therapeutic process is an essential element in the treatment of these patients. As we describe the unfolding of treatment, it will become clear how transference-focused psychotherapy (TFP) provides structure for the patient that begins immediately in the assessment process.

CLINICAL ASSESSMENT

The goal of clinical assessment, generally accomplished in one to three sessions (an initial double session is recommended) prior to treatment contracting, is to ascertain the diagnosis and, if a personality disorder is present, the severity of the disorder and its organization as NPO or high- or low-level

BPO. In addition to providing the therapist with information on the symptoms, critical areas of dysfunction, and level of personality organization, the assessment also has the potential for providing the patient with a careful view of his or her difficulties and a beginning experience of the interaction with a helping other. Most relevant to subsequent articulation of a treatment contract, the clinician must elicit information concerning prior treatment attempts, with particular attention to the quality of the relationship the patient developed with previous therapists and the ways the prior treatments ended. It is useful to contact previous therapists (with the patient's permission), especially to discuss issues of how the treatment was disrupted and/or discontinued and what the therapist would do differently if another opportunity arose.

The clinical usefulness of the personality disorder criteria of DSM-5 (American Psychiatric Association 2013) is limited,[1] and therefore we emphasize an assessment that captures current symptoms and mental status, level of personality organization, and current functioning in key areas of adjustment (work, social and intimate life, and creativity) that are crucial to the psychological investments that constitute identity.

THE STRUCTURAL INTERVIEW

The structural interview (Kernberg 1984) is a method of clinical assessment that focuses on the patient's symptomatology, present and past; the patient's personality organization, including conception of self and others; and the quality of here-and-now interaction between patient and interviewer. The interviewer focuses on the patient's main difficulties with tactful assessment of the variables central to structural diagnosis: 1) identity integration versus diffusion, 2) characteristic defenses, and 3) level of reality testing. The interviewer also assesses any awareness of internal conflict—in contrast to externalization—within the patient. It is assumed this exploration creates enough tension so that the patient's predominant defensive or "structural" organization of mental functioning will emerge. The structural interview focuses more on the patient's psychological functioning in the here-and-now than the traditional psychiatric anamnesis although it also includes a review of the patient's personal history. The structural diagnosis depends in a major way on how the patient handles the exploration of his or her areas of difficulties in the interview.

---

[1]However, Section III of DSM-5 introduces considerations that have long been central to our understanding of personality disorders and structural diagnostic system, such as experience of self and others.

In contrast to the structured or semistructured psychiatric interviews used for research, the structural interview does not follow a totally predetermined order: it is called structural because it seeks to determine the psychological structure. Although the beginning and end are clear, the ways in which the interview develops and the diagnostic elements emerge are less rigidly established; they depend on what emerges in the patient's self presentation and response to the interviewer. A cyclical process is a significant feature of the structural interviewing (see Figure 4–1). In this model, the positioning of anchoring symptoms along the perimeter of a circle makes it possible for the interviewer to proceed from one cardinal symptom to the next and return eventually to the starting point and reinitiate a new cycle of inquiry if necessary. This is in contrast to a "decision tree" model of inquiry, which has a fixed pattern of progression. Recycling along the anchoring symptoms enables the interviewer to return as often as necessary to the same issues in different contexts, retesting preliminary findings at later stages of the interview. It is not intended that the anchoring symptoms invariably be explored systematically. Depending on early findings, different approaches to this cycling of inquiry are recommended.

There are three parts of the structural interview, each one framed by a crucial lead-in question or questions. The first part begins with the interviewer asking four questions:

1. What brings you here?
2. What is the overall extent of your problems and difficulties? (The therapist is seeking a complete inventory of the patient's problems, including ones that might not have been the reason for the current consultation.)
3. How do you understand your problems?
4. What do you expect from treatment?

In addition to seeking information, the fact of asking about these areas all at once at the beginning of the interview serves as a means of assessing cognitive function and possible deficits. A patient with memory or concentration difficulties will have trouble taking in these questions at one time. If the patient does have difficulty, the therapist should tactfully explore the difficulty. The reader should keep in mind that patients may present with problems that have not yet been diagnosed and the assessment should screen for possible problems such as affective illness and cognitive or organic problems as well as personality disorder.

The opening questions provide the patient with an opportunity to discuss his or her symptoms, chief reasons for coming for treatment, and other difficulties that he or she is experiencing in present life. In listening to the patient's

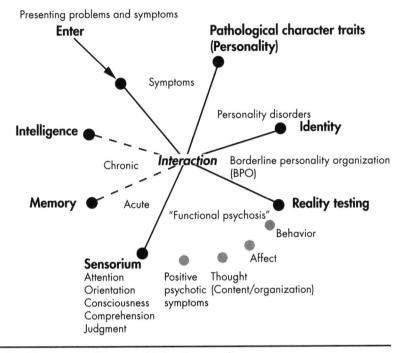

Presenting problems and symptoms

Enter

Pathological character traits (Personality)

Symptoms

Personality disorders

Intelligence

Identity

Chronic   *Interaction*   Borderline personality organization (BPO)

Memory   Acute

Reality testing

"Functional psychosis"

Behavior

Affect

Sensorium
Attention
Orientation
Consciousness
Comprehension
Judgment

Positive
psychotic
symptoms

Thought
(Content/organization)

FIGURE 4–1.   Structural interview cycle.

Note.   Review any symptoms suggesting major affective, anxiety, or psychotic disorders.

response, the interviewer can evaluate the patient's awareness of pathology and need for treatment, as well as the patient's expectations (realistic or unrealistic) of treatment. Patients without psychotic or organic difficulties often talk about difficulties in their interpersonal life that would suggest pathological character traits and give evidence for generally adequate reality testing.

The patient's understanding of his or her problems may suggest the use of primitive defense mechanisms that externalize responsibility and project aspects of the patient's internal world onto the surrounding world. For example, one patient stated that the suicide attempt that brought her to treatment was not an indication of any psychiatric illness or problem in her but was a rational response to living with a husband who was "a monster." The therapist is not in a position of knowing the real situation at this point and should maintain a neutral stance. In this case, the neutral stance would be to consider that the patient's husband may indeed be a monster but also to consider the possibility that the patient may be projecting elements of her internal world onto her husband (i.e., the therapist is considering what characteristic defenses the patient may be using). The developments in the transference after treatment begins can help sort out these issues (see Chapter 6, "Techniques of Treatment," for a full discussion of the therapist's neutrality). The position of neutrality, in contrast to overt support of the patient's position ("It must be terrible to have a husband like that") may lead to some increase in anxiety because it may connect with the side of the patient that questions her projection and the role it plays in decreasing her internal conflict. The therapist's neutrality is part of a subtle assessment of the patient's capacity to be aware of internal conflict in contrast to being in a completely rigid defensive system or frame of mind.

The patient's manner of listening to and responding to the interviewer's questions also provides indirect evidence of sensorium and memory, as well as some indication of intelligence. For example, the patient may show memory deficits or limited capacity for abstraction, or the patient may be overly concrete. The patient may respond appropriately to the questions but, in the process of clarifying answers, become lost in details. In patients with borderline organization, careful evaluation of suicidal and other self-destructive behaviors, eating disorders, substance abuse, and the nature and extent of depression can be complicated because those topics both stir up affects and defend against affects.

In a second part, the interviewer asks the patient to first describe himself or herself as fully as possible, then to describe someone important in his or her life as fully as possible. This is helpful in the evaluation of identity or identity diffusion. The request is not a simple one. It calls on self-reflection and self-understanding. A person with an integrated identity will be able to provide a rich and complex self-description, whereas someone with identity diffusion will give a limited and superficial description of self and others. Video 1–1 shows Dr. Otto Kernberg carrying out this part of the structural interview with an actor playing the role of a patient. The patient, Albert, has come for treatment because Saskia, his girlfriend of 4 years, has abruptly left him. He is depressed and lost at this point in his life. Dr. Kernberg's effort in the interview is to get a diagnostic picture that includes getting Albert's understanding of the events that transpired. Dr. Kernberg also elicits Albert's descriptions of himself and of Saskia. As seen in the video, Albert provides superficial and one-dimensional descriptions that are characteristic of people who do not have an integrated sense of self and others. He describes himself as a very loving person, leaving out any mention of his angry outbursts. When asked to describe Saskia, he begins with a description of her physical appearance, followed by a superficial idealized picture. Readers are encouraged to view the full structural interview in *Psychoanalytic Psychotherapy*, which can be found at http://www.psychotherapy.net/video/psychoanalytic-psychotherapy-otto-kernberg.

 Video 1–1: Description of Self and Description of Other (4:24)

In the final part of the interview, there is an exploration of the past as it relates to current difficulties. While the TFP therapist focuses attention on the patient's internal world as it unfolds in the here and now, it is essential to have information about the patient's family and developmental history to have an idea of the interaction between external reality, as best as it can be discerned, and the patient's internal world. In each section of the interview, the interviewer is interested not only in the content of the patient's answers (e.g., patient is depressed, describes self as without intimate relations) but most importantly the form (manner) of the answers, the way the patient relates to the interviewer in answering, and any difficulties in responding that the patient demonstrates.

A SEMISTRUCTURED INTERVIEW

For clinicians who have not been trained in administering the structural interview and/or for readers interested in doing clinical research, we have included a semistructured interview, the Structured Interview for Personality Organization—Revised (STIPO-R), which can be accessed online at http://www.personalitystudiesinstitute.com/pdf/Structured-Interview-of-Personality-Organization.pdf. With its structured questions and probes, the STIPO-R provides the clinician with a guide to the assessment of key areas needed for a psychodynamic diagnosis distinguishing patients with BPO from patients with NPO (see Table 1–1 in Chapter 1). Although the STIPO-R lacks the clinical intuitiveness and subtlety of the structural interview, it provides a standardized way to gather information and score it objectively, which is very helpful for research purposes. The goal of the STIPO-R is to arrive at a structural diagnosis (of NPO or high- or low-level BPO) through the thorough assessment of seven essential constructs: identity, coping and rigidity, primitive defenses, reality testing, quality of object relations, aggression, and moral values.

The individual with NPO manifests a consolidated identity, relatively stable and enduring interpersonal/object relations,[2] and an absence of

_____

[2]The reader is reminded that *quality of object relations* refers to the expectations (internal, organizing principles) and capacities that organize interpersonal relationships.

primitive defenses with varying degrees of rigidity in coping. Moral values may be overly harsh and rigid, and reality testing is intact.

The patient with high-level BPO has mild to moderate identity diffusion, split and superficial interpersonal/object relations with some degree of stability, and impaired empathy. This individual has primitive defenses and maladaptive coping, with aggression directed against self and others, but also a desire for love and intimacy. Moral values are variable, and there are moderate difficulties in reality testing.

The patient with low-level BPO is somewhat more severe than the patient with high-level BPO on all seven dimensions, most prominently in poor quality of object relations (no empathy, no capacity to maintain consistent interpersonal relations), aggression (dangerous levels of aggression toward self and others), and absence of an organized value system (antisocial features, behavior).

Others have been concerned about the diagnostic issues of assessing patients with personality difficulties. The Quality of Object Relations Scale, an established interview measure, has been used to assess patients for differential response to brief psychotherapy (Piper and Duncan 1999). Most particularly, Shedler and Westen (2010) have pointed out that clinicians often evaluate by obtaining patients' descriptions of themselves and others, captured in interpersonal narratives. These interviews can be structured and then rated reliably with Q-sort techniques.

TREATMENT INDICATIONS

Within the range of BPO diagnoses, clinicians can consider psychoanalysis for some patients at the higher level of the range (e.g., narcissistic patients organized at a high level). However, models of therapy developed specifically for BPD are generally indicated for patients with the disorder who, historically, were often found to become disorganized in the relatively unstructured setting of the analytic couch. TFP, mentalization-based therapy (MBT; Bateman and Fonagy 2004), and psychodynamic supportive psychotherapy (Kernberg 1984; Rockland 1992) are based to varying degrees on psychoanalytic concepts. Dialectical behavioral therapy (DBT; Linehan 1993) and schema-focused therapy (Beck et al. 2004) are integrated methods based on principles of cognitive-behavioral therapy and behavioral therapy. The research that exists to date suggests that DBT and MBT may be initially indicated for the subgroup of patients with BPO who are actively suicidal or parasuicidal, although TFP also addresses these issues in the contracting phase and consequent limit setting. There is some research that finds that working with the transference is especially beneficial in patients with a low quality of interpersonal relations (Høglend et al. 2008) and some that finds that patients with a low initial level of reflective functioning remain in treatment longer in TFP than in DBT or psychodynamic supportive therapy (Levy et al. 2011).

We have noted that some patients who have been helped with behavioral control of symptoms by DBT then seek TFP because of continued difficulties in relationships, especially of an intimate nature. More narcissistic patients who have difficulty accepting advice may do better in TFP than DBT. For those BPO patients with multiple symptoms, a negativistic attitude toward treatment, and few resources for therapy, a supportive approach can be utilized (Rockland, 1992). A history of lack of motivation and poor treatment adherence may also indicate supportive psychotherapy. Good Psychiatric Management (GPM; Gunderson 2014) is a treatment approach that provides basic treatment management principles for BPD patients to clinicians. It can be used to treat more straightforward higher-level BPO cases and can provide stabilization for complicated cases that can then be referred to TFP for more in-depth treatment.

It is usually not one patient characteristic but rather a constellation of characteristics that is crucial for treatment selection. Patient characteristics that suggest that treatment will be difficult include antisocial personality disorder or behavior, severe arrogance that would interfere with learning from the therapist, secondary gain, poor quality of object relations, significant disruptions in life caused by drug and/or alcohol use, and a horrible life situation that cannot be changed. Patient characteristics that are positive for most treatments include motivation for change and realistic time to invest in doing something toward self-improvement, taking responsibility for treatment, intelligence, some real talent, and attractiveness as a person.

TFP is indicated for those patients with BPO who possess at least an average intelligence and have moderate to severe symptoms with serious compromise to their functioning in work or profession, love and sex, or social life and creativity (Table 4–1). Interestingly, patients are sometimes high in professional functioning but extremely compromised in the area of relationships. The ability and extent of self-reflection shown in the structural interview is an asset in TFP, but we have also had successful outcomes with patients showing minimal self-reflection on initial evaluation.

Psychoanalysis and TFP (Caligor et al. 2007) are appropriate treatments for patients with NPO—that is, those with hysterical personality, obsessive-compulsive personality, or depressive-masochistic personality. Either may also be indicated for those with a mixture of infantile and hysterical features. Patients with narcissistic personality disorder (NPO) in the high-level BPO range may respond to psychoanalysis if overt borderline features of impul-

TABLE 4–1.   Patient heterogeneity and treatment planning

Comorbid personality disorders	Comorbid antisocial personality disorder may preclude psychodynamic treatment
Symptoms	The treatment should be structured for controlling substance abuse or eating disorders (see Chapter 5); treatment includes possible medication treatment for major depression or other biological disorders
Structural differences	Identity diffusion can be masked by the pathological grandiose self, a structure that characterizes narcissistic personality disorder and requires special treatment consideration[a]
Sexuality and intimacy	Patients with attachment longings, some ability to fall in love, and some integration of eroticism with tenderness have better prognosis

Source.   [a]Diamond et al. 2011; Stern et al. 2013.

sive behavior are absent and the patient demonstrates anxiety tolerance and sublimatory channeling. Otherwise, patients with NPO should be referred to TFP (Diamond et al. 2001, Stern et al. 2013).

We will illustrate the principal elements of the structural interview as seen in the case of Betty, whose case we will refer to in Chapter 8, "Early Treatment Phase," as an example of TFP with a high-level BPO patient.

CLINICAL ILLUSTRATION: THE CASE OF BETTY

Early Part of the Interview

Betty, a 33-year-old single woman, presented for therapy because of frustration that she was not getting better in other treatments. She had been in numerous therapies since age 16 when she took an overdose. Her initial diagnosis was major depressive episode. Over the years, this was changed to bipolar disorder. She had been hospitalized twice: after the first overdose and then in her early 30s when she felt that life was hopeless and she took a second overdose. Over the years, Betty had been prescribed tricyclic antidepressants and selective serotonin reuptake inhibitors, low-dose neuroleptics, anxiolytics, mood stabilizers, and electroconvulsive therapy. At the time of evaluation, she was taking gabapentin 1,200 mg/day. Her treatments had included many trials of individual therapy (supportive and cognitive-behavioral), group therapy, and day hospital stays, as well as the two hospitalizations that followed each overdose. In response to the initial questions in the structural interview, Betty said, "I get so depressed, I can't get out of bed. I have no energy, no interest in anything. Sometimes I almost get dehydrated because I can't get up and get a glass of water. This can go on for weeks. I've been that way most of the past 6 months. Getting up to get here today is the most I've been able to do since I don't know when."

Betty's therapist, Dr. Em, inquired appropriately about Betty's neurovegetative symptoms of depression (problems with sleep, appetite, concentration, sex drive, etc.) and about her prior treatments (described in preceding paragraph). He then asked what kind of thoughts were on Betty's mind as she lay in bed in this depressed state. Betty replied that she thought of all the success and fame she could have as an author if she were not afflicted with this "incurable depression." She compared her writing abilities to those of the most successful author of the day. This material alerted Dr. Em to important information about Betty's self representations and about the likely role of narcissistic character pathology in her depressive symptoms.

Middle Part of the Interview

Dr. Em then asked Betty about her vocational, social, and interpersonal functioning and about what impact, if any, her symptoms had on these areas of functioning. It is essential for the interviewer to acquire a comprehensive and in-depth vision of the patient's present-life situation and functioning. Betty reported that she had left college after 1½ years because of difficulty concentrating and difficulty getting along with her classmates. Specifically, she felt that they were always excluding her from things, which she explained by saying "they resented my talent"—evidence of the defense of projection and externalization. Since leaving college, she had been fired from every job she had. She attributed this to a similar resentment and to her often understanding things better than her boss. With regard to social functioning, she had no friends and had never had an intimate relationship. Her sexual experiences were limited to one-night stands. She maintained intense and conflictual relations with many members of her family. Betty lived by herself in a small apartment and had spent the last 6 months isolated in the apartment watching television. When her earnings were exhausted, she turned to her parents for help with the rent. She expressed no interest in any activities, including living. She did not see this as a problem and stated her lack of interest in living in a provocative way, as though it should be the therapist's problem rather than hers and even though this attitude was in contradiction with her coming for therapy.

Dr. Em then sought information regarding a significant other in Betty's life in an effort to understand her level of conceptualizing others: "I would now like to ask you something about the people who are most important in your present life. Please describe someone to me so that I might form a real, live impression of that person." This exploration may reveal both the extent of integration or diffusion of identity cross-sectionally at one point in time and the longitudinal, historical relationships with others across time.

Betty described her father: "He's like Stalin. I know you don't believe me, but he's like Stalin. I'm not exaggerating. He doesn't care about people. All he cared about was grades. It didn't matter if I was crying in my room. I never saw him. You said I could ask him for help paying for therapy! You don't know him. He's never lifted a finger for me. He just wants his family to perform. He doesn't care about what you feel. All he ever did was perform. He wants us to be just like him."

A few minutes later, when describing her mother, Betty returned to the topic of her father: "He cares about her a lot. She's had these crises. Maybe that's why she couldn't be there for us. But when she goes into a crisis, he does what he can. He doesn't really know what to do. He's not that kind of guy. She's really hard to deal with. I don't know how to deal with her."

Dr. Em took note of these discrepant descriptions of Betty's father, and the extremity of the first description, and considered them evidence of identity diffusion insofar as they offered two partial and unconnected internal representations of her father. He addressed this discrepancy to see if Betty could integrate it to any degree.

> **Dr. Em:** At this point, you're telling me that your father did the best he could, while you told me before that he was like Stalin. What do you make of that?
> **Betty:** He *was* like Stalin. Can't you see? Maybe that's why my mother was depressed in the first place.

Betty's reverting to an all-negative view of her father without demonstrating any capacity to integrate his good and bad qualities is further evidence of a split internal psychological structure and identity diffusion.

In order to further assess the patient's identity, Dr. Em next asked Betty to describe herself: "You have told me about your symptoms and difficulties, and I would now like to hear more about you as a person. Describe yourself, your personality, what you think is important for me to know to get a real feeling for you as a person."

This question requires the patient to adopt a self-reflective mode and construct a coherent, verbal description of self that may involve various layers of description and abstraction. In clinically evaluating the patient's response, the interviewer attends not only to the content of what is said but also to the process of thinking and articulation that the patient engages in. The extent to which the patient can engage in lucid, detailed, multilayered construction of a description of self is an indication of identity integration versus diffusion and helps determine the level of personality pathology. The patient's intelligence and education will influence the level and style of self-reflection, but a high level of intelligence does not necessarily correlate with a good reflective capacity.

Betty responded to the request to describe herself as follows:

> **Betty:** I'm depressed. I told you that. And people don't like me. I don't know why. Maybe because I'm fat. As soon as I get on the bus, I see everyone staring at me. Sometimes they talk about me. That's another reason I can't get out.
> **Dr. Em:** Is there anything else you could tell me about yourself?
> **Betty:** I had a boyfriend once. We went out a few times. Then he tried to rape me.
> **Dr. Em:** Rape you?

Betty: Yes, we got home from the movies and he wanted to have sex, but I chased him away.

This information opened the topic of sexual relations and attachment issues, about which Betty was very conflicted. In addition, Dr. Em thought of the earlier information Betty had given about her aspirations as a writer, noting that she made no note of this in her self-description. This omission added to his sense of the impoverished and fragmented quality of her self-description, which, along with the basic difficulty of staying on the topic of describing herself, provided further evidence of identity diffusion.

Third Part of the Interview

The relevant information about a patient's past often flows naturally from the questions asked about the patient's current personality and relationships with others. Especially with patients with BPO, for whom the details of the past are contaminated by the difficulties of the present and may be distorted by the unintegrated internal representations, it is preferable to explore the past only along general lines. The most important elements of the past to evaluate are any history of meaningful interpersonal relations, including relations with previous therapists and any history of antisocial behavior.

Betty gave a history of generally poor and adversarial interpersonal relations. She had no friends. She had been fired from every job she had had. She had never had sexual relations. Her only relationship with a "boyfriend" ended as soon as he tried to initiate sex. Her description of earlier therapists focused on their incompetence. She had registered a complaint against one of them for mismanaging her treatment. The only people with whom she had regular contact were family members. Betty described the contact as negative, emphasizing her family's criticism and rejection of her. The one person she described with positive feelings was an elderly therapist whom she felt truly tried to understand her. However, even though she appreciated his efforts, she felt that they did not help her change. Even so, she regretted that his retirement ended their work together. This example of a relationship in which negative feelings did not predominate was the only note that suggested a capacity to form an attachment, a quality that Dr. Em appreciated as evidence she was not at the lowest level of the BPO spectrum.

Betty's developmental history was intertwined with her description of relations with others. Her family moved often because her father was an army officer. She described him as having no concern about his children except regarding their academic performance and added that she and her brothers could never do well enough to please him. She always felt like an outsider in school. Her mother was inconsistent in taking care of her children because she would go in and out of "moods." Even though Betty appeared to be bright, she dropped out of college after the second year because of difficulties getting along with others and because she isolated herself in her room and did not study. Through her father's influence, Betty managed to get jobs but, as stated earlier, was always fired from them, leading to a period of nonfunctioning, such as the one that preceded the current evaluation.

After evaluating identity, particularly with cases of severe identity diffusion, the therapist should explore those aspects of the patient's behavior, thought processes and contents, and affects that seem to be strange or bizarre or out of context with the general direction of the patient's interaction with the therapist. If the therapist finds such behaviors, thoughts, or affects, he or she should tactfully confront the patient with his or her puzzlement, raising the question of whether the patient can understand this puzzlement in the diagnostician's mind and provide an explanation that would make the patient's expressions more understandable to the therapist.

The patient's capacity to provide such an explanation—in other words, the capacity to empathize with ordinary criteria of social reality as represented, at this point, by the therapist—indicates good reality testing and points in the direction of the diagnosis of personality disorder. The patient's lack of capacity to empathize with the tactful confrontation of what seemed strange to the therapist in the patient's behavior, thinking, or affects indicates loss of reality testing and therefore the likelihood that the patient presents with a psychotic illness or an organic mental disorder. This is a practical and relatively simple way to differentiate BPO from these more severe and regressive conditions.

> Dr. Em returned to a comment by Betty that he thought might reflect a problem with reality testing:
>
> **Dr. Em:** You said that when you get on the bus everyone stares at you and talks about you. Are you totally convinced of this, or is this more like a possibility that may or may not be happening?
> **Betty:** It seems to me that they're talking about me, but how do I know? You think I can read minds?
>
> Although somewhat aggressive, this response reflected Betty's capacity to consider alternative points of view and showed that, at least at this point in time, she did not exhibit a complete breakdown in reality testing.
>
> ### Conclusion of the Interview
>
> Dr. Em concludes the structural interview by acknowledging that he has completed his task and asking Betty whether she wishes to provide information or raise issues that have not come up thus far. One helpful question is the following: "What do you think I should have asked you and have not yet asked?" Betty's response to this was a terse "You're the expert."

SUMMARY OF THE DIAGNOSTIC TASK

TFP carries a dual focus that addresses both the in-session behavior of the patient in relation to the therapist and also the patient's current functioning outside the session in daily life. Therefore, the therapist's diagnostic task is to simultaneously explore the patient's subjective experience and world, observe the patient's behavior and interaction with the interviewer, and use his or her own affective reaction to the patient in order to understand the underlying activated object relations the patient brings to the interview. The interviewer is constructing a model of the patient's self image(s) (self representations) and of the extent to which the patient is aware of and capable of communicating such view(s). Likewise, the interviewer is building a model of the significant others in the patient's life, as well as a representation of the interaction between self and other. In this sense, the interview is a precursor of the process in TFP treatment.

In addition, the interviewer obtains a detailed view of current functioning in work, social relations, intimate relations, and areas of investment in creativity and cultural pursuits.

Summary of the Evaluation: Case Conceptualization

In contrast to Betty's earlier diagnoses of recurrent major depressive episodes and bipolar disorder, the structural interview led to a diagnosis of BPO with narcissistic features and characterological depression. The diagnosis of BPO was based on the evidence of identity diffusion and primitive defenses—especially splitting and projective identification (inducing projected anger and aggressive feelings in others)—and on the grandiose quality of some of her self representations. Betty's depression was considered characterological because of its clinical features and the links to her internal object relations (grandiose self image alternating with harsh self-criticism and rejection in her attitude toward herself), the lack of *consistent* neurovegetative symptoms, and her poor response to repeated medication trials. Betty was dysfunctional in all areas of life: work, social life, love life, and creative pursuits.

TFP was recommended as indicated for Betty. The diagnosis and proposed treatment were discussed in tandem with her. Specifically, Dr. Em first explained to Betty that although she may well have a biological vulnerability to emotional distress, it was possible to understand the symptoms and dysfunction she was experiencing as based in an underlying psychological condition that could be understood and could be changed through in-depth psychotherapy. Dr. Em included a layman's description of the concept of personality disorder in this discussion, describing personality disorder as a rigid and limited set of reactions to self and others that leads to difficulty adapting to the complexities of life and exacerbates tendencies to emotional reactivity. Betty felt that this understanding of her problems might make sense and agreed to move on to establishing the treatment contract. The plan was to continue her medication while she settled into the treatment frame and then to taper her off it.

Key Clinical Concepts

- An object relations nosology of personality pathology conceptualizes both dimensions of dysfunction (identity, defenses, reality testing, aggression, and moral values), and constellations of organization (neurotic, high-level borderline, and low-level borderline).

- Clinical assessment combines both an assessment of symptoms and an assessment of identity, level of defense mechanisms, and quality of reality testing, with a focus on internal representations of self, others, and relationship patterns.

- A constellation of factors leads to the recommendation of TFP, including borderline personality organization, average intelligence, and moderate to severe symptoms. A major contraindication is comorbid antisocial personality disorder.

SELECTED READINGS

Caligor E, Clarkin JF: An object relations model of personality and personality pathology, in Psychodynamic Psychotherapy for Personality Disorders: A Clinical Handbook. Edited by Clarkin JF, Fonagy P, Gabbard GO. Washington, DC, American Psychiatric Publishing, 2010, pp 3–36

Hörz S, Clarkin JF, Stern BL, et al: The Structured Interview of Personality Organization (STIPO): An instrument to assess severity and change of personality pathology, in Psychodynamic Psychotherapy Research. Edited by Levy R, Ablon J, Kachele H. New York, Springer, 2012, pp 571–592

Kernberg OF: Structural diagnosis and the structural interview, in Severe Personality Disorders. New Haven, CT, Yale University Press, 1984, pp 3–51

PDM Task Force: Psychodynamic Diagnostic Manual, Personality Patterns and Disorders. Silver Spring, MD, Alliance of Psychoanalytic Organizations, 2006

5

ESTABLISHING THE TREATMENT FRAME

Contracting, Medication, and Adjunctive Treatments

THE INITIAL treatment task after assessment is setting the frame of treatment, the first of a series of tactics of transference-focused psychotherapy (TFP; other tactics are described in Chapter 7, "Tactics of Treatment and Clinical Challenges"). Both the assessment and contract setting precede the initiation of therapy because therapy cannot proceed until clear conditions of treatment are in place (Yeomans et al. 1992). Treatment contracting is carried out by the negotiation of a verbal treatment contract or understanding between the therapist and patient. The contract details the *least restrictive* set of conditions necessary to ensure an environment in which the psychotherapeutic process can unfold. A treatment contract establishes the frame of the treatment, defines the responsibilities of each participant, and sets the stage for observing the patient's dynamics in a defined "space." In essence, the contract defines what the reality of the therapeutic relationship is. It is important that the therapist keep this in mind because the patient's inner world of object relations will be evident in pressures to distort the real relationship. Because the distortions may be subtle, the therapist must have the reality of the relations anchored in his or her mind as the reference point against which any deviations may be understood. A simple example is the therapist who begins to feel (countertransference) that he is selfish and withholding because he is not available to the patient by phone when the patient is upset at night. Checking his reaction against the part of the contract about communication outside of sessions can remind him that he is not in fact negligent but rather is following the treatment agreement. This reminder can help the therapist understand that his countertransference corresponds to an element in the patient's internal world that should be discussed.

INITIATION OF THERAPY

The initiation of therapy has the following sequence: assessment (one to three sessions on average, as discussed in Chapter 4, "Assessment Phase"), setting of the treatment contract (two to three sessions on average but may require more in complicated cases), and the beginning of therapy (if patient and therapist agree on the contract). Creating conditions in which a psychodynamic exploration can take place involves 1) agreeing that the patient's difficulties may benefit from deeper understanding of the self (in contrast to a purely biological view of the problems), 2) containing acting-out behaviors so that the exploratory work is not interrupted repeatedly by "putting out fires," and 3) defining what the treatment and treatment relationship are.

A guiding principle in setting up the conditions of treatment is that the therapist must feel comfortable and safe enough to think clearly. This is no small matter in the treatment of patients who often create a level of anxiety that can lead the therapist either to abandon psychodynamic techniques in favor of whatever measures seem to meet the need of the moment or, much worse, to abandon the case. In so doing, therapists are usually participating in acting out the primitive dynamics of the patient rather than helping the patient understand and resolve them. Another guiding principle in setting the frame of treatment is to limit the patient's secondary gain of illness (use of symptoms to obtain extra benefits, such as more access to the therapist or medical disability). A summary of the essential functions of the treatment contract is provided in Table 5–1.

DISCUSSION OF DIAGNOSIS: AN ELEMENT OF PSYCHOEDUCATION

In entering the description of the conditions of treatment with the patient, the therapist should refer to his or her diagnostic impression because the con-

---

TABLE 5-1. Functions of the treatment contract

---

1. Establish a mutual understanding of problem(s) to address in treatment
2. Define the reality of the treatment relationship
3. Define patient and therapist responsibilities to the treatment
4. Protect the patient, the therapist, and the therapy, including protecting the therapist's ability to think clearly
5. Minimize secondary gains of illness
6. Provide a safe place for the patient's dynamics to unfold
7. Set the stage for interpreting the meaning of deviations from the treatment frame established by the contract
8. Provide an organizing therapeutic frame that permits therapy to become an anchor in the patient's life; internalization of the contract discussions often becomes a first internal link with the therapist
9. Begin to define patient's choices; discussion of possible life activities begins to clarify elements of identity and conflicts therein

---

ditions of the recommended treatment stem from the understanding of the illness. Because of the unfortunate stigma that has been attached to borderline personality disorder (BPD), many therapists are hesitant to name and discuss the diagnosis. However, the therapist's explanation to a patient who believes that he or she is suffering from anxiety and depression and who has no understanding of the deeper psychological issues involved that the diagnosis appears be a personality disorder, and then an explanation of that concept in layman's terms, can be reassuring to a patient who does not understand the source of the chaos in his or her life. It is helpful to explain that BPD involves 1) intense and quickly changing emotions ("life as an emotional roller coaster"), 2) unstable and stormy interpersonal relations, 3) impulsive actions that can be of a destructive nature,[1] and 4) an underlying lack of clarity about the patient's sense of who he or she is and difficulties assessing others realistically that generally is the root of the other problems. It is important to emphasize that although acting-out behaviors may be the most dramatic manifestation of the illness, they do not constitute the illness. Rather, it is the fragmented and confusing sense of self that is at the core.

In discussing the treatment contract, the therapist must address 1) universal and essential parameters of treatment that apply to all cases in psy-

---

[1]The reader should be aware that although impulsive aggression characterizes the actions of many BPD patients, some patients act aggressively in a controlled way, as in the case of a patient who methodically cut himself over a period of 2 hours.

chodynamic therapy (Table 5–2) and 2) resistances that can appear in the form of specific behaviors that could threaten the treatment. These behavioral resistances stem from the fact that exploratory therapy threatens the patient's fragile homeostasis. Even though splitting-based defense mechanisms do not provide for good adaptation to the complexities of life, they do provide some relief from anxiety insofar as they order the patient's world around externalization via projection. Any questioning of this system—any change in a person's defensive structure—causes anxiety until the new structure is in place. Behavioral resistances require the establishment of specific parameters that go beyond the universal parameters of psychodynamic treatment and that vary according to the individual patient; an example is the need for the therapist to set up contingencies that clarify his or her position vis-à-vis a patient whose previous therapist was so involved in the emergency management of the patient's suicide attempts that the therapist was unable to carry out any meaningful psychological exploration.

Although the patient must make a commitment to try from the start to work within the parameters of treatment, the therapist should understand that difficulty following the contract may constitute a primary topic in therapy before full adherence is achieved. Even though the contract is set up before the therapy begins, the work of therapy often involves referring back to the contract and sometimes involves revising it or adding to it during the course of treatment.

The therapist should not feel an obligation to work with a particular patient if that patient does not accept fundamental aspects of the treatment. It is the therapist's job to make sure that he or she is providing proper treatment. This is analogous to the situation of a surgeon who will not proceed with an operation unless essential conditions, such as a sterile operating field, are in place. If the patient does not accept the essential conditions of exploratory therapy, the therapist should either offer or refer the patient to a less structured, more supportive treatment. TFP is an intensive treatment with ambitious goals requiring major input from both patient and therapist. If a patient is not ready or able to commit to or is not interested in committing to the conditions of treatment, a less intense and less ambitious treatment is indicated, at least for the moment.

The contracting stage may include a meeting with the patient's parents, spouse, or partner if the therapist deems it necessary to discuss the nature of the patient's condition and the nature and limits of the therapy. This meeting generally occurs when the patient is very dependent on these others in his or her life and when there is a risk that they do not understand either the nature of the illness or the fact that the treatment offers no guarantee that a self-destructive patient will not harm or possibly kill himself or

---

TABLE 5–2. Essential elements in treatment contracting

---

1. The patient's responsibilities:
   - Attending on a regular basis
   - Paying the fee
   - Free association (making the effort to report thoughts and feelings freely, without censoring) in relation to the problems for which the patient sought therapy[a]
   - Making the effort to reflect on what he or she is reporting, on the therapist's comments, and on the interaction
2. The therapist's responsibilities:
   - Attending to the schedule
   - Evenly suspended attention to patient material
   - Making every effort to help the patient gain understanding about himself or herself and deeper aspects of his or her personality and difficulties
   - Clarifying the limits of his or her involvement, if necessary

---

Note. [a]This "modified" free association stems from the fact that patients may use the process of free association as a resistance to accessing difficult, dissociated internal states. This issue is explored further in Chapter 7 in the discussion of addressing "trivialization" in the patient's discourse.

herself even in the context of treatment. The therapist who proceeds without such an understanding in place generally experiences a pressure to "cure" the patient that is counterproductive and that leads to deviations from adhering to the role of exploratory therapist; this is most common when close family members have the impression that the patient is suffering from an exclusively biological condition that should respond to medication. In cases where the patient has been misdiagnosed for years with more biologically based conditions (generally treatment-resistant depression or bipolar disorder) and has gone through multiple treatments without benefit, families are often relieved to learn about the nature of personality disorder and the possibility of effective therapy. In cases of young adults with severe antisocial traits and dishonesty, it may be necessary to establish treatment parameters that include communication with the parents or other third parties (e.g., substance abuse counselor) to try to ensure that the therapist has accurate information.

PROCESS OF NEGOTIATING THE CONTRACT

The contracting process is not a unilateral statement by the therapist but rather a dialogue in which the therapist pays careful attention to the patient's reaction to the description of the conditions of treatment. This attention is geared both to avoid superficial meaningless agreement and to discern early transference patterns as they emerge in this process.[2] It is important that the therapist not agree to treatment arrangements that require unusual efforts or heroic measures. The temptation to provide heroic treatment provides a clue to the beginning of countertransference difficulties. When the therapist accepts more than would be reasonable in the average therapeutic treatment, the end result can be a reinforcement of the patient's self-destructive potential as the therapist assumes responsibilities that should lie with the patient, as well as an increase in the likelihood of unmanageable countertransference developments as the therapist becomes exhausted, overwhelmed, and/or harassed (Carsky and Yeomans 2012). The therapist should keep in mind what the "good-enough" therapist would be likely to do and, if there is an inner compulsion to go beyond that, examine his or her own motives.

PATIENT RESPONSIBILITIES

The areas of patient responsibility that should be routinely discussed with every patient include attendance, participation in the form of reporting thoughts and feelings without censoring, fees, and making the effort to reflect. The idea of having responsibilities in treatment may be foreign to some borderline patients who feel that they have no control over their actions and that the therapist's role is to take care of them. These patients may feel that lack of control is the essence of their illness. This attitude may be supported by family members and therapists who view borderline patients as incapable of controlling their actions and who feel it is the therapist's role to "take over" for the patient. Our substantial clinical experience suggests that these patients are generally capable of both a higher level of control and a higher level of activity than is often assumed and that approaching them with this understanding is beneficial for progress in therapy and appeals to the patient's potential. It can be helpful for the therapist to explain that he or she sees the patient's acting-out behaviors not as the essence of his or her illness but rather as a manifestation of underlying psychological difficulties that can be understood and changed. Furthermore, the therapist should indicate that if the diagnosis of borderline personality is correct, the patient should be able, with

---

[2]The Contract Rating Scale is provided on our Web site (http://www.borderline-disorders.com/images/RITCS.pdf). The reader can examine this rating scale to obtain a more detailed conception of what behaviors (by both therapist and patient) are rated in order to gain a qualitative understanding of the contract rating process. In fact, the outline of this chapter is congruent with the sequence of ratings in this instrument.

effort, to control his or her impulses to act out a good deal of the time and to seek help appropriately when he or she cannot. It may be that the patient had never made the necessary effort before because neither the patient nor his or her treaters believed that the patient was capable of it.

Therapy Attendance

The patient is expected to arrive at every session on time and to leave at the scheduled end of the session. If the patient is not able to come to a session, he or she is responsible for informing the therapist as early as possible and, if possible, rescheduling. For example, the clinician might say to the patient, "It is your responsibility to come on time to every session and to leave when the time is up. If you know in advance that you will be unable to come to a session, please let me know as early as possible. Though there may be a variety of issues that could make coming to session difficult, it is important that you try to come to each scheduled session."

Although the therapist may view these conditions regarding attendance as reasonable and obvious, patients may see them otherwise. For example, these conditions could be perceived as a threat to the patient's belief in an omnipotent other: the fact that the therapist clarifies that he or she cannot help the patient if the patient is not there may challenge the patient's primitive notion that there is an all-powerful savior who can solve all of his or her problems by magic. Another possibility is that the patient will experience this responsibility as confining or as being controlled by the therapist. Yet another possibility is that the patent may argue that there are days when he or she simply does not have the energy to get out of the house. If, for any reason, the patient objects to the expectations concerning attendance in therapy, the therapist makes it clear that he or she is not making a judgment but is simply referring to the reality that treatment requires attendance. Although we emphasize the need for discussion of the conditions of the contract in order to understand the patient's position in relation to them, the basic parameters are a *sine qua non* for this type of therapy. Therefore, should the patient object, the therapist notes the objection and points out that understanding the patient's objection might provide valuable information for the therapy. However, for the purposes of beginning therapy, the therapist would then review the requirement for attendance, explaining that attendance is a necessity for treatment to take place. We repeat that if the therapist and patient do not agree on the conditions of treatment, a perfectly valid outcome of the contract setting phase is for the therapist and patient to agree not to work together. In our clinical experience, it is rare that patients reject the contract if the therapist engages in a clear discussion of the reasons behind the conditions of treatment.

Because the contract setting phase is designed to determine whether treatment can begin, interpretations during this phase are premature and are generally avoided. The issue at this point is not a full understanding of why the patient objects to the conditions but, because they are essential, whether the patient is willing to work within these conditions and explore the meaning of objections in the course of the work. A matter-of-fact statement is in order: "I understand that there are many reasons why this might appear difficult for you. Indeed, I expect that looking at some of these reasons will form important aspects of our work together if we proceed. However, at this point what is important to note is that if you are not here, no work can go on. From time to time it may be difficult for you to come to or stay in the sessions, but it is essential that we discuss those difficulties rather than having you acting on them by not appearing."

Responsibility Regarding Fees

The patient and therapist must agree on the fee per session, a policy on when bills should be paid, and a policy on payment for missed appointments. If the therapist works within a range, there may be a discussion of the fee depending on the patient's means. Different therapists may employ different policies regarding missed sessions, rescheduling, and payment due dates. The essential point is that the therapist should describe a consistent policy and be prepared to follow through on it. Establishing the ground rules regarding the fee at the outset establishes an anchoring point to which the therapist can return if the situation warrants.

For example, a patient began therapy and failed to pay her bill within the contracted time (by the end of the month). At the same time, in session, she was communicating that given her history of early deprivation, she felt she should be exempt from certain responsibilities in life: "I'm just not prepared to do everything others do. It's just not fair to expect me to. If someone could give me a break, then I might get over my anger."

The therapist might be tempted to forgo discussion of the errant bill for fear that the anger would be focused on him or her. However, to acknowledge that the patient's affect is directly tied to the here and now of the transference is crucial to the treatment, and the contract is a reminder of the responsibility to raise the issue with the patient in spite of any reluctance the therapist may experience. In fact, it is likely that such reluctance corresponds directly to the affective significance of this material within the transference and that the therapist's reluctance is a manifestation of the impact of the patient's attempts to control others—an attribute that probably contributes to the patient's failure with relationships outside of therapy. In this example, the patient's not paying is an enactment within the transference of the theme she is discussing. In other cases, nonpayment may occur without such a clear connection to the verbal content of sessions, but it should always be considered as acting out in relation to the treatment frame.

Patient's Role in Therapy

Every type of psychiatric treatment requires some form of patient participation if the treatment is to be effective. However, patients often approach treatment expecting to passively receive treatment as the therapist works on them. In borderline patients, this expectation is often especially intense because of the primitive nature of the patients' internal object world. Pointing out to the patient the need to participate in his or her own treatment and, more importantly, telling the patient that the outcome depends on his or her active participation touches on many themes common in borderline patients, such as the expectation of an omnipotent other and the wish for and/or fear of dependency.

TFP modifies the general psychoanalytic rule of free association by asking the person to report everything that comes to mind—all thoughts and feelings—in relation to the problems that brought him or her to treatment. The stable conditions of the sessions should help the patient access deeper aspects of his or her internal world. Although the rule of free association is generally followed in TFP, we have also noticed that the associative process can sometimes be used as a defense against access to dissociated material. Thus, the therapist must continually pay attention to the other two channels of communication—the nonverbal and the countertransference—to assess whether the verbal channel is in sync with the others and is affectively laden or whether it represents a defensive trivialization.

The following is a typical informational statement to a patient regarding the method of treatment:

> Your role in therapy is to speak freely about whatever is on your mind, particularly in relation to the main problems that brought you here, with the goal of understanding the unknown motivations for your emotions and behavior. Although at times it may feel difficult for you to do this, it is important to speak your mind without censoring yourself; this can include thoughts, feelings, dreams, fantasies, and so on. Your thought may take the form of a question for me; should that be the case, I may or may not answer depending on what I feel to be most therapeutic in that instance. Because our goal is to increase your understanding, it may be more helpful for me to encourage your own reflection than to answer directly.
>
> Beyond the general rule of speaking freely in session, if something is happening in your life where you run the risk of harming yourself or others or that might affect the continuity of the treatment, then you should bring that issue up before anything else. For example, if you got a bad report at

work that threatened your job, and thus your means for affording therapy, it would be important to bring that up for discussion before talking about whatever else might come into your mind.

THERAPIST RESPONSIBILITIES

The very fact that the therapist enunciates his or her responsibilities concretizes the therapist's belief that therapy is a two-way process. Responsibility defines involvement. The therapist's central responsibility is helping the patient achieve more understanding about himself or herself, his or her personality, and his or her difficulties, with the goal of helping to resolve these problems. The therapist's other responsibilities have to do with the scheduling of regular appointments, attending to the work of therapy during the sessions, limiting his or her involvement with the patient to the work of exploratory therapy, and maintaining confidentiality.

Therapist Responsibilities Regarding the Schedule

The clinician discusses with the patient the scheduling of appointments, including time arrangements and the therapist's procedure for notifying the patient when he or she will be away. The therapist should state clearly and succinctly both his or her proposal for the schedule and what would happen should he or she have to cancel. For example, the clinician might say, "I'll arrange for you two regular sessions a week at times we will work out jointly. The meetings will be 45 minutes each. Unless I have an emergency, I will tell you at least 1 month in advance when I am planning not to be in the office. If I have to cancel a session on a particular day when I will be in the office the rest of the week, I'll do my best to reschedule that session for another day of the week. I am committed to working with you on a regular twice-a-week basis."

Therapist Attitude Regarding the Fee

The therapist's statement about fees has important clinical implications. In discussing the payment, the clinician is declaring that the service provided has a value for which compensation is expected. Although the statement about fees can be made in a few words, much is communicated attitudinally. The clinician who coughs, lowers his or her voice, or looks away while stating the fee is making an important statement. A therapist who experiences doubts about his or her ability to help the patient may discuss the fee in an apologetic tone, suggesting that he or she may not be able to provide the patient with "his or her money's worth." In short, many countertransference issues are touched on by discussion of the fee, as are many transference issues in this group of patients who are generally characterized by an insecure internal model of attachment.

Ideally, the clinician will discuss fees just as he or she would any other subject. This is especially important given the borderline patient's tendency to distort the meaning of the fee to the therapist. The therapist is informing the patient that his or her efforts are being compensated for by the money received and that he or she requires from the patient nothing more and nothing less for his or her services. The patient's beliefs about and attitudes toward the therapist's perceived position in relation to the therapy and in relation to the fee can then be analyzed for their transference implications.

Therapist Role in the Method of Treatment

One of the aims of the discussion of the contract is to educate the patient about the nature of the therapy being recommended. It would be naïve to assume that even patients who have been in treatment in the past have a clear understanding of the responsibilities of each of the participants. The statement regarding the therapist's role should include some discussion of his or her focus on listening and trying to help the patient gain understanding, the rules that he or she uses to guide his or her choice of when to speak, the fact that there will be no physical contact, and the nature of confidentiality. The following is an example:

> My responsibility is to listen as attentively as I can to what you are saying and to make comments when I feel they might be helpful to furthering our understanding of you. There may be times when you will ask questions that I may not answer, or there may be times when you want me to speak and I may not have anything to say at the moment. Whatever the situation, I will always be interested in your experience of what is going on. There may well be times when you want me to give advice or tell you what to do. The form of therapy I'm recommending for you is meant to foster your own ability to reflect successfully on yourself, on interactions, and on situations. It is also meant to foster your autonomy and independent functioning. Therefore, in most cases, my providing you with direct answers or advice (as though I *had* all the answers) would not be as useful as my helping you arrive at your own decisions. In addition, it would be presumptuous of me to pretend to know what you want and what is best for you. Because of all of this, my position will be to try to help you to understand what it is that you want, and what conflicts you have around what you want, rather than for me to tell you what to do. With regard to confidentiality, what we say here is a private matter between us. I will provide no information to others unless we first discuss it here and agree on it, and then I will ask you for a written authorization before releasing the information.

It may be necessary, with patients who have a previous history of suicide or violent outbursts, to add, "The only exception to this rule would be if you pose a threat to your life or anyone else's, in which case I will be obliged to take whatever steps are necessary, which may include violating confidentiality, to protect you or whoever else might be involved."

It is important for the therapist to feel comfortable with the role he or she is describing. Novice therapists sometimes fail to appreciate how important it is, and how difficult, to maintain the listening role of the exploratory therapist. These therapists may take to heart the common criticism that they are "sitting there doing nothing" in the face of the patient's pain and chaotic life. This form of criticism is the counterpart to the patient's primitive belief that an all-powerful other could magically fix him or her and is not doing so only because of sadistic withholding. The novice therapist may be vulnerable to abandoning the position of neutrality in response to such criticism. In reality, however, devoting one's attention and concentration to the intense and chaotic unfolding of a patient's inner world is a major undertaking, and the therapist is likely to be the only person in the patient's life who is capable of taking on that role and willing to become immersed in the intense affects of the patient's internal world.

Depending on the patient's history and presentation, the therapist may want to delineate more explicitly the limits of his or her involvement with the patient, specifically that the therapy is restricted to verbal interaction within an office setting during the established session times except in cases of true emergencies. The following is an example of such a communication:

> You've told me that in the past you called your therapist whenever you felt upset and anxious. Although that made you feel better in the short term, it did not help resolve your problems in any lasting way. The work we will do in this therapy will take place during our regularly scheduled sessions and within the time frame we have agreed on. There may be times when you will want to communicate with me outside the sessions either by phone, mail, e-mail, or in person. In most instances, I will keep such discussion for the office at our regular times. As I said before, this form of therapy is geared to fostering your own reflection, your independent functioning, and your arriving at your own decisions. That may mean, for example, that I will not return your phone call except in the case of a practical matter, such as rescheduling, or a true emergency.

The limits of the therapist's involvement in the treatment may have to be elaborated in more detail if, for example, the patient has a history of intruding on prior therapists' privacy.

At this stage of discussing the contract, there is often confusion as to the nature of an emergency. The patient may believe that it is an emergency any time he or she is feeling upset, anxious, or suicidal. The patient may have had therapists in the past who agreed with this understanding of emergencies. In TFP, the therapist distinguishes between chronic, ongoing conditions and emergencies, as in the following example:

In the past you called your therapist whenever you were upset and/or had suicidal thoughts. I do not consider those to be times of emergency because, unfortunately, such feelings represent a chronic way of being for you at this point in time. Whenever you experience a stress, your habitual response is to become upset and, often, suicidal. This is one of the principal reasons you're seeking therapy here—to change those habitual responses. In the meantime, however, we can predict that you will experience such feelings. In the past a long-term hospital stay may have been an option to treat your condition. Such treatment is not available now, so we need an arrangement to allow for treatment on an outpatient basis. We know you will continue to experience times of feeling upset, anxious, and suicidal. It will be your responsibility to deal with these feelings as they come up outside of sessions. It might help, at those times, to think of our discussions here. It might help, at times, to call on family or friends. And, if you feel you are at a risk you cannot control, you will have to go to a hospital emergency room or call 911.

Nevertheless, there could be times of emergency when it would be appropriate to call between sessions. I consider an emergency a major, unforeseen stressful event, something that would have a major impact in a person's life, such as if you learned your husband was diagnosed with cancer, or you had a fire at your house. In such cases of stressful events, it would be appropriate to call. I might be able to help you with certain aspects of your reaction; it might be appropriate to schedule an extra session. Even in such cases, however, you should remember that I do not carry a beeper and that it might be a number of hours before I get your message and get back to you. It is important to be clear that I am providing an ongoing therapy that I believe will help you in the long run, but I am not in a position to provide emergency services around the clock and, given the nature of our work and our goals, I don't think that my doing so would be helpful for you even if I could.

As a technical point, so that the patient will know what to realistically expect, it is important that the therapist make his or her actual availability clear (e.g., "I check my messages around 9 A.M., noon, 5 P.M., and 9 P.M. on weekdays and in the afternoon on weekends").

The therapist's description of his or her availability is important both to establish what the patient can realistically expect and to provide a model of measured consistency as opposed to impulse-driven erratic contact. Patients may complain that the therapist offers them nothing to help with their distress between sessions. However, the therapy being offered will help the patient develop the capacity to maintain a consistent positive internal image of, and sense of attachment to, the other as the interpretive work (see Chapter 6, "Techniques of Treatment") helps the patient understand how his or her internal affects tend to destroy the stability of such images.

The position that the therapist takes regarding patient phone calls may vary according to the dynamics of the situation. The example of the therapist's comments above involved a patient whose calls were motivated by the secondary gain of extra therapist contact, which felt gratifying but did not help in the process of change. As the therapist explained, calls are justified in cases of emergency. One type of emergency is when a patient, usually one without a history of calling between sessions, begins to experience severe distress and anxiety when the work in therapy begins to challenge his or her characterological defensive structure. An example of this is the narcissistic borderline patient whose internal structure is based on a grandiose, albeit fragile, sense of self and a devaluing dismissing of others. The dismissing of others usually involves a fundamental mistrust, a belief that depending on others can only lead to abandonment and hurt. When such a patient begins to sense a dependency (usually covert at first) on the therapist, he or she generally experiences increased anxiety. This may be manifested by wishes to drop out of treatment, or even by suicidal ideation.

In a situation like this—in which necessary shifts in the patient's internal world (in this case, the experience of dependency in an internal world that does not allow for it) are so distressing to the patient that they seem intolerable for a period of time—the therapist may take an active role in the following way: 1) by communicating that he or she understands the acute difficulty the patient is experiencing; 2) by confirming that, as difficult as this experience is, it may be necessary for meaningful change to take place; and 3) by letting the patient know that during this time of feeling that he or she is in frightening "unknown territory," the patient *can* call the therapist at times when he or she feels the urge to end the therapy or end his or her life. At that point, the therapist can reconfirm that the patient's anxiety is understandable at a time of a shift in the patient's internal world. The therapist may also offer an additional session to work on the anxiety aroused by the developments in the treatment.

Although this message may appear to contradict the general policy that phone calls are appropriate only in times of emergency, the fact is that as the therapy develops, emergencies can occur in the transference. Most typically, these occur when a patient develops a feeling of dependency in the context of a chronic narcissistic ("You don't matter to me") or chronic paranoid ("You're going to harm me") transference. If the patient continues to call after the crisis has calmed down (although such crises may recur before being finally resolved), the therapist should explore whether the motivation of the calls has become the secondary gain of increased contact with the therapist and set limits appropriately.

THERAPIST-PATIENT DIALOGUE IN THE CONTRACTING PROCESS

Setting the treatment contract is an interactive process. Whereas many points in the contract are non-negotiable because they are the *minimum* conditions required for the therapy to occur, the setting of the contract is a dialogue. The therapist must inquire about the patient's reaction to the treatment parameters. If the patient has objections to the parameters, the therapist asks the patient to explain those objections and attempts to see if the patient can come to understand why the parameters are necessary.

Evaluation of Patient's Hearing and Accepting the Contract

After the clinician has presented any part of the treatment contract, he or she must then observe the patient's response in order to evaluate the significance of these issues to the patient and to begin to observe transference patterns. First, the therapist needs to be certain that the patient has listened to and heard what the clinician has said, as opposed to impatiently waiting for the clinician to finish so the patient can go ahead with getting the therapy. Second, if the patient has heard, the clinician needs to determine what the patient's reaction is.

The clinician also needs to consider the patient's willingness to accept the terms of the contract. Both the willingness to hear and the willingness to accept occur along a continuum. Once the patient has clearly heard and understood the conditions of the contract, he or she may decide to reject it. Rejection of the contract is more common with narcissistic borderline patients who find the very idea of a contract offensive to their sense of importance and entitlement. The contract setting process may stir up a massive refusal to cooperate by such patients. At times the objection is presented in a challenging way: "If I have to say that I agree to these things, then you're not the therapist for me." Or the challenge to the contract may be less overtly aggressive: "I think we'd do better without these rules. Why don't we just start meeting and see how we work together?" See D. Diamond, F.E. Yeomans, and B.L. Stern, A Clinical Guide for Treating Narcissistic Pathology: A Transference Focused Psychotherapy (in preparation) for a discussion of modifications that can be useful in the contracting process with narcissistic patients.

Another variant of rejecting the contract is that the patient may superficially agree but signal that he or she is dismissing any real acceptance of the contract by the facile nature of his or her agreement to it. For example, the patient may interrupt the clinician before he or she has even completed presenting the contract and say, "Oh yes, I'll give it a shot. Let's stop obsessing about details and get to work."

A more promising position along the continuum of accepting the treatment is represented by the patient who does *not* claim to agree with all aspects but presents no major objections to the basic conditions and shows that he or she has considered them; there is a "yes, but" quality to the agreement: "I understand what you are saying about reporting whatever comes to mind here, but I'm not sure I can do it." The patient who is able to present objections in a thoughtful fashion is more likely to collaborate with the therapy than one who initially endorses every aspect without any sense of reservation. In fact, if the latter were the case, the diagnostician should wonder aloud, "How is it that you have no questions or reservations whatsoever to any part of what I have said?"

Given the choice of therapies for borderline personality, patients sometimes ask why a psychodynamic approach would be preferable to other approaches. If the therapist has considered the indications for therapy, as presented in Chapter 4, he or she can respond that the recommendation for TFP is based on his or her belief that the most complete resolution of the patient's problems will come from addressing the psychological makeup that underlies the patient's specific symptoms and that work on this level is most likely to lead to achieving normal functioning in the areas of work, love, interpersonal relations, and creative and leisure activities.

Reacting to the Patient's Response

The contracting process is subject to the dynamics of the patient-therapist dyad. There is far more to the creation of the frame than simply reciting a checklist of mutual responsibilities. The clinician, having presented the general conditions for the treatment and listened carefully to the patient's reaction, must decide whether to accept the patient's response as adequate to begin the therapy or to pursue exploration of the patient's implicit or explicit opposition to the contract. The skill of the therapist's pursuit of the patient's responses to the different parts of the contract is a major factor in establishing an adequate treatment frame. An unskilled therapist might react to the patient's objections by apologizing, withdrawing certain conditions of treatment, or abdicating his or her role and letting the patient determine the conditions.

For example, a clinician who is confronted by a challenging, devaluing patient may choose to postpone mentioning all of the patient's responsibilities, telling himself or herself that the patient needs to be eased into therapy. Whenever the clinician avoids discussing an aspect of the contract, he or she is indicating a countertransference issue. If the clinician cannot allow himself or herself to describe what is required for treatment to take place, then that difficulty in articulation will most likely manifest itself later in treatment in the clinician's avoiding confronting or interpreting the patient's grandiosity or aggression or entitlement. This is why the therapist must have a clear, internalized sense of the contract and frame of treatment when entering into the process. The therapist will then be sensitive to any deviation on his or her part and will see this as a red flag indicating the need to examine his or her countertransference at that point, whether it be fear, pity, or another uncomfortable emotional response.

In a different version of this problem, a clinician may articulate fully the areas of responsibility but then undo his or her statements in various ways. The following are examples:

1. After having agreed that one of the patient's responsibilities is to come to the session on time, the therapist might add, "Of course there will be days when you can't get to session on time, and in those cases I'll try to make up for the lost time at the end of the session."
2. In response to a patient's vehement denunciation of the idea of any contract at all, the clinician might say, "Well, this may be too much to ask all at once. We can see if we can work toward it."

Another possibility is that the therapist's words can be letter perfect, but the "melody" may present an altogether different picture. For example, a therapist who is anxious about what he or she is doing might race through the presentation of the patient's responsibilities, including all the appropriate items but without allowing the patient any time to reflect and respond.

A different version of the diagnostician's withdrawing from the conditions of the contract would be to ignore the patient's objections and act as if an agreement to begin the treatment had been reached. Accepting a pseudo agreement sidesteps confrontation but leads to difficulties later in the treatment. A better but still incomplete position is represented by the clinician who responds to the patient's objection by asking for further clarification but fails to return to the fact that the condition of treatment being discussed is a necessary condition of treatment.[3] For example, the therapist might say, "Tell me more about why you may not be able to come to sessions regularly," but after the patient replies that she may need extra hours for

---

[3] We are not, for the moment, considering those aspects of the treatment contract that are designed in response to particular treatment-interfering behaviors specific to a given patient. Rather, the discussion thus far has centered on the *minimal* requirements for conducting an exploratory psychotherapy. These are conditions determined by the nature of the therapy, not by the therapist, although the patient often responds as if the latter were the case and accuses the therapist of imposing arbitrary rules that serve the sole purpose of making the therapist's life easy.

her studies, the therapist makes no further comment and moves on to another issue.

The therapist may have to return several times to the need for a particular condition of treatment—each time explaining the reason for it (e.g., "Therapy can't happen if you're not here"), reviewing the patient's objection, and seeing whether the patient can understand that although he or she may have strong feelings about the issues involved, the therapy is a specific process with certain requirements. Patience, persistence, and repetition are hallmarks of a therapist's work with a borderline patient.

On the other end of the spectrum, an unskilled therapist may require such rigid and "letter-perfect" agreement to the contract as to be unrealistic (and probably to enact a harsh punitive object in the countertransference). The clinician needs to strive for appropriate flexibility in addressing the patient's response to the contract.

There will certainly be patients who, despite not fully endorsing what has been recommended, indicate enough willingness to comply that the clinician feels that the treatment can begin. In fact, clinical judgment is essential to knowing when there is good enough agreement to proceed with the therapy. It would be naïve to expect that most borderline patients would come to the point of offering wholehearted, unambivalent agreement to all aspects of the contract. The therapist must assess when the patient has gotten the gist of the terms and seems willing to try, albeit somewhat grudgingly. It is important for the clinician to indicate his or her awareness that the patient continues to experience some ambivalence and to mention that if this ambivalence should grow into a major objection, it would constitute a priority issue for discussion.

A patient's behavior during contracting sessions may be at odds with his or her verbal agreement. If so, the clinician needs to address the apparent contradiction: "Even though you've agreed to come twice a week if we decide to begin treatment, you've already missed two sessions during our discussion of the conditions of treatment." Although it is important not to shift imperceptibly from contract setting into doing therapy, the therapist must address the patient's behavior related to contract issues as they are being discussed. Otherwise, the therapist would be ignoring an important source of information. In such an instance, the therapist might say, "It's not the time to try to understand the deeper motivation of why you've missed these sessions. For now, our task is to make our agreement about the arrangements for treatment clear. Your missing two sessions is a sign to me that you're not as fully in agreement with coming to this therapy as you've said. It would be important to tell me about your reservations openly. Otherwise, they are likely to continue to get expressed as actions, and that would put the therapy at risk."

In brief, although the contracting process precedes the therapy, it is subject to the impact of the intense affects and forces to be dealt with in the therapy. Therapists engaging in this work should, therefore, be comfortable enough with borderline pathology to be able to carry out the establishing of the contract without feeling intimidated or deskilled.

TREATMENT CONTRACTING: INDIVIDUALIZED ASPECTS

In addition to the general arrangements required for any patient to engage in TFP, a major goal of setting up the contract is to anticipate which forms of resistance to exploration a particular patient is likely to create that could threaten the continuation of the treatment and to devise parameters to address and reduce that threat. This process is individualized for each patient and can be subtle and complex. The type of reasoning involved in this part of the contract setting is important for the therapist to master because the need to set up specific parameters around threats to the treatment is not limited to this preliminary stage of the treatment. In many cases, patients present new resistances and threats to the treatment during the course of the therapy. At such times, the therapist must be prepared to return to the process that is described in this chapter.

POSSIBLE BEHAVIORAL FORMS OF RESISTANCE TO THE TREATMENT

Potential threats to treatment range from patients' serious suicidal and self-destructive behaviors to more indirect things such as patients enraging parents who are paying for the treatment (see Table 5–3). Resistances may consist of behaviors that have a direct impact on the therapy and/or the therapist or of behaviors that create external situations that endanger the therapy. Examples of the latter would be the patient's alienating a family member whose financial support is necessary for the treatment, the patient's endangering (e.g., through chronic tardiness) the job that allows him or her to afford therapy, or the patient's stirring up animosity against the therapist in a family member to the extent that the family member threatens the therapist.

Threats to treatment are generally grounded in resistance—the result of primitive defense mechanisms working to maintain a brittle status quo in which conflicting parts of the patient's internal world are kept split off and are acted out—and efforts to maintain the secondary gain of illness. The elimination of the latter is one of the tasks of the first phase of treatment. In the overall course of treatment, the elimination of secondary gain

---

TABLE 5–3.   Examples of resistances/threats to the treatment

1. Suicidal and major self-destructive behaviors
2. Homicidal impulses or actions, including threatening the therapist
3. Lying or withholding of information
4. Substance dependence and substance abuse
5. Eating disorder behaviors
6. Minor self-destructive behaviors (scratching, in contrast to cutting)
7. Poor attendance
8. Excessive phone calls or other intrusions into the therapist's life
9. Not paying the fee or creating circumstances that interfere with payment
10. Creating problems outside of therapy that interfere with continuing therapy
11. Maintaining a chronically passive lifestyle, favoring secondary gain of illness

---

generally leads to the patient's engaging more fully in treatment and clears the field for effective interpretation of primitive defense mechanisms.

A patient's talk of harming self, or sometimes others, creates a tension and a distraction that can inhibit the therapist from thinking freely and spontaneously within the session, which can lead to the therapist's getting involved in the actions of the patient's life (taking the patient to the emergency room, sending the police to his or her home, etc.). The therapist who begins to take an active role in the patient's life generally enacts a role from the patient's internal world of object relations and loses the capacity to help the patient observe, reflect on, and understand the makeup of that internal world and its impact on the patient's functioning.

Not all threats to effective treatment are active behaviors. If the patient's lifestyle is so chronically passive or socially withdrawn that the treatment is the patient's only activity in life, the therapist may discuss with the patient the need for some form of work or study as a condition of treatment. For the therapist to accept that the patient will go on indefinitely doing nothing except attending treatment is to collude with a view that the patient is helpless and must exist forever as a passive, dependent recipient of caregiving. Our experience is that it is very rare that a borderline patient is not able to improve and achieve a level of independent functioning. This is a more optimistic view than many clinicians have. In fact, the pessimism of many therapists who do not expect the patient to develop a level of independence, as well as the associated possibility that disability benefits will be extended indefinitely, hampers the progress of many patients. The prospect of continuing in a dependent position can be attractive; however, in our experience, many patients demonstrate a side of themselves that is interested in functioning at a higher level and respond, albeit often with a degree of conflict and struggle, to the message that they are probably capable of doing more.

ASSESSMENT OF SPECIFIC THREATS TO TREATMENT

Diagnostic Impression

It is important to keep in mind that the treatment plan is predicated on an adequate diagnostic impression. *Before* setting up the contract, the therapist should be comfortable that the patient is organized at a borderline level and is not currently experiencing another major pathology, such as a major depressive episode or psychotic illness. If the therapist begins to set up the contract with a patient and then begins to change course because of emerging suspicions that the patient may be experiencing other major pathology, the therapist must establish whether his or her doubts about the diagnosis are grounded in reality or whether it is a countertransference issue (e.g., is the patient eliciting doubt in the therapist involving guilt that the therapist is asking too much of the patient?). An appropriate technique at that point would be to make a clear shift to reassessing the diagnostic question and holding the establishment of the contract in abeyance until this question is resolved. If, however, the therapist acted on his or her doubts about diagnosis by changing the conditions being set up as if those doubts immediately required a change in the conditions of the contract, he or she would be at risk of acting out the countertransference. A more therapeutic approach, demonstrated in the following case example, would be for the therapist to examine his or her reaction, as well as the emerging picture of the patient, to see what further information about the patient's inner world of affects and object relations can be ascertained from it.

CASE EXAMPLE

A patient with narcissistic personality disorder (NPD) at a borderline level of organization presented with antisocial traits that included receiving disability payments for "treatment-refractory depression." In the assessment, the patient's mood did not appear depressed. The therapist's diagnosis of NPD was based, among other things, on the impression that the patient's history of depression seemed related to a discrepancy between her image of what her role in life should be (famous writer) and the reality of her life, a low-functioning status that she attributed to depression. The patient was willing to consider the new diagnosis of personality disorder and readily agreed to the general conditions of treatment (attending, speaking without censoring, etc.). However, when the therapist discussed the need for her to engage in some form of work or study, the patient responded, in a menacing way, that any such activity would assuredly lead to relapsing to a thoroughly depressed, life-threatening state. The therapist's initial countertransference was to feel guilt for proposing a harmful condition of treatment. However, as he internally reviewed the basis for his diagnostic impression, he returned to a calmer affective state and proceeded with the discussion of the patient's need to work with his understanding that the patient's passive antisocial features were behind her allegation that this parameter of treatment would harm her. With the idea that the patient was attempting to safeguard a secondary gain of illness, the therapist continued discussing active engagement in a structured activity, reminding the patient that the decision as to whether or not to enter into this treatment was in her hands.

The importance of the diagnostic conclusion cannot be overestimated because borderline patients may be subject to brief psychotic episodes and also to episodes of transference psychosis and/or episodes of affective illness. Some of the most difficult moments later on in the treatment may involve how to understand and deal with such phenomena. These eventualities bear directly on issues of contract setting because the expectations of the contract imply that the patient is able to take responsibility for himself or herself rather than shift it to someone else.

Attention to Prior Therapies and to the Here-and-Now Interaction

In deciding which specific issues need to be addressed with an individual patient, the therapist needs to pay particular attention both to what transpired in the patient's previous therapies—especially those factors that resulted in disruptions and/or terminations of the treatment—and to the patient's here-and-now interactions with the clinician. The patient's attitudes and behaviors in the sessions are especially useful because they are not reports from someone else (patient, previous therapist, family, etc.) but are what the therapist observes occurring between himself or herself and the patient. In theory, both participants can agree on the information, although the extent to which they disagree provides valuable information about the status of the agreement and about the dynamics unfolding in the patient-therapist dyad. For example, if the patient has been late for three diagnostic interviews, the clinician would be remiss if he or she failed to mention that lateness might be an issue in the treatment and to discuss how they might plan together for that possibility. It is an advantage when potentially treatment-threatening behaviors surface in the diagnostic phase because, presumably, patient and therapist can agree that these activities have occurred even though they may differ as to the implications for the work that is to follow. For example, although patient and evaluator may agree that the patient has come late for several sessions, the patient may argue that this behavior in no way prognosticates his or her behavior "once the therapy begins." At the very least, the clinician needs to explore the basis for the patient's reassurance and, unless it makes sense to the evaluator to do otherwise, to include the risk of chronic lateness as an issue to discuss in the contract.

Learning about the patient's prior treatment history is second only to the study of the patient's behavior with the clinician in yielding data about likely threats to the treatment. Borderline patients, even at a relatively young age, often have an extensive treatment history. It is particularly important to learn a number of things: 1) what the patient expected of his or her treatment(s), treater(s), and himself or herself; 2) how, if at all, the patient's experience resulted in modifying his or her understanding, behavior, and desires or expectations regarding treatment; 3) in what way he or she would have liked the treatment to have been done differently; 4) what role, if any, the patient felt he or she played in the ending of any prior treatment; and 5) how he or she would incorporate that knowledge into the construction of a new treatment setting. Obviously, it is important to obtain the patient's permission to contact prior therapists to gather their perceptions of the situation. It is also important to share those prior therapists' perceptions with the patient, paying particular attention to how the patient deals with any discrepancies between his or her perception and that of previous therapists.

The clinician should clearly explain to the patient the reasons for his or her particular concerns, citing the exact information the patient has provided that signaled the need for discussion and a plan of intervention: "Because you have told me that three earlier therapies ended because you called the therapists at home late at night, we need to discuss a policy on phone calls before we start so that we can protect this treatment from what happened in those earlier ones." The clinician then observes the patient's response to his or her comment to determine how seriously the patient takes his or her own behaviors.

By focusing on the patient's past or present behavior, the clinician communicates that his or her decision about what constitutes a threat to the treatment derives *directly* from the patient's own actions rather than from the therapist's being arbitrary or capricious. The patient often experiences the establishment of a parameter in terms of a negative internal object representation—as a harmful action instigated by a self-serving or punitive person. The therapist should challenge this representation by making clear to the patient that his or her intention is to help the patient and that his or her help includes setting up parameters to safeguard the treatment. The therapist is able to deal with the patient's challenge—"Why do we need all this?" or "Why are you insisting on these things?"—by explaining that it is the patient who is determining the need for these conditions to protect the treatment rather than the clinician who is imposing his or her will on the patient. For example, the clinician might say, "Since you have come drunk to the last two sessions and, by your own admission, have not been able to think clearly, it is not that I am arbitrarily saying drinking is a problem but rather you are telling me that drinking is interfering with your thinking and therefore with your sessions. Because you want help with how you think about yourself, you are telling me that you cannot be drinking and come to sessions." (Further discussion would include specifics about participating in a sobriety program, such as attending Alcoholics Anonymous [AA] meetings, and the possible use of random testing for alcohol as a parameter of treatment.)

In assessing what might constitute a threat to the therapy, the clinician needs to remember that the fundamental task of the contract is to establish a frame within which the treatment process can unfold, to create and preserve an environment in which clinician and patient are sufficiently protected so that each can carry on his or her respective tasks. The patient must be able to keep himself or herself and the clinician apprised, as much as possible, of all that is going on within him or her, as well as to be open to the impact of the therapist and the therapeutic process on his or her beliefs, feelings, and reactions. The therapist must be able, in relative comfort, to listen as openly as possible; must be able to freely make use of his or her own knowledge, past experience, and emotional as well as rational experience of the therapy; and must be willing to change his or her mind on the basis of evolving material so as to comment therapeutically. Nothing within the treatment process should threaten either the patient or the clinician to the extent that either is no longer able to participate in a spontaneous, thoughtful, and imaginative fashion.

It is no coincidence that the list of threats to the treatment (see Table 5–3) is somewhat homologous to the hierarchy of priorities that the therapist is instructed to address (see Chapter 7) because the first issues to be addressed in a session, should they be present, are threats to the treatment. In setting up the contract around specific threats to the treatment, the clinician must be alert to the wide range of acting-out behaviors. In addition to the most common forms of these—cutting and overdosing—patients may be self-destructive by burning themselves, driving recklessly, engaging in promiscuous sex, abusing drugs or alcohol, and so on. Treatment-threatening behaviors include in-session behaviors as well as behaviors in the patient's life outside of therapy.

PROCEDURE FOR CONTRACTING AROUND SPECIFIC THREATS TO TREATMENT

In principle, the procedure for setting up a treatment contract around specific threats is the same as that regarding the universal conditions of treatment. However, there are some differences. First, contracting around specific threats calls more actively on the therapist's judgment because it requires the therapist to decide 1) which aspects of a particular patient's behavior and history may present a threat to the treatment and 2) whether the threat is so serious that a strict parameter must be in place before therapy can begin (e.g., "You will have to stop all drug use and regularly attend a 12-step meeting for therapy to begin") or whether the therapy can begin while the threatening behavior is being worked on (e.g., "I know you are still struggling with your anorexic behaviors, but as long as you agree to meet regularly with the dietician and stay above the minimum weight, we will be able to proceed with our treatment"). Second, contracting around specific elements often elicits more resistance from the patient than the universal conditions of treatment. Patients may feel that the behaviors designated by the therapist as threats to the treatment are precisely those coping mechanisms that help them find relief or even survive. They may therefore be reluctant to give them up, such as in the case of a patient who insisted she could not tolerate the stress of therapy, and of life in general, without continuing her daily use of addictive tranquilizers. Patients may deny the seriousness of the behaviors designated as threats by the therapist; they may claim that their past behavior has been exaggerated or misrepresented or is no longer valid.

Therefore, the therapist's first order of business is to articulate what he or she sees as the particular threat to the treatment and to ask the patient whether he or she can empathize with this concern. If the patient can understand the therapist's concern, then the clinician should proceed to examine what steps might be taken to safeguard the treatment as much as possible. If, however, the patient cannot appreciate the therapist's concern, the clinician should then present the evidence on which it is based. For example, a therapist might say, "Two of your previous therapists said that the reason treatment ended was because you began to attend sessions so infrequently that they felt they could not carry out the work; in addition to this, you missed two of the evaluation sessions we scheduled. That is why I am concerned about your attendance and why I feel we have to think about ways to address the possibility that this behavior will undermine yet another treatment." Should the patient fail to acknowledge the validity of the basis for concern after the data have been presented, then the therapist has no choice but to point out that a treatment contract is not possible if the two parties cannot agree on what poses a threat to the treatment.

Although the majority of patients will agree to a contract, some patients make clear during the contract setting phase that they are opposed to acknowledging the ways in which their behaviors may threaten the feasibility of treatment or to doing anything to reduce the power of that threat. In such instances, the patient's position effectively renders successful treatment impossible. In those cases, it is preferable that the therapist frame his or her comment in such a way as to keep open the possibility that the patient might at a later date seek therapy when he or she is more willing to consider the relevance of the disputed issues. The following is an example of such a communication:

> It is clear at this point that you and I cannot agree that your drinking poses a threat to the treatment. From your perspective, I am exaggerating the facts. However, my own experience of your having come drunk to one of our evaluation sessions, combined with the history other therapists have reported to me, makes it clear to me that any treatment effort begun with this much risk not only is likely to fail but also would put me in a position of supporting what I view as an unrealistic assumption of yours—that you can continue to drink heavily and at the same time fully participate in your treatment. I do not know why you insist on maintaining this belief, and, indeed, if you were to be in treatment, that would be an issue that would be very important to investigate. At this point, however, effective treatment is not possible under these conditions. If, in the future, what I am saying to you makes sense and you would like to contact me about the possibility of treatment, I would be happy to continue our discussions.

Pursuing a Plan to Safeguard the Treatment

In the case of a patient who appreciates the therapist's concern, the clinician's next step is to invite the patient to participate in a plan to safeguard the treatment against the particular threat—for example, by asking, "How might we protect the treatment against the danger of your suicide threats, a danger that has resulted thus far in the end of three treatment efforts and your nearly losing your life?" The most reassuring evidence of the patient's cooperation at this point would be active participation in the development of the plan and voicing concerns and objections regarding what the therapist is saying while at the same time revealing the capacity to consider alternatives to his or her own ideas.

Contracting Around Suicidal Behaviors

The risk of suicide is likely the aspect of treating borderline patients that creates the most difficulty for therapists. Therefore, it is important for the

If the patient feels the urge to kill self between sessions,
there are three possible scenarios:

Scenario 1

The patient experiences suicidal ideation and feels she can
control her behavior, then:

(in accordance with the contract)
Patient does not call the therapist but
rather discusses the impulse in the
next session.

Scenario 2

The patient feels she cannot control the impulse, then either:

(in accordance with the contract)   or
Patient goes to the ER, then either:
• Patient is discharged from ER and
  comes to next session, or
• Hospitalization is recommended.

If hospitalization recommended, either:
• Patient agrees and returns to therapy
  upon discharge, or
• Patient refuses, requiring referral to a
  different outpatient therapy.

(noncompliant with the contract)
Patient calls therapist, who reminds
him or her of the contract, then
either:
• Patient goes to ER, or
• Patient refuses to go. Then
  therapist does what is necessary
  for the safety of the patient and,
  when safe conditions are in place,
  discusses with the patient whether
  the therapy can continue.

Scenario 3

The patient has taken suicidal action, then either:

(in accordance with the contract)   or
Patient calls family, friend, or 911
to get to hospital for evaluation.
Decision is made to admit patient
to hospital or to return to therapy.

(noncompliant with the contract)
Patient calls therapist, who does all
he or she can to help save patient's
life. Then, when calm and neutrality
are reinstituted, therapist addresses
question of whether or not therapy
of this type can continue.

FIGURE 5–1.   Contract around suicidality in a chronically suicidal
borderline patient not experiencing a major depressive episode.

therapist to have a clear plan for how to address this issue. The following
discussion is summarized in Figure 5–1.

In formulating the treatment of a patient whose history includes self-
destructive actions that have led to disruptions in the frame of past therapies,
the therapist should make clear to the patient how self-destructive actions

will be viewed and treated in the context of the therapy under discussion. The following is an example of such a discussion.

> **Therapist:** In the past, your suicide attempts and gestures became the focus of your interactions with your therapists. In your most recent therapy, you would call Dr. Black at night saying you felt suicidal, or you would say that you could not leave her office at the end of a session because you felt like killing yourself. She would extend sessions or call the crisis team for you or take you to the emergency room. One might say that she became your around-the-clock emergency service. This approach is one option to try to help you deal with your self-destructiveness.
>
> However, a serious disadvantage of this approach is that, as happened in your treatment with Dr. Black, the treatment tends to dwell so much on your actions that it is difficult to work on understanding what deeper feelings underlie and motivate your actions. In addition, there was no improvement with regard to your being suicidal. My evaluation leads me to believe that the kind of therapy with the greatest potential for helping you move beyond the problems you describe is a therapy based on trying to understand the feelings and conflicts currently *outside of your awareness* that lead to your repeatedly breaking off relationships, losing jobs, feeling angry, getting desperate, making suicide attempts, and so on.
>
> Although you may say you agree with my comments but see no conflict between this point of view and your behavior in therapy with Dr. Black, I see it differently. If we engage in a therapy aimed at exploring your inner feelings and conflicts, any active involvement on my part in your life would impair my ability to observe and reflect on and try to understand what underlies your actions. I cannot get caught up in the action of your life and carry out exploratory therapy with you at the same time. [Authors' note: The therapist is describing in layman's terms the need to observe therapeutic neutrality.]
>
> Therefore, if you are interested, I would like to describe to you the approach to your suicidal feelings required by this kind of therapy. [The patient expresses interest.] When you feel suicidal, it will be your responsibility to evaluate your ability to control and contain that feeling. [Authors' note: Our clinical experience is that patients are generally able to diagnose when they can no longer control themselves. That is the time for going to an emergency room.]
>
> If you feel you can control the feeling, you can then discuss it in the next session. If you feel you cannot control the feeling, it will be your responsibility to take whatever steps are necessary to safeguard your life. This could include calling family or friends or the county crisis team or 911. It might be a question of your going directly to a hospital emergency room or admitting office for an evaluation. Whoever is evaluating you may try to contact me for information, but it will be up to him or her—not me—to make the final decision as to whether you need to be hospitalized because that person will have the most immediate information regarding your current state.

Defining the arrangements this way decreases the patient's secondary gain of involving the therapist in her life by removing the therapist from the decision-making and action-taking "loop." Although the hospital doctor may speak with the therapist to obtain information, the therapist does not otherwise get involved in the situation.

> **Therapist:** In such a case, your responsibility would be to accept the recommendation coming out of the evaluation. If hospital admission were recommended and you refused it, I would not be able to continue therapy with you because you would be placing yourself in a situation judged by the physician evaluating you to be dangerous. This therapy requires that we feel safe to explore whatever is on your mind. This would not be the case if we both knew that you had rejected a recommendation to be in the hospital when that was determined to be the necessary level of care.
>
> Once in the hospital you would be in the care of the hospital team, and I would not have an active role in your treatment until it was time to discuss discharge plans. At that time I would be a part of the discussion with you and your inpatient therapist about the indications regarding our resuming therapy. That would be an important moment for reflection on both of our parts—for you to reflect again on the kind of therapy you think would be most helpful for you, and for me to review our treatment arrangements to see if any changes would be necessary. How does this sound to you so far?
>
> **Patient:** Well, it sure sounds different. On the one hand, it just sounds like you don't want to be bothered by any real problems I might have—like you want to be the kind of therapist who just likes to sit and eat bonbons and thinks about saying smart things. On the other hand, since I've been through 3 years of therapy, going in and out of the hospital, with a wonderful therapist I thought would have given her life for me, but I don't think I'm any better, maybe you know what you're talking about.
>
> **Therapist:** Okay, I'll go on, but if you change your mind and begin to think that I don't know what I'm talking about, it would be important to tell me about that. What I've described so far assumes that you got yourself to an emergency room before taking any self-destructive action. The situation may arise in which you have acted in a suicidal way before contacting anyone else. This possibility is, of course, a reflection of the real risk that you could actually take your life. As I said before, your life is ultimately in your hands; although I can try to help you gain more mastery over your self-destructiveness, I cannot guarantee your safety—only you can do that. If you have taken suicidal action, such as an overdose, and then decide to try to save your life, your responsibility would be to get to an emergency room for a medical evaluation and subsequent psychiatric evaluation. Once again, it is up to you to decide whether to call family, friends, 911, or the crisis team. If you are found to be medically unstable, you would be admitted to

a medical unit before you could decide about your further psychiatric care. If you refuse to be admitted, you would put me in a position of having to end the therapy rather than cooperating with your putting yourself in an unsafe situation, as in the case I described above if you were to reject the recommendation for psychiatric admission.

Having described the above expectations with regard to the patient's management of her suicidal impulses, the therapist would ask for the patient's further reaction to and thoughts about these conditions of therapy. After discussing the patient's reaction to the conditions described thus far, the therapist goes on to describe the parameters he would follow in response to deviations from the expected management of these impulses.

Therapist: If you call me between sessions with questions about your self-destructiveness, I will suggest that you discuss these feelings in our next session. If you say you cannot wait until then, I will remind you that it is your responsibility to get to the emergency room. If you say you will not do that, I will do everything I can at that time to help you get the crisis intervention you need, and then, after the crisis is over, we will have to meet to discuss the meaning of what happened and talk about whether this therapy, which puts an emphasis on increasing your autonomy, is the right therapy for you. Similarly, if you call me to announce that you are about to take or have taken suicidal action such as an overdose and have not taken the responsibility to get to an emergency room, I will do everything I can on that occasion to help try to save your life. Then, when the situation is stable, we will meet to consider whether it is advisable to continue the therapy under those circumstances, or whether your actions reflect a rejection of the type of treatment we had agreed on, which would call for referral to another therapy.

At this point, the patient may accuse the therapist of negligence:

Patient: So, you're not really offering to help me; you're setting up a situation where I pay you to take care of me, and your main concern is that I won't bother you.

Clarification of the nature of the therapy under discussion and the need to frame the therapy so that it stands a chance of surviving where other therapies have failed may have to be repeated a number of times for the patient to understand that the conditions being presented flow from the requirements of the treatment rather than from the personal wishes of the therapist. The patient's perception of the contracting process will be influenced by her internal object representations, and she may perceive the therapist as an indifferent, neglectful figure. It is appropriate for the therapist to specifically state that his wish is to help the patient and to indicate how he proposes going about that, adding that this can only be done if the necessary conditions are in place.

> **Therapist:** My reason for being here is to try to help you. I'm discussing our treatment arrangements for that reason. The plan I'm proposing for therapy is based on what I know of you from our evaluation sessions, your history, and the history of your prior therapies. But before we get to that, I would also like to explain again that the type of treatment I'm recommending is a therapy focusing on the exploration of your inner feelings and conflicts. Your idea that you would be paying me to "take care of you" suggests that you have a different kind of treatment in mind—something like case management with a counselor who would help you make decisions and get through your life on a day-to-day basis because you both agreed that you were not able to function independently. Although that kind of treatment is an option for you, I have not recommended it for you because you have had that kind of help in the past without experiencing any long-term improvement in your ability to cope with life and get any satisfaction from it. In fact, one of the reasons you gave for seeking out an exploratory form of therapy at this point was that you repeatedly disrupted your relations with a number of case managers because of recurrent angry arguments in which you accused them of intentionally working against you. You still have the option of trying to work with a case manager again, and we can discuss that possibility. However, the immediate issue with regard to the subject of case management is the question of why you have not been able to use that kind of help to make changes in your behavior patterns. If you are convinced that what you need now is further case management or any other form of treatment different from the one I am recommending for you, it would be important for you to make that clear right now.
>
> I have a feeling that one aspect of what's going on here is that you're experiencing me as an indifferent, neglectful, and self-serving individual who is only pretending to offer you help. My point of view on this is different; I feel I'm doing the best I can to try to help you. If we agree on doing therapy, it would be helpful to understand this difference in perspectives. However, we can't really get involved in therapy unless we agree on the problems and how to approach them. If you would like to hear more about this treatment, I can respond to your concern that the conditions of treatment I am outlining might have the purpose of serving my interests at the expense of yours. [Patient expresses interest in hearing more.]
>
> As I said, these conditions are based on what we know of you and your history. We know that in your prior therapy, you called Dr. Black so often between sessions to report suicidal impulses that she could no longer distinguish between a situation of true seriousness and one of "crying wolf." Under these circumstances she did not feel that it was safe for

her to continue to treat you. She also reported that it was hard for her to remain neutral and objective while listening to you in sessions because of all the times your late-night calls left her tired the next day. One impact of these calls was to impair her ability to listen to you with full attention, concentration, and objectivity. All therapists are human, and I am no exception. In that sense there is a grain of truth when you say that I am defining these conditions to "keep you from bothering me." Insofar as your behavior in between sessions with Dr. Black bothered her to the point that she could no longer work with you, I am proposing conditions to protect the treatment, which include protecting my ability to work in a therapeutic way with you.

Contracting Around Substance Abuse or Dependence

When assessing a patient who uses alcohol or drugs, the therapist must establish whether the behavior constitutes abuse or dependence. Meaningful involvement in TFP requires sobriety. In our experience, a period of at least 3 months of sobriety is advisable before starting TFP. This period of time provides an indication that the patient can make a commitment to sobriety and whatever external supports are needed to help him or her maintain it. The most common external support is participation in a 12-step program. Patients whose alcohol or drug dependence is severe at the time of evaluation may require inpatient detoxification and rehabilitation programs before being able to participate in outpatient treatment. Referring the patient to a substance abuse specialist may be helpful in addressing the alcohol or drug problem.

If sobriety is in place, the therapist must discuss parameters of treatment that support avoiding relapse. These parameters always include a commitment to remain sober and usually include continuing in or initiating a 12-step program. In cases where the patient has a history of frequent relapse or the therapist questions the patient's honest reporting of alcohol or drug use, the therapist may include random screening for alcohol or drug use as a necessary parameter of treatment.

Contracting Around Eating Disorders

Like alcohol and substance use, eating disorders may present with varying degrees of severity. In the most severe cases, anorexia can be life threatening. When the patient has a history of going below a healthy body weight, consultation with a dietician, nutritionist, or internist is necessary before TFP can be started. The consultant establishes what the patient's minimal healthy weight is. If the patient is not at that weight, a behavioral eating disorders treatment is indicated before the patient starts TFP. This treatment could be on an inpatient or outpatient basis, according to the severity of the case. Once the patient's weight is above the minimum acceptable level, the

TFP therapist can go on with setting up the therapy. A parameter of treatment is that for the initial phase of treatment the patient be weighed on a periodic basis by the dietician, nutritionist, or internist. If the patient's weight falls below the minimum healthy level, the TFP is suspended and the patient returns to behavioral eating disorders treatment until her weight returns to the acceptable range.

In general, bulimia presents a less immediate risk to health than anorexia. Most binge eating and vomiting constitute a slow, chronic type of self-destructive behavior that can be addressed in the therapy. However, if a patient is vomiting multiple times each day, consultation with an internist is necessary to determine whether the vomiting is creating a medical risk, such as electrolyte imbalance. In such cases, ongoing medical monitoring may be a necessary parameter of the early phase of treatment. In general, progress in the therapy leads to a phasing out of this, and other, forms of acting out.

Contracting Around Issues of Social Dependency

Prior to coming to treatment, many borderline patients are deemed to be disabled, unable to work, and therefore entitled to public assistance. This situation may be brought to the therapist's attention immediately or may remain undisclosed for a period of time if the patient chooses not to bring up this issue. Therefore, the therapist must always inquire as to the patient's source of financial support. If the patient is receiving disability payments, the clinician needs to 1) assess whether the patient is able to work and 2) evaluate the patient's willingness to act on his or her capacity to work versus resistance to work because of the psychological and financial secondary gain that promotes maintaining a nonfunctional lifestyle.

We do not intend to imply that all borderline patients are not functioning in any capacity at the point of starting therapy; many are in school or have a job or career. Even those who are living a dependent life often experience ambivalence and internal conflict regarding their passive, dependent status. However, patients come for treatment manifesting different sides of the conflict. Although some patients leave therapy when it is made clear that functioning at an appropriate level is an expectation of the treatment, others may find this expectation appealing because of some frustration with their nonfunctioning and an urge to take on a more active role. There is a certain irony that some patients whose illness is expressed primarily as immature dependency and pursuit of secondary gain, and who do not appear "as sick" as patients who manifest severe self-destructive behaviors, do not do as well as this latter group because it is easier for them to be comfortable in their pathology. It is more difficult for the patient with severe self-destructive behaviors to deny the severity of his or her illness. The pathologically dependent patient is more likely to avoid or drop out of a treatment that tries to get at the root of his or her illness and that attempts to effect fundamental change. This type of patient is more likely to settle into the status of chronic patient, especially in social settings where alternative treatments and social benefit systems support this status. The best strategy for the TFP therapist is to question this choice of chronic dependency and to support the patient's strivings for more autonomous functioning.

In establishing the conditions of treatment, the therapist should always consider the patient's current level of day-to-day functioning and discuss a realistic level of structured activity. Activities could range from attending a day program to obtaining meaningful employment. The therapist needs to consider a variety of scenarios:

1. For patients who are not working and for whom there are no clear psychological or physical reasons why they cannot work, the goal of obtaining work within a specified period of time must be negotiated in the contract setting phase of treatment. Patients with borderline personality organization (BPO) generally are capable of functioning either at a job or at school. Nevertheless, patients with BPO who have passive, infantile, dependent, and/or antisocial traits often avoid the challenge of work despite the potential for functioning and instead exploit the social system—that is, either government aid or family aid. This behavior may stem from the combination of an internal conflict around functioning (a patient's internal world often includes a defective, incompetent self representation subjected to merciless harsh criticism from an object representation), emotional reactivity to others (based on a combination of genetic loading and the internal representations), and a wish to have the external world compensate for a history of real or perceived neglect or mistreatment. Even if these problems are present, our experience is that most patients are capable of functioning and that functioning is essential to any real improvement and has important psychological benefits (such as helping the person address choices in life and thereby helping resolving identity diffusion and supporting the patient's being in an interpersonal situation in which stresses can be experienced, discussed, and understood).

2. For patients who are not working because of symptoms such as depression and anxiety, an assessment must be made of the nature of the symptoms. If the patient is experiencing a major depressive episode, treatment with antidepressant medication may be necessary before the patient is able to start increasing his or her level of functioning. With regard to

anxiety, some patients are helped by low doses of atypical antipsychotic medication. However, it is also helpful to address the nature of the anxiety that interferes with functioning. We have found that the anxiety often involves a paranoid position in relation to others—the expectation that others in the school or work setting will be critical of the patient, resent him or her, talk behind his or her back, and so on. Discussion of such fears, as well as of the fact that this anxiety usually corresponds to a harsh internal object representation that is being projected, can help the patient begin to take on a functioning role. However, this discussion often becomes most meaningful when those dynamics have been experienced and explored in the relationship with the therapist.

3. When patients are working below their potential, the therapist should explain that this issue would be addressed in therapy both to understand why this is the case and, if the patient is interested, with the concrete expectation that the patient will take action to improve his or her level of functioning.

4. A variant of problems with level of functioning involves patients who are active but are involved in activities with dangerous or antisocial aspects (e.g., working as a prostitute). In such cases, the therapist should take the position that progression to work of a less dangerous and/or less antisocial nature would be a goal of treatment.

LIMITS OF INITIAL CONTRACT SETTING

The contract spells out those issues that appear to pose a threat to the treatment process and proposes a plan to prevent the therapy from being derailed. It would be naïve to assume that establishing a contract requires that all the patient's reservations be abolished before treatment can begin. Somewhere between one extreme—a blanket refusal to modify any behavior (e.g., "But doctor, if I could do that already, I wouldn't need to be here")—and the other—an expectation of the immediate eradication of the problem by setting up a parameter—is the point at which the contract phase is over and the treatment begins.

Deviations From the Contract or Treatment Frame as Signals to the Therapist

Setting the contract defines the limits of responsibility for each participant; it defines the reality of the therapeutic relationship. As the therapy develops, the therapist will repeatedly experience moments in which he or she is not clear whether his or her experience of the moment corresponds to an accurate objective appreciation of the interaction or whether it is being determined by projected elements from within the patient's internal world. The therapist caught up in possible countertransference reactions can use the contract to monitor whether his or her reactions are appropriate to the treatment method and goals or are motivated by the power of the patient's influence on his or her internal responses. For example, if in the course of treatment the patient addresses the therapist with accusations of coldness and insensitivity, arousing countertransference fears in the therapist that the patient's condemnations are accurate, the clinician may have a hard time assessing whether not answering the patient's nonemergency phone calls is proof of the validity of the accusation. However, if this is a patient whose prior history included excessive calling to previous therapists and if the issue had been discussed as a potential threat to the current treatment, the therapist, at the moment of doubt as to his or her motivation, can reflect on the contract and recognize that the thought that he or she may be harming the patient by refusing to answer the phone calls runs counter to the agreement and therefore signals a countertransference issue. This reflection helps the therapist avoid acting out by getting involved in phone conversations rather than exploring the dyad that is active.

Setting the contract gives the therapist bearings for the exploratory therapy that is to follow. Should the patient begin to deviate from the agreement, the therapist can refer to that agreement and search for an understanding of what in the current situation might be responsible for the patient's deviation. This is a way of approaching important dynamic material before it "erupts" into more major acting out. The therapist might say, "Before the treatment began we agreed that your ambivalence about therapy might surface in the form of dropping out of school, resulting in your father's no longer paying the bill. Now you tell me you're not studying and are thinking of not taking the exams. If you are having second thoughts about the therapy, it's better for us to discuss them than for you to act on them in a nonreflective way."

The potential for threats to the treatment also calls on the clinician's efforts to include both an adequate articulation of the nature of the problem and sensitive and judicious responsiveness to the patient's reactions. Contract setting *does not* eradicate the problem; it *does* alert both patient and therapist to the nature of the threat as well as to the need to construct a plan to contain the danger. It provides the clinician with a reference point to return to should the threat emerge in the ensuing treatment: "As we had talked about prior to beginning our work together, your tendency to [behave in this way] has surfaced. We will need to find out why this is occurring at this time, but first we must address the part of you that is challenging the treatment and expressing itself through action and try to understand it in a way that will, hopefully, prevent you from acting on it." If an element of the contract has been breached after the therapy has started, the general principle is to address the situation with a combination of limit setting and an interpretive stance as to the reason and significance of the contract breach and consequent limit setting.

If a patient breaks the contract, it is important for the therapist to give the patient a second chance. The issue is the need to confront the patient consistently, from this point on, with the risk of a sudden and unexpected end to the treatment if there is another break to the contract. The meaning of such a risk, particularly the patient's severe self-defeating impulses, needs to be integrated into the interpretive work. Otherwise, there could be a cycle of repeated acting out of unexamined aggressive and self-aggressive impulses. Although this may appear obvious, in clinical practice the therapist may join with the patient in avoiding full exploration of episodes of acting out; this is a form of collusion with dissociative defenses that protect against conscious awareness of the disturbing and uncomfortable affects underlying severe acting out.

Common Therapist Problems in Contract Setting

Setting up the contract represents a microcosm of the dynamics that will unfold in the treatment. Therefore, the therapist must appreciate the complexities that can develop around establishing the contract and avoid moving prematurely from the contract phase to the therapy. To prevent a premature shift into therapy, the therapist should avoid the temptation of beginning to interpret resistances before the conditions of treatment have been agreed on. The therapist should focus instead on the techniques of the contract phase, which are primarily repeated clarifications of the conditions of treatment and of the patient's response to these conditions. However, there are exceptions to every rule, and the possibility of an interpretation during the contracting phase is not excluded if it might make the difference in the patient's staying or going. For example, a therapist might say the following:

> After I discussed the importance of reporting what's on your mind without censoring, I heard you say "I'm out of here" under your breath, and you looked anxious. Although we can only understand things fully once therapy has begun, I'm wondering if your reaction represents a fear. It could be a fear that what you would say would meet with disapproval from me. It could be a fear that speaking openly would create a closeness here that might make you anxious. It could be something else. If you continue in therapy here, we can explore all the possibilities. But for the moment, we might consider them as reasons for seeming anxious and possibly not returning to continue our discussion.

Failure to Pursue Patient's Response

A deficiency in setting up the contract may result if a therapist did an adequate job of presenting the conditions of treatment in each area but then failed to adequately explore the patient's response. This type of error is common because patients often reply with a superficial compliance, saying little or nothing about their deeper thoughts. A superficial response, such as "That sounds okay to me," should be explored to make sure that the patient actually heard, took in, and considered the therapist's words. The therapist might say, "Could you tell me your understanding of the conditions you are agreeing to?" Another reason this type of error is common is that therapists may prefer to avoid the difficulties and resistance that may emerge if a thorough pursuit of the patient's response is carried out. This constitutes a naïve "looking the other way" regarding issues that are sure to emerge eventually in the treatment. A principle of TFP is that it is better to have those issues on the table as soon as possible rather than have them acted out later in treatment.

A therapist might be reluctant to pursue the patient's understanding, fearing that exploration would elicit underlying objection or anger from the patient. The fear that the patient might object to the terms of treatment is often based on the therapist's concern that the patient might, in fact, not accept the therapy being offered. This concern is most typical of beginning therapists, who often judge their success or failure by whether they can keep the patient in treatment. It is important for the therapist to keep in mind that the most essential part of the work at this stage is to establish conditions of treatment that will allow exploratory therapy to happen. It does not help patients to participate in a treatment whose lack of a clear frame allows them to continue to avoid experiencing—and to continue to put into action—the conflicts and affects that are at the root of maladaptive behaviors. Some authors would argue that it is most important to meet patients "where they are" and to work from there. In our experience, borderline patients, whose histories are often replete with multiple failed treatments, generally show that they are able to comply with expectations of taking responsibility even though they, and their previous therapists, may have thought they were incapable of this change. Often, no therapist has previously approached these patients with the belief that they are capable of exercising a measure of responsibility and control over their behaviors. Our clinical experience has shown that such a belief is not unreasonable.

In addition to having concern that the patient might not accept the treatment, the therapist might fear that uncovering strong patient objections to the conditions of the contract would provoke negative transference.

It is essential to keep in mind the role of transference and countertransference issues during the contract setting phase, especially because the very term *contract* suggests a fundamentally cognitive process. However, the difficulties that typically surface during contract setting are illustrative of how even the most cognitive and rational element of the treatment can become a field in which intrapsychic dynamics are played out. Our emphasis at this point is on *awareness* of transference and countertransference within the contract setting process, without yet entering into analysis of it. An awareness of these issues is important to guide the interventions of the therapist during this phase of treatment while keeping interpretation to a minimum in favor of an emphasis on clarification with appropriate confrontation of inconsistencies. If the patient should begin to communicate a negative transference (e.g., "I'm beginning to see that you don't give a damn about me, only about the 'purity' of your treatment"), the therapist should communicate his or her appreciation of what the patient is feeling and an interest in understanding more about it when the therapy begins but must make clear that the task for now is to explain the rationale for the treatment conditions to see if the patient would like to begin. To nondefensively express interest in any negative reaction the patient has to the therapist may reassure the patient; an important initial function of the therapist is to communicate that he or she can contain the patient's negative affects.

The therapist who fears encountering major objections to the conditions of the contract may sense the potential for an angry and devaluing response from the patient and may shy away from any exploration or confrontation for fear of unleashing that response. This reaction would be an error on two scores. First, the therapist would be working under the illusion of being able to control what comes out of the patient. This would be an illusion not only because the therapist cannot exert this type of control but also because it would be the patient in this case who is controlling the therapist's behavior in the session. Second, the therapist is attempting to avoid the emergence of the negative transference. Transference and countertransference emerge very early in the therapy of borderline patients. Working with the negative transference is essential with this population. In our experience, the sooner the negative transference emerges in the treatment and the sooner the therapist indicates that it can be contained in the treatment, the more likely the treatment is to continue and to approach the central issues.

Aggressive Pursuit of Patient's Response

A therapist pursuing the patient's response to the conditions of the contract also could err in the *opposite* direction: instead of avoiding exploration of the patient's response, the therapist might address the patient with a tenacity and assiduousness that take on an aggressive quality. The therapist might begin by appropriately inquiring about the patient's response but then might continue to ask again and again for further reactions from the patient and further assurances that he or she indeed understands and accepts the contract. This situation exemplifies how any material that comes up in therapy, whatever its manifest content, can be used in a defensive manner by either the therapist or the patient. In this case, one possibility is that the therapist may already be caught up in a projective identification and may be acting out through bearing down on the patient when aggression originates within the patient. Another possibility is that the therapist could be enacting aggression of his or her own, whether it is primary or in reaction to anxiety evoked by the prospect of working with a potentially difficult patient. Therapists are not immune to blindness regarding their own resistance around accepting a case and subsequent actions that may contribute to the patient's leaving treatment. Attention to the treatment contract, meant to strengthen and advance the treatment, could turn into overbearingness and become the arena in which a therapist's ambivalence gets played out. Thus, a therapist's attention must be directed as much to his or her own participation in the contract setting process as to the patient's. If a therapist has reservations about treating a particular patient or borderline patients in general, he or she should address this issue directly and avoid turning the contract setting into a way to dispatch an unwelcome patient. One of the main rationales for the treatment contract and frame is to make the therapy feel safe enough for the therapist to not feel this kind of anxiety.

Therapist Ambivalence About the Contract

A more complicated form of difficulty with the contract arises when the therapist has adequately studied the contract setting procedure and is able to carry it out but inwardly harbors objections to it as a technique of therapy. This problem is most typical of clinicians who feel that therapy should not include expectations of the patient but should follow the patient's lead within the context of a loosely established treatment frame. On the one hand, the therapist's objections could be based on an honest difference of opinion regarding this approach to treatment, in which case the therapist should hold off applying it. On the other hand, the objections could be based on the therapist's understanding of borderline pathology. For example, a therapist might base his or her understanding of a patient's borderline pathology on the patient's status as a victim of abuse. This understanding might stress the view that borderline patients are unfairly scapegoated as difficult patients and consequently might lead to the opinion that a special focus on setting up the contract perpetuates this scapegoating and humiliates the patient by "requiring" him or her to agree to a particularly rigid treatment frame. Different understandings of borderline pathology have stimulated much interesting debate. We would see the therapist's position that the patient is exclusively in a victim role as representing a particular countertransference position in which the therapist was fixed in a concordant countertransference with the patient's self representation as weak victim, leaving the internal representation invested with aggression split off and likely to be expressed in action and/or fixated on an external object. The relevance of this attitude to the contract setting process is that therapists who focus on the patient's victim status have often demonstrated objections to or difficulty with this aspect of the treatment.

Another example of countertransference is exemplified by the therapist who views borderline patients as so marked by constitutional deficit that the demands of the contract are unrealistic: "If the patient could follow these expectations, he wouldn't need therapy; he'd be at the end of his treatment." Of course, the establishment of the treatment contract is a challenging task. It requires skill on the part of the therapist and effort by the patient to agree to responsibilities that he or she may never have accepted before. The therapist who feels that the demands of the contract are unrealistic for the patient might wonder about his or her anxiety with regard to setting up an expectation or a limit with patients characterized by impulsive and sometimes rageful reactions. Some therapists feel that it is the limit that they set, rather than the patient, that is responsible for the patient's action. We are again dealing with the subtle question of the boundary between the patient's internal world and a more objective external reality.

SHIFTING FROM THE CONTRACT TO THERAPY AND RETURNING TO CONTRACTING ISSUES

With an understanding of the contracting process described above, the therapist must decide when he or she and the patient have achieved a good enough agreement to end the discussion of the conditions of treatment and move on to therapy. The therapist then proceeds with a statement such as, "It seems we have a good enough understanding about working together to begin the work. At this stage, if you do not have any more questions, let's start, as we discussed, with your reporting what is on your mind."

As careful as the contracting process may have been, the therapist may have to return to contracting issues during the course of the therapy. This necessity could originate because either 1) a new problem arises that was not present at the beginning of treatment (e.g., first onset of self-cutting or of substance abuse) or 2) the patient does not adhere to the conditions discussed in the initial contract. In the first case, the therapist should feel free to take time to address the need for new parameters: "Since we have this new problem in front of us, we should discuss how it affects our therapy and what conditions of therapy would make the most sense in dealing with it."

The second problem, nonadherence, is a common form of resistance. Dealing with such breaks in the contract is discussed in Chapter 7. In brief, the therapist works with a combination of reestablishing the parameter of treatment and interpreting the meaning of the patient's breaking of the contract. It is advisable for the therapist to give the patient a second chance and to consider the possibility that the patient is provoking the enactment of a harsh punitive object representation. For example, the therapist might say, "We had a clear understanding that therapy can work only if you maintain sobriety. This news that you have stopped going to AA meetings and started drinking again is an emergency signal. To get back to our work, you will have to recommit yourself to our initial agreement. Only then can we have a hope of figuring out what is behind this return to self-destructive actions." In a situation like this, the therapist alerts the patient that the latter has created a situation in which the treatment is at immediate risk. By returning to the parameters, the patient can reestablish the treatment and move on, but a repeat of breaking the contract could well signal the patient's unwillingness or inability to work in this form of treatment and could lead to referral elsewhere.

COMBINATIONS OF TFP AND OTHER INTERVENTIONS

TFP can be combined with other interventions, including medication for specific symptom constellations, and more behavioral treatments for specific symptomatic behaviors, such as eating disorders or substance abuse, or skill deficits (see Koenigsberg et al. 2000b).

TFP AND MEDICATION TREATMENT

The combination of psychotherapy and medication has the potential for substantial synergism in the treatment of borderline patients. Medications may help the patient to be better able to utilize psychotherapy. For example, the impact of interpretations is strongly influenced by the patient's affective state at the time they are delivered. With a borderline patient, affective intensity and instability often give rise to periods when the patient is not receptive to verbal interventions. Medications that moderate the extremes of borderline affect could increase the patient's accessibility (although overmedicating the patient could diminish his or her accessibility). Transient psychotic phenomena such as reality distortions or disordered thinking also may interfere with the psychotherapeutic process. A low-dose neuroleptic medication could be of potential benefit in this situation. A medication that improves impulse control could reduce acting out that might disrupt the treatment itself.

Because no specific medication regimen exists for BPO or for BPD, the current standard of practice is to consider a patient's specific target symptoms and to use medication in an attempt to achieve some degree of symptom alleviation. Despite some divergent findings (explainable in part by differences in subject selection criteria across studies), a number of patterns of symptom response appear.

Although specific symptoms of BPD may be targeted for pharmacological treatment—affective dysregulation, impulsive-behavioral dyscontrol, and cognitive-perceptual difficulties—there is no clear treatment of choice for a given symptom. In addition, the effects of drug treatment for patients with BPD are found to be, overall, weak and nonspecific, and they may diminish over time. In addition, patients with BPD seem particularly sensitive to side effects (Silk and Friedel, in press). If the clinician believes that medication may be indicated in patients with BPD, Silk and Friedel recommend systematic, successive, response-based trials of only one medication at a time. Adhering to such a plan is not always easy with patients who may pressure the clinician for quick relief and whose experience and reporting of symptoms can change rapidly. Because of the frequent pattern of an initial medication response that then diminishes over time, Silk and Friedel recommend keeping a patient on a medication only if there is clear evidence that the patient is continuing to do better on it after 3 months or more. Current trends in medicating specific symptoms of BPD include a greater role for mood stabilizers and low-dose antipsychotics and a diminished but still significant role for the antidepressive medications that had long been considered the first line of medication (Silk and Friedel, in press; Stoffers et al. 2010).

Because medications do not provide a cure for character pathology, it is important that clinicians be aware of the limitations of this approach and avoid the temptation to seek a cure by continuously escalating the medication strategy. There is a risk that the clinician who expects too much from medications may lose a psychodynamic focus by engaging in serial medication trials, even as important dynamics may be getting played out in the interactions around medication (see section "Meaning(s) of Medication Treatment to the Patient and to the Therapist").

Most patients who enter therapy are already taking medication. It may be clinically useful to continue the medication as the patient engages in therapy if there is a good rationale for the medication and the patient reports a positive response; however, a goal of the treatment is generally to attempt to taper the medication when the patient has engaged in treatment. The decision to taper involves careful diagnostic differentiation between, for instance, characterological depression and the possibility of periods of major depressive episodes. It may be possible to taper some patients off medication during the course of therapy, although other patients may benefit from continued medication; the difference between the two groups may have to do with the degree that biological versus developmental factors play a role in the specific patient's illness.

Symptoms That Arise in the Course of Psychotherapy

During the course of treatment, a borderline patient may experience a major depressive episode, a manic episode, or a psychotic episode. These comorbid conditions require appropriate biological interventions. However, depressive mood, transient psychotic symptoms, panic, impulsivity, or labile moods may represent manifestations of the personality pathology itself rather than comorbid conditions. Therefore, it is essential for the therapist to fully evaluate the symptoms and to understand them in the context of the treatment. If such symptoms represent responses to developments in the transference or to events in the patient's life, the most effective treatment is to help the patient understand the origin and meaning of the symptom.

Combining Psychotherapy and Medication

Attention to the psychotherapeutic process could do much to improve medication compliance and to maintain the patient in treatment long enough for the medication to take effect. Effective pharmacotherapy requires an alliance in which the patient accurately reports the positive and negative effects of medication. The subjective experience of borderline patients includes rapid shifts of cognitive and mood states as the patient's internal world is dominated by alternating split-off object representations. Consequently, these patients may provide distorted reports of medication effects. Concurrent psychotherapy provides an opportunity to diagnose the presence of such distortions and to reduce them by using interpretation to understand the patient's internal object world.

Meaning(s) of Medication Treatment to the Patient and to the Therapist

The meaning the patient attributes to medication is of paramount importance. Most basically, studies continue to show the importance of the placebo effect. When medication is introduced into the treatment, the therapist should determine its meaning from three vantage points: 1) the patient's conscious beliefs and fantasies about the medication and its effects, 2) the meaning(s) of the medication to the patient in the context of the current state of the transference, and 3) the meaning of medicating the patient in the countertransference.

The patient's reaction to medication will be strongly colored by the current state of the transference. Medication may be seen as an agent of the therapist's control, as a sign of nurturance, as a gift, as proof of the therapist's intolerance of the patient's affective states, or as confirmation of the therapist's desperation. Understanding the transference meaning of the medication can help the therapist to understand shifts and intensifications in the transference and can also help him or her understand and interpret unconscious motivations for noncompliance. If serious acting out around medication is expected, the therapist might choose to predict and interpret this in advance.

When considering medication, the therapist should also examine the state of the countertransference. For example, therapists may turn to medication when they are feeling particularly powerless with respect to a patient's behavior or attitude. Therapists may be tempted to turn to medication at times when they are feeling hopeless about the treatment or have been made to feel less deskilled as a psychotherapist by a patient. Medication may also be used to distance oneself from the patient.

Symptoms, Side Effects, and Medication as Defenses Against Exploration

Although symptoms may serve as a channel for interpersonal communication for patients from any diagnostic group, borderline patients are especially prone to use reports of symptoms to elicit particular reactions in the therapist. Changes in symptom intensity or the advent of disturbing side effects may reflect transference shifts as much as they reflect genuine drug effect. It is important to try to understand the dynamic meaning, if present, of symptoms and side effects. Patients may attempt to control the actions of the therapist through the way they report symptoms or side effects—usually as a defense against pursuing the exploratory enterprise. Therapists who are not confident in the focus on exploratory work and/or in the management of medication may allow the patient to set the pace in determining changes of dose or of medication. Consequently, patients with BPD often receive inadequate trials of medication or may be maintained either on homeopathic doses or on excessive doses for long periods.

An essential principle in using medication with borderline patients is to pursue accepted guidelines in terms of length of medication trials and to avoid the temptation to make abrupt medication changes. Because affective and behavioral instability are characteristic of these patients, it can be difficult for clinicians to determine whether symptomatic improvement or worsening is a medication effect. To determine the genuine effects of medication, the therapist should wait to identify long-term trends above the background of shifting affective states and transferences.

Complications With Combined Treatment in Borderline Patients

The form of treatment a patient receives (psychotherapy and/or medication) may encourage him or her to cling to a self representation as either a biological self or a psychological self. If the biological view of the self predominates, impulse and feeling states are attributed to chemical and physiological events. If the psychological view of the self predominates, these states are attributed to conscious or unconscious desires, fears, and values. When combined treatment is carried out, both models are evoked. Borderline patients may enlist these two frames of reference for defensive purposes. They may defend against the implications of intrapsychic conflicts or interpersonal experiences by attributing their feeling states exclusively to biology. Alternatively, they may defend against recognition of the role of medication through noncompliance, minimizing the improvement due to medication or attributing true physiological effects to psychological processes. This is especially true in patients with narcissistic traits who experience the need for medication as a sign of weakness and imperfection. One of the therapist's tasks in medication-supplemented intensive psychotherapy is to interpret such defensive positions.

Question of Who Provides Medication Management

If a patient is deemed to need pharmacotherapy, the next issue is to determine who should provide the medication management: If the therapist providing psychodynamic treatment is a psychiatrist, should that individual also manage the medication? Under what conditions would it be best for a second individual to be in charge of prescribing? If the psychodynamic therapist is not a physician, what are the principles of communication between therapist and psychopharmacologist? There is no absolute right or wrong answer to the question of who should manage the medication, but certain principles apply.

1. If the treatment is divided, the doctor responsible for medication management *must* be familiar with the psychodynamic model of therapy. Although this familiarity does not guarantee that there will be no splits between the treaters, it at least creates a situation in which such developments can be discussed in the framework of the treatment. One essential aspect of the treatment that must be accepted by the doctor providing

the medication is that symptoms—especially depressive feelings, anxiety, and mood lability—can represent internal affect states catalyzed by developments in the transference or other events in the patient's life.

2. If the treatment is not divided, the therapist—psychiatrist or not—should be knowledgeable enough about medications to know what can realistically be expected from them. If not, the therapist may find himself or herself appealing to medication to resolve treatment impasses that may actually be the province of psychotherapeutic intervention.

Advantages and Disadvantages of Combining the Two Roles

The question of whether to separate a patient's medication management from therapy depends on the clinical judgment of the therapist. The roles were traditionally separated because of the view that evaluating and monitoring symptoms, along with prescribing, took the therapist out of the exploratory role; however, it has become increasingly clear that a well-trained therapist can be aware of the dynamics that develop around including those elements in the exploratory therapy. A possible risk has to do with the fact that the pharmacotherapist must sometimes be directive, both actively inquiring about symptom change and side effects and also recommending dosage changes. This task might be a challenge for the psychodynamic psychotherapist who wishes to have a less directive role and who is trying to avoid deviation from technical neutrality.

The therapist who chooses the double role must decide how discussion of medication issues fits into the frame. The therapist might choose to adhere to the principle of letting the patient begin the session and bringing up medication issues when appropriate. If an appropriate moment does not come up during the session, the therapist might say a few minutes before the end of the session that it is necessary to check on medication issues. An alternative approach is to allocate a fixed time at the beginning of a session (once a week perhaps) for medication questions, prescription writing, and brief reviews of medication effects and side effects.

Advantages and Risks of Separating the Two Roles

The therapist and psychopharmacologist roles are most often separate. This arrangement requires careful coordination and vigilance for splitting. Often, the patient treats the pharmacologist as the "good object," facilitated by the fact that the pharmacologist may be less strict about boundaries and technical neutrality, therefore appearing to be more open, available, and warm to the patient. The patient may complain that, in contrast, the therapist is cold and depriving. The therapist can explore and work with this set of split object representations.

Alternatively, the pharmacologist can be perceived as the "bad object," who creates difficulties in scheduling, does not return calls, speaks rudely, does not listen or pay attention, and so on. This perception can create a dilemma for the therapist, who may wonder about the validity of these complaints and may begin to doubt the professionalism of his or her colleague. It is essential that the therapist 1) know the pharmacologist well enough to have a basic trust in his or her professionalism and 2) understand that clarifying and exploring the patient's negative experience of the pharmacologist is not to accuse the patient of misrepresenting or lying (although the patient may claim that it is) but rather is intended to help understand what may be a transference-based distortion (of the pharmacologist) so as to better describe an object representation in the patient's inner world.

TFP COMBINED WITH SKILLS APPROACHES

TFP has the ultimate goal of achieving integrated concepts of self and others, with related changes in mood stability, self concept, interpersonal relations, and satisfaction in love and work. Although elements of TFP such as the treatment contract have a powerful impact on helping the patient control problem behaviors and generally create adequate conditions for exploratory work, there may be particular situations in which TFP can be combined with supportive, informative, and skill-enhancing individual and group approaches carried out by auxiliary or supplementary therapists (see Koenigsberg et al. 2000b). Specific examples of appropriate ancillary treatments include 12-step programs (e.g., AA, Narcotics Anonymous), Weight Watchers, a nutritionist, an internist, skills training, couples treatment, and—for the lowest functioning patients— day hospital programs. It is increasingly common that patients who have benefited symptomatically from more cognitive-behavioral treatments such as dialectical behavioral therapy (Linehan 1993) then seek TFP to address identity and interpersonal and engagement-in-life issues in more depth. This sequence of treatment has often proved beneficial.

Key Clinical Concepts

- The treatment contract establishes parameters that protect the patient, the therapist, and the therapy and that help the therapist understand the patient's internal world as the therapy moves forward.

- The verbal contract between patient and therapist specifies the responsibilities of each party with regard to the treatment.

- The contracting process establishes the reality of the therapeutic relationship; it helps the therapist understand the patient's internal world when, in sessions, the patient's attitude and behaviors toward the therapist and the treatment inevitably deviate from the relationship as defined by the contract.

- A careful review of the patient's history and prior treatments provides information about behavioral resistances that the patient may present to the therapeutic process. Treatment parameters anticipate and address these possible resistances in ways that channel the underlying affects into the therapy.

- Depending on the specific patient's symptoms and areas of dysfunction, TFP can be combined with medication and other ancillary treatments.

SELECTED READINGS

Silk KR, Friedel RO: Medication in the context of integrated treatment, in An Integrated Modular Treatment for the Personality Disorders. Edited by Livesley WJ, DiMaggio G, Clarkin JF. New York, Guilford, in press.

Yeomans FE, Selzer MA, Clarkin JF. Treating the Borderline Patient: A Contract-Based Approach. New York, Basic Books, 1992

6

TECHNIQUES OF TREATMENT

Moment-to-Moment Interventions and Mechanisms of Change

THE TECHNIQUES of transference-focused psychotherapy (TFP) are the moment-to-moment interventions the therapist addresses to the patient in the therapy session. In this chapter, we describe in detail the four basic techniques used in TFP: interpretation, transference analysis, technical neutrality, and countertransference. We discuss the techniques individually, but the reader must remember that there is a constant interplay of the techniques and their relation to the treatment frame in the therapist's mind.

The borderline patient's experience of the therapist in the moment-to-moment interaction is determined by his or her fragmented internal world and can change dramatically from one moment to the next. In this transference relationship with the therapist, the patient experiences perceptions, attitudes, affects, and fantasies that are unconscious repetitions of internalized perceptions. Transferences are repetitions in the present of internalized object relations patterns that have become the structures that determine the individual's experience of the present reality and, in particular, of relationships. In the case of borderline patients, these internalized relationship paradigms retain primitive characteristics derived from unresolved conflicts between love and hatred from infancy and childhood and result in pathological relations to self and others in the present. The unfolding of these internal paradigms in the patient's reactions to the therapist will become the principal means of understanding and intervening in the patient's internal world.

Object relations theory emphasizes that the transference activation involves basic dyadic units of both a self and a related object representation linked by a distinctive affect. These dyadic units play important roles in determining the expression of drives and the experience of affects in an individual. These dyads are the means through which the different drives are experienced and also the means through which the inhibition to the drive is experienced. The object relations dyads therefore are the vehicle for the experience of intrapsychic conflict. These dyadic units of earliest affective experiences become, under normal circumstances of psychological development, triadic ones as the child becomes aware of the relationship between the parents. This capacity for the development of triadic units initiates the capacity for reflection on the nature of internal units, an essential element of mentalization. In the therapeutic relationship, that capacity is tested in the therapist's interpretive clarification and interpretation of dyadic units in the transference. Borderline patients have different degrees of limitation in identification with such a "third-person's" view. Intolerance to triangulation, to an observing perspective (Britton 2004), refers to a particularly severe distortion of internalized object relations, a regression within which the patient cannot tolerate any thoughts that are different from his or her own, and the *initial* role of the therapist may be to confirm that view of the patient and to assure the patient of the reality and stability of that shared experience, in contrast to starting with a threatening world of difference in viewpoints that immediately heightens anxiety.

Here we introduce an important addition to the concept of *activated dyads* in the transference. Insofar as the patient expresses a relationship to the therapist, there is still a potential, implicit hope—mostly unconscious at that point—that the therapist will not perpetuate the problems of the past but will instead introduce a new "actor" into the relationship. By the same token, the therapist's role is both to experience his or her transitory identification with the self representation or the object representation that the patient has projected onto the therapist and to take an observing distance from that part of himself or herself involved in the reexperience of that emotional relationship. The therapist acts as an excluded third party that disrupts the primitive object relation by means of his or her interpretive interventions that incorporate the knowledge gained from listening to the patient's verbal discourse, observing his or her nonverbal behavior, and analyzing the countertransference. The dyadic relationships in the transference are thus continuously exposed to a potentially triadic one.

The dyads that are activated in the transference may represent the expression of drives or defenses against them. It is typical in the patient's transference reaction to the therapist that the impulse-defense organization is activated first in the form of an object relation that represents the defensive side of the conflict. For example, a patient whose initial response to the therapist consists of angry depreciation of the therapist as a cold, uncaring person may be defending against a libidinal impulse rooted in a split-off dyad in which the therapist is imagined as the wished-for nurturing other. An alternative example would be that of a patient who initially idealized the therapist in a way that defends against split-off paranoid and aggressive feelings. Later, the object relation reflecting the impulsive side of the conflict emerges in the transference. An object relations point of view enables the therapist to have a framework to understand what at first looks like a chaotic relationship and to begin to perceive the pattern in the oscillations and alternations of the relationships dyads as they are reenacted in the transference. This understanding provides the basis from which the therapist intervenes with the techniques to be described in this chapter.

The object relations stimulated in borderline patients' transferences are best conceived of as a combination of realistic and fantasized, distorted representations of past relations with important others. Therefore, transference interpretation is different with borderline patients than with patients who are organized at a neurotic level. In neurotic patients, the more primitive, caricatured, split-off internal representations of early developmental stages have been integrated into more complex, coherent intrapsychic structures constituting the self and the internal object world (with a relatively clear sense of identity) and the superego (with a relatively consistent sense of moral values and internal prohibitions). In therapy with neurotic patients, the analysis of resistance activates in the transference relatively global and consistent characteristics of these structures (e.g., superego prohibitions against id drives). These structures have a coherent quality because in a neurotic individual the self aspects are linked together and the object aspects are linked together. In other words, a self representation "sticks" to the rest of the self, and the same is true for object representations. In the neurotic individual, interchanges between split-off, unintegrated representations of self and others occur only at times of extreme regression.

In contrast, in borderline patients, primitive internal representations remain split off from other representations of self and others, all of which are unintegrated into any larger, more coherent structure on a chronic basis. The results are a more chaotic subjective experience, more erratic behavior, and more disturbed interpersonal relations. Internal conflicts are not expressed in a consistent pattern with fixed impulsive and inhibiting forces but are expressed in dissociated ego states based on the primitive defense of splitting. These dissociated ego states may shift abruptly, with the patient identifying exclusively with one side of a conflict at one moment only to shift to identifying exclusively with the other side of the conflict at the next moment.

TECHNIQUES OF TFP

There are four basic techniques in TFP: the interpretive process, transference analysis, utilization of technical neutrality, and countertransference utilization.

INTERPRETIVE PROCESS

Interpretation is a process of uncovering unconscious conflicts, whether predominantly repressed or dissociated/split off. In borderline patients, the unconscious conflicts reactivated in the transference include relatively typical oedipal developments, with themes of desire, competitive strivings and rivalry, and guilt and anxiety, condensed with pre-oedipal themes of intense desire for nurturing, fears of abandonment, and rage against perceived persecutors. Although oedipal conflicts, especially aggressively laden ones, are pervasive, it is the pre-oedipal ones that tend to be prevalent, with very early attachment conflicts sometimes masking severe condensed conflicts that will become apparent later.

In the early phase of TFP, the interpretive process has a different quality from traditional psychoanalytic work. This stems from the nature of the borderline patient's initial experience of the transference. The primitive object relations that are activated in the transference may first be experienced as strong affects only (usually a variant of hatred or idealization) that flood the clinical interaction. Thus, the patient's experience of the therapist is concrete, and the patient has limited capacity to appreciate the distinction between internal and external reality. The therapist is not *like* a rejecting other—the therapist *is* a rejecting other. There is experience without cognitive representation of the object relation that is activated. The patient may initially be unable to establish any observing distance from or perspective on his or her immediate experience in the transference. Both therapist and patient experience an initial sense of confusion and anxiety. Transference dispositions may be most clearly expressed in the patient's behavior and/or in the countertransference. Because of the lack of observing distance, the patient is not able, at first, to make use of traditional interpretations of underlying anxieties and defenses organizing his or her experience. In addition, the patient may experience any sort of intervention as a criticism or an assault. In this situation, the patient may be able to use more basic interventions to contain and hold the affective experience and to promote the emergence of the capacity to cognitively represent it. The therapist's ability to contain the affect serves the purpose of communicating that the affect *can* be experienced without disaster striking. In such situations, the first step of the interpretive process is simply to *name* what is present before there can be any *explanation* as to what underlies the experience.

An example of this naming process is seen with Betty in Video 2, "Prevacation Session." The therapist, Dr. Em, first attempts a more classical interpretation, saying that Betty's anger and devaluing attitude are her response to his not being the ideal caretaker she seeks. When this does not seem to advance understanding, he says more simply, "What's going on now [anger and devaluing] is a real dramatic reaction to feeling like you're getting attached to someone, and this is apparently what happens when that process begins." The intervention is based on elements of Betty's nonverbal communication—in prior sessions an unspoken warmth had emerged at times—and on Dr. Em's countertransference that included libidinal elements in spite of the patient's angry barrage at the moment. This comment by Dr. Em is an interpretation because although it does not offer an explanation, it brings Betty's awareness one step beyond what she could currently see—it brings her in touch with the defended-against libidinal dyad that Dr. Em senses through the other channels of communication. Dr. Em's holding of the affect and then helping Betty name it can gradually lead to her capacity to symbolically manage and reflect on experience in the transference that had previously only been acted out (Winnicott 1949).

 Video 2–1: Prevacation Session, Part 1 (9:24)

 Video 2–2: Prevacation Session, Part 2 (6:12)

Before providing a more detailed description of the interpretive process, we describe the broad strokes of our understanding of how to use this technique with borderline patients. Because of the predominance of splitting-based defensive operations (rather than repression-based defenses) in patients with borderline personality disorder, interpretation focuses on mutually dissociated aspects of experience that are accessible to consciousness (rather than consistently repressed), although at different times. As treatment progresses and the internal psychological structure becomes more integrated, dissociative defenses give way to repressive defenses, when interpretations can shift to focus on repressed mental contents. The interpretive process follows the basic strategies of TFP (discussed in Chapter 3, "Strategies of Transference-Focused Psychotherapy") in attempting to help the patient achieve identity integration. On the broadest level, interpretation first spells out the nature of the dominant object relation and the patient's difficulty identifying with both poles of that dyad. Therefore, in its earliest phase, interpretation focuses on one dyad at a time and the reversals within it. The process then goes on to address the defensive split between persecutory dyads and idealized dyads and to explore the reasons that keep them separate.

Clarifying, Confronting, and Interpreting

It is possible to roughly break down the interpretive process into four steps (Caligor et al. 2009):

1. Identify and understand the patient's self state in the moment and elaborate the corresponding understanding of the other/therapist
2. Consider the other's/therapist's possible experience of the moment and realize that it may be different from the patient's as part of the process of observing reversals in the dyad
3. Put the moment that has been explored in a broader context and contrast the immediate experiences of self and of therapist with those experienced at other times
4. Address the layering of dyads (the split keeping them separated), splits, and conflicts by interpreting the motivation of the split between dyads with opposite affective valences

Clarification and confrontation are the parts of the interpretive process that prepare for interpretation per se. Interpretation is often considered the fundamental technique in psychoanalytically based therapy; it can be carried out in different ways. In our work with borderline patients, we emphasize interpretation of the here-and-now transference interaction over "genetic" interpretation of historical developmental material. We also emphasize that interpretive work is a process moving from clarification to confrontation to the interpretation itself.

Listening to the three channels of communication.   Effective clarifications, confrontations, and interpretations require careful attention to the three channels of communication: the patient communicates through what he or she says directly, through actions and other nonverbal communications, and through projective processes that provide data via the therapist's countertransference. The discrepancies, conflicts, or contradictions in communication that are to be confronted often are observed by contrasting what is being communicated through one channel with what is being communicated through another.

Clarification.   Clarification is the first step in the interpretive process. It consists of the therapist's invitation to the patient to explore and explain any information that is unclear, vague, puzzling, or contradictory. Clarification may focus on elements of external reality, the patient's past, or the experience of the moment, but it always has the goal of elaborating an understanding of the patient's subjective experience to the fullest. Clarification has the dual functions of elucidating specific data and of discovering how the patient experiences things and the extent to which he or she understands the material. The process of clarification helps the patient bring out new elements of the selected communication, which may throw light on previously obscure or unknown aspects.

Generally, the initial subjective experience of the therapist concerning the borderline patient is one of confusion. This stems from the unintegrated state of the patient's internal world and the fact that the patient is experiencing external reality according to an internal object relation that may not correspond well to the outside reality and the fact that the internal object relations that determine the patient's view of reality can shift abruptly from one moment to the next. In addition to these sources of confusion, the communication style of borderline patients may be confusing because they are unclear about what they are trying to communicate, because they may speak with the narcissistic assumption that the listener will be able to understand them without their providing a full explanation, or simply because they are anxious.

Therapists often hesitate to pursue clarification sufficiently. Patients often explicitly or implicitly demand immediate understanding and devalue a therapist who indicates that he or she does not have such an understanding but must work toward it. Despite these pressures, the therapist should never hesitate to ask the patient to clarify what he or she is saying. This is often the dominant intervention during the first phase of therapy. The therapist's feeling that he or she should understand the patient right from the start and the related hesitancy to seek clarification reflect not only fear of the patient's devaluation but also the therapist's unconscious attempt to assume the primitive role of the omniscient other that the patient may be projecting on the therapist. It is inevitable, however, that at the beginning of therapy the therapist will share the patient's state of confusion. In fact, the therapist may be more aware of the confusion than the patient because the dissociated nature of the patient's different states insulates him or her, to some degree, from experiencing the confusion arising from the contrast between them. In any case, the therapist who finds himself or herself hesitating to ask the patient for clarification on any point of unclarity, no matter how simple, should explore his or her countertransference at that point.

The following are examples of clarification seeking by a therapist:

- "You referred to someone named John, but it's not clear to me who that is." (The therapist might hesitate to seek even as simple a clarification as this. He or she might fear that the patient had mentioned John before and that asking who John is would reveal having forgotten. The therapist's fear of being a normal human, capable of forgetting, corresponds to the patient's implicit demand for a perfect other.)
- "Could you explain in more detail what you meant when you said you were 'an average teenager'?"
- "Could you explain to me what goes on at the clubs you mention?"
- "What did you mean when you said your mother was 'a saint'?"
- "You've said that whatever sexual problems you have with your boyfriend, it's 'the greatest sex ever.' Could you give me an idea of what that is for you?"
- "You said that whenever you visit your mother, you get 'too confused to think clearly.' Could you give me a sense of what the elements of the confusion are?"

Confrontation.   Like clarification, confrontation is a precursor to interpretation. Also like clarification, it often is used more frequently than interpretation in the early stages of therapy (except at times of crisis in the treatment, when the therapist may have to move quickly to deep interpretations in an attempt to save the therapy). The aim of confrontation is to encourage the patient to reflect on incongruous aspects of the material he or she is communicating verbally and nonverbally, with the goal of increasing awareness of internal inconsistencies and conflicts. The technique of confrontation also could be called an "invitation to reflect." As the second step toward interpretation, confrontation brings together conscious and preconscious or unconscious material that the patient experiences separately, or, in the case of unconscious material, does not experience but acts out, because the different elements of the material are split off from each other. Confrontation draws the patient's attention to data that either have been outside awareness or are assumed to be perfectly natural but that are discrepant with other ideas, attitudes, or actions of the patient. In essence, it brings the patient's attention to dissociated aspects of the self.

Confrontation generally involves pointing out discrepancies in what is being communicated through the different channels of communication. Although in plain English the word *confrontation* has a connotation of adversarial belligerence, confrontation as a therapeutic technique should be carried out with courtesy and tact and, above all, with genuine curiosity. Nevertheless, even a tactful confrontation is sometimes experienced by a patient as hostile because the intervention questions the patient's defensive system of splitting off conflicting images and affects. Whereas clarification is purely elucidative, confrontation implies a therapist's decision that certain observed facts are dynamically and therapeutically significant. Confrontation can occur in relation to material from any aspect of the patient's communication, including affects, external reality, the transference, or the patient's past. If the patient is able to respond to the confrontation with reflection, he or she may be able to accomplish some interpretive work himself or herself. For example, a patient might say, "You're right; I seem to have come in 'loaded for bear' today, whereas I was feeling good about therapy last week. I guess maybe I'm wrong that your going away next week means nothing to me, but it's hard for me to acknowledge that openly."

The following are some examples of confrontation by a therapist:

- "As you were describing how you were feeling so terrible that you had to cut yourself to relieve the pain, you had a distinct smile. What do you make of that?"
- "Earlier in this session, you were thanking me for having agreed to be your therapist, and now you are telling me that I'm useless to you and that it's a waste of your time to come here. How do you put those two things together?"

Interpretation.   In interpretation, the therapist utilizes and integrates the information stemming from clarification and confrontation to link material the patient is conscious of with inferred, hypothesized unconscious material believed to be exerting an impact on the patient's motivation and functioning. The therapist formulates a hypothesis about unconscious or dissociated intrapsychic conflicts that may explain what he or she is observing in the patient's words and behaviors. The aim of interpretation is to resolve the conflictual nature of material and, especially in the case of borderline patients, of behaviors rooted in conflicts between split-off intrapsychic parts. The process assumes that the patient's understanding of underlying unconscious motives and defenses will make previous apparent contradictions and maladaptive behaviors resolvable. The therapist may direct interpretations toward the here and now of the transference, the patient's current or past external reality, or the patient's characteristic defenses or may link these elements with the assumed unconscious past (so-called genetic interpretations, which are used principally in the later stages of treatment).

Making effective interpretations is central to the success of therapy, and an effective therapist must be skilled in this technique. A therapist's competence with regard to making interpretations in TFP involves the following elements: 1) the clarity of the interpretation, 2) the speed or tempo of the interpretive intervention, 3) the pertinence of the interpretation, and 4) the appropriate depth of interpretation.

In preparing for interpretations, the therapist must be aware of the conscious communication of the patient, of what within his or her internal world is intolerable to the patient, and of the defensive mechanism(s) by which the patient protects himself or herself from what is intolerable. The therapist gains awareness of what the patient cannot tolerate by listening to the other channels of communication—that is, the patient's nonverbal behavior and the countertransference. In this process, the therapist must analyze his or her countertransference at deeper levels in order to have access to material beyond the patient's awareness. When equipped with adequate data, the therapist must feel comfortable to spell out his or her interpretation in detail. Although it is true that an interpretation is a hypothesis and the therapist should acknowledge this, the therapist is generally advised to deliver it with conviction, both because it is based on his or her careful analysis of the data and because the interpretation will often be met by strong resistance grounded in the patient's primitive defenses. The therapist's work in Video 2 reflects this.

It can be helpful for the therapist to introduce an interpretation with a statement that demonstrates empathy with the patient's internal split and resistance to awareness. For example, in a situation in which the therapist is about to comment on a part of the patient's inner world (e.g., aggression) that is split off and that the patient would likely condemn if it were brought into his or her awareness, the therapist might begin by saying, "You may well hear what I'm about to say as a criticism, but it might be worth a moment's reflection, even if it's painful to consider."

TRANSFERENCE ANALYSIS

Transference analysis is the ongoing analysis of distortions of the "normal," "real" therapeutic relationship that is defined in the treatment contract (see Chapter 5, "Establishing the Treatment Frame"). Any deviation from the relationship as initially defined provides information about the patient's internal world. The deviations could be in the form of specific comments or actions or in the form of general attitudes in the sessions. The therapist explores these developments in the treatment relationship and eventually links them with similar distortions in the patient's relations outside therapy. Transference analysis is very similar to character analysis as described by Reich (1972) in the first six chapters of his book.

The following dialogue is an example of transference analysis regarding a specific comment:

> **Patient:** But you've *got* to tell me if I should marry him! You know I can't decide, and I need help with this.
>
> **Therapist:** Of course I could give you my opinion, but let's think back to how we set up this therapy. We agreed to work together in a way that would help you grow and become more in charge of your life. We agreed that it would be best to try to understand what's behind the difficulties you have sorting things out in your life. This is one of those moments when the way you are feeling in relation to me could be part of the problem. You seem to feel I have access to some knowledge that would provide the guaranteed right answer to this complicated question [making reference to the internal ideal object]. We should consider this and the other elements that contribute to your difficulty making a decision on your own.

This example shows how the work of transference analysis depends on the therapist's attitude of technical neutrality that will be discussed in the subsection "Utilization of Technical Neutrality."

The following dialogue is an example of transference analysis around a general attitude:

> **Patient** [beginning with a comment similar to one made in each Monday session]: How was your weekend? Did you play a few rounds of golf?
>
> **Therapist:** I can understand that you may be interested in whether I share your interest in golf, and we can talk about that. However, there could be some therapeutic value in thinking about how you begin the Monday sessions. When we began therapy, we agreed that your role would be to come to sessions and report everything on your mind in relation to the problems that brought you to therapy. Now, of course, there may be some connection between your problems and your questions

about my weekend, but it's not clear to me at this point what that might be. Do you have any thoughts about that?

With her question, the therapist is beginning the interpretive process with a request for clarification. She is exploring how far the patient can go in understanding what might motivate his behavior. Depending on the extent of the patient's understanding, the therapist would continue with the interpretive process. It is likely that the exploration would relate to narcissistic traits of difficulty tolerating a difference in status (a difference the patient may actually exaggerate at a deeper level of his mind) and the need to try to equalize the relation or possibly subtly devalue the therapist.

A simple frame of mind to facilitate transference analysis is for the therapist, while listening to and observing the material, always to be asking in the back of his or her mind, "How does this compare to what a 'normal' reaction/response would be in this situation (i.e., the therapy session as defined by the contract)?" Another helpful internal question is "What relation is being created by the patient choosing to discuss this particular material with me at this time?"

Transference interpretations, including interpretation in the treatment of borderline patients (Bateman and Fonagy 2004; Gabbard 1991), continue to be a controversial issue in the psychotherapy literature. The number of research studies on this topic is small, those that have been done typically have a small number of subjects, and the results are not consistent (Crits-Christoph et al. 2013). Most informative are the studies on the influence of transference interpretations as influenced by patient moderator variables. In a study of brief psychodynamic therapy, high levels of transference interpretations were associated with poor treatment outcome only with patients with high quality of object relations at treatment baseline (Piper et al. 1991). Yet in another study of brief dynamic treatment, high levels of transference interpretations were associated with poor treatment outcome for those patients with poor quality of relationships at treatment baseline (Connolly et al. 1999).

More recent studies have begun to portray a more consistent picture. In a study of a 1-year psychodynamic treatment (Høglend et al. 2008), patients with poor quality of object relations had better outcomes as measured by psychodynamic functioning in therapies with high levels of transference interpretations in comparison with patients in therapies that avoided use of transference interpretations. Although this result goes against a long-standing belief that only higher functioning, "psychologically minded" patients can benefit from transference interpretation, one could argue that the patients with a poor quality of object relations do better with transference interpretations precisely because those interpretations are less abstract. Transference interpretations offer the immediate data—the patient's experience in the here and now with the therapist—that link with the patient's affect and the attempt to explain and understand it.

From our point of view, transference interpretations should neither be conceptualized clinically or in a research study as an isolated therapeutic event separated from the process of therapy nor be judged in isolation. As this manual makes clear, we embed interpretations in the context of an interactional sequence between therapist and patient—a sequence that includes the full extent of the patient's understanding (aided by the therapist's work toward clarification of the patient's mental states) and the emergence of contradictory elements in the patient's presentation, which the therapist encourages the patient to reflect on (confrontation), and only then a hypothesis by the therapist (interpretation) as to possible meanings and motivations of the thought, emotion, or behavior in question.

Analyzing Negative and Positive Transferences

One simple classification of transference developments divides them into positive and negative transferences. Both positive and negative transferences must be interpreted because, in the borderline organization, they correspond to the idealized and persecutory segments of the internal world. Dealing directly with the borderline patient's primitive conflicts about aggression and intolerance of ambivalent feelings is the major vehicle for indirectly strengthening the therapeutic alliance. In other words, a meaningful therapeutic alliance is not simply a positive feeling between patient and therapist but rather the patient's confidence that he or she is welcome to participate in the therapy no matter how intense and negative the emotions that emerge may be. The transference as dominant affective material usually starts with the very beginning of treatment and therefore can be addressed early. The negative transference should be experienced, explored, and interpreted as fully as possible. The analysis of the negative transference generally allows for the emergence of more positive feelings in the transference and for the development of ambivalence. If the patient senses that the therapist is avoiding the negative transference, the patient's fear or belief that his or her affects are too destructive to be tolerated will be reinforced. The patient may then react by attempting to either suppress or displace his or her negative feelings or by "blowing the therapist away" in a triumphant and/or destructive outburst.

It is important to be alert to the beginnings of patient ambivalence in the face of what may appear to be unambivalent hostility. Generally, the more positive aspects are first demonstrated in the patient's behavior and, because of the effectiveness of the splitting, do not create any sense of conflict about the seemingly absolute negative position the patient may be taking more overtly. Pointing to any positive developments, such as moments of a feeling of good mutual working together, may mitigate the patient's sense of being all bad and may become the object of curiosity and exploration—that is, attempting to understand the hidden and fragile nature of this set of affects. If positive aspects are not perceived or acknowledged, the emphasis on the negative transference may perpetuate the patient's perception of the self as relentlessly bad.[1] Thus, the therapist might point out, "Even though you say I'm a useless therapist, you have started coming to sessions regularly and on time. This suggests that, somewhere within you, you may feel that I am not the totally cold and ungiving person you describe me as."

With regard to the positive transference, the focus of interpretation should be on the primitive, exaggerated idealizations that reflect the splitting of all-good from all-bad object relations. It is important to distinguish the idealized positive transference from the more integrated and realistic positive working alliance that is a goal of treatment. The idealized representations must be interpreted systematically as part of the effort to work through the primitive defenses and to integrate self and object representations. The counterpart of primitive idealization is a sense of persecution. In contrast to the idealized elements, the less primitively determined, more modulated aspects of the positive transference should not be interpreted in the early phase but should be accepted as evidence of some degree of ego function. Respecting these aspects of the transference fosters gradual development of the therapeutic alliance. For example, indications that the patient views the therapist as a helpful, interested person should not be interpreted; however, if the patient treats the therapist with gross idealization, then a statement such as "You treat me as if I can do no wrong" or "You seem to feel I have some magic I could offer you" is appropriate and necessary.

In the later stages of the treatment, after the intense negative transference has been analyzed, therapists often err by being less vigorous in their analysis of an idealized positive transference and its interference with the integration process. An idealized transference, which may include dependent and/or eroticized features, can function as a defense against advancing to the depressive position with its acceptance of the mixture of good and bad—and limitations—that can be realistically expected from the world. An

---

[1]If no explicit or implicit positive aspects of the relation emerge over time, the therapist should consider the diagnosis of antisocial personality disorder, a condition that seems to lack any attachment longings based on affection.

example is that of a young woman who began therapy very defensive against—but yearning for—the possibility of a positive relationship with her therapist because of her suspicions rooted in her fundamentally paranoid transference. After this transference had been analyzed in the first year of therapy, the patient's predominant transference became an idealizing one—she saw her therapist as flawless: intelligent, educated, and cultured, with perfect taste in all areas and a perfect life. She contrasted him to her husband, whom she found increasingly intolerable in his shortcomings and limitations. It was clear that although the negative transference had been analyzed at length, this patient had not yet advanced to integration in her internal world. She continued to demonstrate splitting, with the bad object externalized onto her husband and the therapist representing an unrealistically perfect good object. The therapist consistently pointed out that the patient's image of him was based on what she imagined, because she did not know a great deal about him in reality. The patient was eventually able to understand the unreal nature of her view of him, and, as she came to this understanding, her view of and relationship with her husband, whom she ceased to describe as the world's worst oaf, improved.

Analyzing Primitive Defenses in the Context of Transference Analysis

Primitive defense mechanisms determine the subjective experience of the borderline patient. One goal of therapy is to help the patient become aware of these mechanisms and the reasons they are present. The basic primitive defenses are splitting, projective identification, idealization/devaluation, primitive denial, omnipotence, and omnipotent control. Insofar as this technique is the crux of the treatment, the entire description of this treatment deals with how to carry out the analysis of primitive defenses in transference developments. Therefore, in this section, we do not provide an exhaustive commentary on this technique but instead offer some typical examples of analyzing primitive defenses and transference developments when conditions that allow for this level of interpretation have been established.

CASE EXAMPLE: ANALYZING SPLITTING IN THE TRANSFERENCE

A patient had completed the first year of a therapy that had begun with a predominantly negative transference and that had been characterized by many sessions involving intense affect storms. She began a session by stating, "I feel very lucky to have you as a therapist. All my other therapies were of no real help, and I see friends of mine who aren't getting anything out of therapy. As far as I can see, you're just who I need." In the course of the session, the patient brought up the fact that her disability status was about to expire, and she asked the therapist to submit forms attesting to her continued disability. When the therapist questioned whether she suffered a disability at that point, the patient became enraged and stated, "I don't even know why I bother to come here. These sessions are a waste of my time, and I've never gotten anything out of them. You pretend to help patients when you don't do anything at all. The only thing that would make sense for me to do would be to report you to the authorities for being a fraud."

The therapist responded to this by confronting the patient with the two opposing views she had regarding him. He asked the patient whether she recalled the sentiments she had expressed earlier in the session and how she might understand the difference in her feelings now. Resolute in her devaluing view of him, the patient stated that her earlier words represented her attempt to make the best of a bad situation and to convince herself that she was getting something out of a therapy that, in fact, was worthless. She further explained that the change in what she was saying simply reflected the fact that there was no way she could continue to delude herself that there was anything good about the therapy.

The therapist proceeded to analyze the patient's splitting as manifested in the transference: "The feelings toward me that you described at the beginning of the session may reflect the deeply rooted wish you have that I, or someone, could be the perfect nurturing caretaker you secretly desire. Your wish for such a person and your belief that you can find such a person are so important to you that you protect that possibility from the threat of disappointment by generally seeing the world as the opposite—a cold and indifferent place where people either don't care for you or actually wish you harm. The beginning of our work together was characterized by your seeing me that way, even though your behavior—for example, your regularly coming to sessions—reflected that deeper wish or belief that the perfect helper you seek may actually be here. As you have come to feel some connection with me and, I believe, to feel that I may in fact be interested in offering you what help I can, you are very anxious that I will disappoint you. In fact, the way your mind works right now, you perceive any degree of disappointment—any failing on my part to provide what you feel is perfect care—as proof that you can expect nothing from me and that you are right to experience me as the opposite—as cruelly depriving. This retreat on your part into that view of me serves to protect your deep-seated belief that you can find a perfect provider. However, that retreat also prevents you from experiencing and accepting anything good that a relationship, such as ours, could provide. Therefore, in the name of protecting your wish for the perfect provider, you may be depriving yourself of real caring that the world has to offer.

"However, you're at a stage now where you can begin to question this. Your rage and devaluing of me right now seem to be in response to your perception that I am not caring for you. Yet one could question whether supporting your disability status is the most caring attitude to have toward you at this point, and one could wonder if your wish for continued disability is not yet another manifestation of the deep-seated wish for total care that has been one of the reasons it has been hard for you to adapt to life as an adult."

Thus, the therapist not only points out the splitting—the defensive separation of a relationship dyad based on a perfect nurturing object from a dyad based on a cruelly depriving object—but helps the patient understand why this defense is in place: to protect and maintain an internal image of a provider that is deeply wished for but not adaptive to the realities of life.

The following example of analyzing primitive defenses in the transference involves omnipotent control. This defense involves the fantasy of controlling and/or attempting to control the other as an expression of the wish to variously 1) maintain the idealized state of fusion with the good object and 2) dominate and control the bad object both to punish it and to avoid the feared retaliation and persecution from it. Omnipotent control can defend against the depression associated with the loss of the ideal object or can defend against the fear associated with the aggression projected onto the "bad" object (Kernberg 1995).

CASE EXAMPLE: ANALYZING OMNIPOTENT CONTROL IN THE TRANSFERENCE

A patient in her second year of therapy began a session by asking her therapist why he was not able to see her later in the day as she had requested in a phone message. (We should point out that by the second year, enough initial understanding of certain dynamics may have been achieved to add a historical/genetic level to the interpretation.) The therapist repeated, as he had said in a phone message, that he could not meet with the patient later because of other commitments. The patient angrily replied that she had mentioned before that a later session time would be more convenient and that it was "obvious" that the therapist gave preference to other patients. The therapist pointed out to the patient—who had experienced her mother as teasingly withholding love and caring from all the children in the family in order to increase the rivalry among them—that he understood that she perceived him as giving preference to other patients and that she was angry because of this perception.

The patient pursued the issue by asking the therapist to find time to see her again at the end of the day after he had completed his commitments. The therapist pointed out that she was having her session but appeared to be using the time to try to impose her will rather than to explore what she was bringing to the session. She insisted that the time of the current session was so inconvenient that even though she was there, she could not effectively use the time. The therapist commented that the patient's insistence on setting up an additional session, combined with her dismissal of the possibility of using the current session, indicated a wish to punish him. On a superficial level, she was punishing him for not doing what she wanted, but on a deeper level, she was punishing herself as well as him by sacrificing her opportunity to use the time with him and to experience him as someone who could help her.

The patient responded by angrily pursuing the issue of why the therapist would not agree to see her at the end of the day. The therapist explained that to further their therapeutic understanding, it would be most helpful to focus on her view of him as neglectful and uninterested and on her effort to transform him, by force if necessary, into a "giving" therapist who would give her an extra session. The patient did not reflect on the therapist's comments but used them to assert ever more vigorously that he—now, according to her, even by his own admission—was neglectful and indifferent. She ragefully insisted that he give her another session and interrupted his attempts to speak so regularly that he decided to remain silent for a while.

After the patient went on repeating her accusations again and again, the therapist spoke up, wondering what the function of the patient's repeating her accusations was. The patient then became silent. After a few minutes, the therapist noted that the patient was looking at him with a hateful and depreciatory expression. He wondered if her silence served the same purpose as her previous repetition of her accusations: to maintain an adversarial atmosphere that precluded their working together to attempt to understand the activation of her rage. The therapist then noted that the patient's accusations against him reminded him of her descriptions of her mother verbally attacking her as a child, accusing her of terrible misbehavior while the patient experienced herself as the helpless victim of that attack. He went on to propose that the patient's enacting this accusing role gave her a sense of strength and power and that feeling powerful in relation to him might be the real issue motivating her rage. He went on to empathize with the fact that feeling powerful is generally preferable to feeling helpless and victimized but that she seemed able to feel powerful only in an indirect way, maintaining the identity of victim superficially. He suggested that this represented anxiety and ambivalence about power and assertion because she associated these characteristics with the unacceptably extreme version she had repeatedly lived through with her mother. He pointed out that her current system of functioning resulted in creating situations in which it seemed more important to achieve this feeling of power than to achieve her concrete goal (in this case, an extra session). Finally, he suggested that her ambivalence about power made it difficult to consciously reflect on those strivings within her and thus kept her from more effectively applying her strengths to desirable goals. (We should note that this was not a new interpretation but part of a line of interpretations over many sessions of the patient's tendency to enact an aggressive relation in the transference, with alternations in the roles of aggressor and victim.)

The patient responded that although she was still angry, she could hear and think about the therapist's words. The therapist inquired as to whether this comment meant that she was capable of considering the possible validity of his thoughts or whether she was now experiencing him as a powerful mother she must obey and herself as a naughty girl who must make amends. The patient replied that she did not feel that she had to make any amends and left at the end of the session in a markedly more relaxed mood.

In this example the therapist addresses the patient's use of omnipotent control in her insistence on making a demand on him and in her drowning him out so that he could not speak. The therapist interprets this in terms of the powerful-helpless dyad that had been one of the principal transference paradigms in the therapy. Later interpretations more fully addressed the deeper motivations of the omnipotent control—to protect, in the patient's internal world, the connection with the imagined all-providing object and to punish the depriving object and defend against the possibility of retaliation.

UTILIZATION OF TECHNICAL NEUTRALITY

Technical neutrality means maintaining a position that does not ally with any one of the forces involved in internal psychological conflict: the patient's drives, which could be in conflict themselves; prohibitions to drives; or the constraints of external reality. Technical neutrality is a position of equidistance from these competing forces that fosters observation and understanding of them—a process the patient is invited to join in. From this vantage point, the therapist is free to comment on any material provided by the patient, as long as the therapist remains allied with the patient's available or potential observing ego. The observing ego is that part of the individual capable of perceiving and assessing both the internal forces (impulses and prohibitions) and elements of external reality that have an impact on the individual's affects, motivations, and behaviors. The observing ego is distinguished from defensive aspects of the ego—the higher-level defenses such as intellectualization, rationalization, suppression, and reaction formation.

Technical neutrality and expressive psychotherapy in general are frequently misunderstood as requiring the therapist to be passive and to maintain a noncommittal attitude with regard to the patient. However, the effective therapist is always active even when listening in silence; the therapist's alert attentiveness conveys ongoing interest in understanding and a steady intent to observe and clear away obstacles to healthier relationships and greater fulfillment in the patient's life. Because the therapist is clearly allied with the healthy, observing-ego aspect of the patient, we can say that the position of neutrality is within a frame that promotes the patient's well-being.

For borderline patients, the observing ego may, at times, be so overcome by stronger forces that the therapist may seem to be speaking from an outside position, unrelated to any part of the patient. In such situations, the therapist must point out to the patient that he or she is speaking for a part of the patient that is, for the moment, split off. The therapist also enters as an "excluded observing third party," disrupting the total control of the situation by the internal dyadic relationship that keeps the patient from the capacity to enter into deep, mutual, and intimate relationships.

The therapist's ability to diagnose, clarify, and interpret the dominant active transference paradigm at each point in the treatment is dependent on the therapist's position as a neutral observer. Technical neutrality with neurotic patients has been described as a position close to the patient's observing ego and equidistant from the patient's id, superego, defensive aspects of the ego, and external reality. Because the dissociated internal world of borderline patients has not yet consolidated into coherent ego and superego structures, with these patients technical neutrality implies an equidistance between self and object representations in mutual conflict and equidistance between mutually split-off, all-good and all-bad object relations dyads; these representations and dyads are the elements that will come together later to form the more coherent ego, superego, and integrated identity.

In contrast to neutral interventions, those therapist interventions that side with one pole of a patient's conflicts lack neutrality. Transference-focused psychotherapy requires a general stance of neutrality because this position allows the therapist to observe and understand all the forces at play in the patient's conflicts, to analyze the interactions among them, and to engage the patient in observing and reflecting on the parts of his or her conflict with the goal of increasing the patient's ability to resolve emotional conflicts and increase his or her autonomy.

The following case is an example of how to work from a position of technical neutrality and how it may differ from supportive therapy:

CASE EXAMPLE: TECHNICAL NEUTRALITY

A bright young woman banker, at a higher level of borderline personality organization, was repeatedly fired from jobs because she became strident and aggressive with her bosses. Her first therapist, who provided supportive therapy, recommended that the patient find a job in sales with the idea that her "spunk and assertiveness" would fit better in that context. The patient agreed but encountered the same interpersonal difficulties in her new position. The supportive therapist had not maintained neutrality but had sided with defensive aspects of the patient's ego and attempted to accept her aggression by rationalization rather than exploring it and its role in the context of the patient's internal and interpersonal conflicts. The patient then changed to a TFP therapist who chose the latter approach. In exploring the patient's aggression in the context of her overall psychological structure, it emerged that the aggression represented a surface self representation defending against a very dependent deeper self representation. As long as this latter aspect of the self remained hidden, the patient repeated her ineffectual

aggressive behavior because that behavior was based not on an unambivalent competitive striving but on a dependency wish that unconsciously
turned the patient's aggressive assertiveness into failure as a compromise,
which 1) was an indirect and awkward attempt to ask for the help she could
not ask for directly and 2) provided the repeated punishment the patient unconsciously felt she deserved for both her dependency wishes and her aggressive actions. If the therapist had not maintained neutrality, the
complexity of these forces would not have been understood.

A second example illustrates how neutrality emerges as an issue in the
course of therapy and interacts with countertransference:

CASE EXAMPLE: NEUTRALITY AND COUNTERTRANSFERENCE

Maria, a bright 33-year-old patient from an underprivileged background
began therapy with the following goals: improve her chronically depressed
mood, establish a stable relationship with the goal of having a family, stop
all substance abuse, and finish her college education so that she could get a
better-paying and more meaningful job. In line with the last goal, she and
her therapist, Dr. Carla, agreed that part of the treatment plan would be for
her to continue her day job and start attending two college courses in the
evening. The therapy went generally well for 6 months. Maria received
good feedback from her professors, although she was not ranked first in the
class. Then she started a session saying, "I'm dropping out of college [as she
had done three times before] and I'm dropping out of therapy! I'm tired of
all the pressure you're putting on me to go to college."

Dr. Carla's countertransference reaction was reflected in her thinking:
"This is a disaster. How can I stop her from destroying her chances?" She
began to think of arguments to persuade Maria to continue college and
therapy. Then she caught herself and realized that a neutral position would
be more therapeutic. She said, "Do you remember when we started to work
together? It seems to me that the idea of finishing college came from you."
Maria agreed. Dr. Carla continued, "It's interesting then that at this point
you're talking about being tired of 'all that pressure' that I'm putting on
you." Maria was listening, and Dr. Carla continued, "Could it be that you
are divided between a part that wants to finish college and a part that puts
so much pressure on yourself that it becomes 'too much'?" Maria continued
to listen. Dr. Carla went on, "It might be that it's easier to think that the
pressure is coming from outside of you—that way you could escape from it
by leaving therapy. But I wonder if the bigger pressure isn't coming from
you. After all, you seem to be doing well, but it may not be enough to satisfy
your internal demands. Maybe that's why you dropped out the other three
times. You never flunked out, but you may live with such harsh internal demands that you try to escape from them—by dropping out and, when that
doesn't work, by drugs. We may have identified something here that is very
important to continue to work on." Maria agreed, accepted Dr. Carla's resit-

uating the conflict that she tried to externalize between them as being within her, and continued in therapy. If Dr. Carla had not maintained neutrality and had argued for Maria to stay in college, Maria might have ended therapy, thinking that she could leave the pressure she experienced there.

The therapist in this case could have added, "Your pattern of finding a reason to drop the plans we made could put me in a position of being the spokesperson for your engaging in more meaningful activities. However, as you know, it is totally up to you whether you live a passive or an active life. It's true that this therapy favors an active life over a passive one, but you're free to choose, and I could help you find a therapy that would help you adjust better to the life you have been leading, if you would like that." Often, when the therapist points out the patient's projection of one side of a conflict, the patient is able to acknowledge the conflict and work with it.

In summary, technical neutrality allows the therapist to analyze the patient's unconscious conflicts from a position of concerned objectivity without losing perspective by aligning himself or herself with one side of a conflict. A classic example is that the therapist would not say "You seem so guilty about cheating on your wife that I don't think you should do it" but would rather explore the guilt and the various desires involved, as well as their implications.

It is important to stress that *maintaining technical neutrality does not mean communicating in a flat and bland style*. Precisely because the borderline patient's observing ego is so weak, it is incumbent on the therapist to communicate with generally natural affect and, at those times when the healthy, observing part of the patient is being overwhelmed by intense affect, to speak firmly, although with warmth and concern. Having emphasized the role of technical neutrality, we will now discuss times when the therapist will be forced to deviate from neutrality.

Deviation From Technical Neutrality

Although technical neutrality can be maintained consistently in the psychodynamic treatment of healthier patients, the tendency for borderline patients to act out in ways that may be dangerous to themselves, others, or the treatment may require that the therapist strategically deviate from neutrality at times. Technical neutrality is, therefore, a desired baseline from which deviations may occur. When these deviations occur, neutrality must always later be restored by interpretation.

Deviations from neutrality are motivated by the need to firmly address forms of acting out that would threaten the patient, others, or the treatment. The usual supportive aspects of a therapeutic situation (e.g., the therapist's efforts at understanding the patient, the frequency and regularity of sessions, the therapist's warmth and understanding) may not constitute a sufficient holding environment for these patients at times and, in fact, can be experienced by the borderline patient as intrusive, dangerous, and overwhelming. Therefore, the therapist may be forced to deviate from neutrality and introduce structuring parameters to control acting out or the risk of acting out. For example, a therapist might say, stating an opinion, "What looks like a rebellion on the surface may really be a self-defeating punishment for such rebellion, and you should not give in to that temptation to drop out of school."

During the time that these parameters—specific, focused, transitory positions the therapist takes—are in effect, interpretation of the unconscious conflict controlled by the parameters is limited by the need to focus on the parameter itself and on what it means that the patient is putting the therapist in a position of having to act this way. The therapist should go on to explore and interpret the meanings the patient attributes to the therapist's action as well as to explain his or her own understanding of the interaction. This step may initiate the process by which the parameters can gradually be reduced and the interpretation of the original conflict pursued from a new perspective.

Returning to Technical Neutrality

Because technical neutrality facilitates the interpretation of transference, it is essential that the therapist make efforts to reinstate the position of neutrality. In the preceding case example involving Maria, if she had strictly maintained her position that she had no interest in continuing her studies, Dr. Carla might have left her neutral position and stated that she *did* think it was important for Maria not to drop out and explained why. If that had been the case, as soon as Maria had indicated a willingness to continue school, Dr. Carla would acknowledge openly that she had taken sides by supporting one aspect of the conflict and then discuss with Maria why and how this taking of sides had occurred. In this way, the therapist would move back toward a more neutral position, as in the following comment:

> Last week I advised you not to drop out of school because at the time it was as if you had deposited in me your own concern for yourself, while at the same time you were testing me as to whether I would be neglectful and allow you to go down the drain. Now that you're back in school, I think it's important that we discuss *all* your feelings about going back to school, both the positive and the negative ones. And I think we should also discuss what it means to you that I was put in a position of strongly recommending that you stay in school.

When deviating from technical neutrality, the therapist faces the danger that he or she may appear to the patient as prohibitive, judgmental, controlling, and even sadistic, possibly initiating a vicious cycle of projection and reintrojections of the patient's self and object representations. The therapist can counteract this danger by interpreting the transference, then introducing the structuring parameters as needed, and finally interpreting the transference again, without abandoning the parameters. The following is such an interpretation: "I have had to stress the danger to you, in your delicate position in the public eye, of picking up men in your social club. It was necessary for me to warn you about this because at that time you didn't have enough concern for yourself; you needed to test the genuineness of my concern for you and your treatment."

For the therapist to maintain the optimal degree of inner freedom to explore his or her own emotional reactions and fantasy formations in connection with the patient's material, he or she must be particularly careful to move away from technical neutrality only when the patient's intention or behavior constitutes a threat to the treatment that cannot be resolved by clarification, confrontation, and interpretation. Except for such a situation, it is important to maintain a consistent attitude of abstinence—in the sense of not giving in to the patient's demands for immediate gratification of primitive dependent, aggressive, or sexual needs within the transference—and to interpret these demands fully and consistently. The therapist's humanity, warmth, and concern will come through naturally in an ongoing attention to and work with the patient's difficulties in the transference and in his or her ability to absorb and yet not react to the pressures stemming from the patient's primitive needs.

It is important to avoid allowing the therapeutic relationship, with its gratifying and sheltered nature, to replace ordinary life lest the patient gratify primitive needs by living out the transference (e.g., dependency) during and outside the sessions. Although patients usually enter therapy with the stated goal of changing, they often simultaneously have a competing urge—that of using the therapy to gratify needs they are not able to gratify elsewhere. If present, this derailing of the purpose of therapy must be pointed out to the patient:

> At the beginning of therapy, you seemed very concerned about the failure of all your attempts to find a man to have a family with. Somehow, over the months we've been working together, you seem to have settled into a calmer state with less energy—both inside and outside of sessions—directed to working on your relationship issues. While, on the one hand, it's good to be calmer, on the other hand, we might be concerned about a subtle development. Could it be that while you came to therapy to change, you've settled into a relationship with me that seems steady and comfortable and that that

comfort now prevails over the wish to change? It would seem unfair to you
to give up on your goal of having a family of your own and to have the idea
that the most gratifying relationship you can attain in life is the one here.

Thus, the therapist must be alert to this possible secondary gain of treatment and be willing to interpret it.

In some cases, a patient who begins therapy at a very low level of functioning may require practical interventions to start on the road to autonomy. In such cases, the therapist may use auxiliary social support systems
(e.g., case manager, nurse, career counselor) rather than intervene directly
in the patient's outside life and thus lose technical neutrality. The therapist
must then monitor the situation and be alert to the risk that the patient uses
the auxiliary part of the system to gratify dependency needs.

The following case is an example of neutrality in dealing with risk of
self-destructive behavior:

CASE EXAMPLE: NEUTRALITY AND SELF-DESTRUCTIVE BEHAVIOR

A patient reported that she had begun a pattern of not going to work in the
morning and instead going to the subway station where she spent hours
thinking about jumping in front of a train. Her therapist experienced the
urge to institute a system of phone contacts with the patient and with her
husband to attempt to put a stop to this behavior. The therapist did not act
on this urge but rather explored his countertransference reaction and then
made the following interpretation: "You know I want you to be alive [alli-
ance with the healthy part of the patient that is not visible in the current sit-
uation], but I cannot control or guarantee that. What you are doing here is
attempting to put into me the part of you that is for life so that you can identify more fully with the part of you that is attacking yourself and threatening
to destroy you. There are a number of things to understand here. One is
that you seem to have the fantasy that as long as I want you alive, I can somehow save you—no matter what you do. Another is that you are acting as
though the destructive part of you will somehow survive and enjoy your being dead, when in fact that part will be dead too. But before we can explore
any of this, I must emphasize that your attempt to put that part of you that
wants to live into me in order to free yourself to be able to identify fully with
your destructive part is a false position. It denies the fact that you are in conflict. Although the destructive part of you is drowning out the part of you
that wants to live, it is my job to point out that both parts are in you, and
we must address the conflict where it exists in you."

The patient agreed with this interpretation, further clarifying that it was
easier for her to pretend that there was no conflict in her and acknowledging
that there must be some conflict because she had not gone ahead and
thrown herself in front of the train. The therapist and patient went on to
explore the internal dynamics of sadistic attack and how they got played out

in the transference with the patient torturing her therapist with her reports of near-suicide. In this example, while the therapist stated a position ("I want you to be alive"), he maintained neutrality by focusing on the conflict within the patient rather than enacting the conflict between the patient and himself by accepting the role of savior.

Avoiding Taking Sides

The patient frequently attempts to engage the therapist in siding with one aspect of the self against another or, at times, in siding against someone else. In either case, the therapist's going along with such efforts would be in violation of technical neutrality unless the side the therapist is taking is clearly that of the healthy observing ego. As stated before, the therapist is neutral *within a frame that favors the growth and well-being of the patient*. A general principle is to address the patient as if he or she is an adult capable of some reflection. In that way, the therapist communicates with the patient's healthy, observing ego and avoids getting caught up in the enactment of a primitive relationship. In other words, the therapist avoids getting "sucked into" a transference-countertransference enactment, although he or she observes the pull to do so and uses these observations to interpret the dynamics of the interaction. Technical neutrality and awareness of countertransference go hand in hand.

Nevertheless, as stated above, there are some occasions when the therapist *does* take sides when doing so is a clear matter of protecting the patient, someone else, or the treatment from aggressive drives. This is most evident in the initial structuring of the treatment and in any need to set limits that may occur. If, however, the therapist finds himself or herself consistently in a position of taking the side of life over aggression, he or she should consider the need to interpret the externalization of an internal conflict, as described in the discussion of projection (see subsection "Level 1: Interpreting Primitive Defenses").

COUNTERTRANSFERENCE UTILIZATION

The third channel of communication between patient and therapist after the patient's verbal communication and nonverbal behavior is the countertransference. We consider the countertransference to be the totality of the therapist's emotional responses to the patient at any particular point in time; this corresponds to the contemporary understanding of this phenomenon in the psychoanalytic literature (Auchinloss and Samberg 2012). The therapist's countertransference responses are determined by 1) the patient's transferences to the therapist; 2) the reality of the patient's life (the therapist may have his or her personal reactions to the circumstances of the patient's life); 3) the therapist's own transference dispositions, as determined by his or her internal world (it is because of this aspect of countertransference that a therapist must be aware of his or her own habitual reactions and that it is advisable for the therapist to have had his or her own exploratory therapy); and 4) the reality of the therapist's life (e.g., is the therapist frustrated in his marriage in a way that might affect his responses to the patient's seductiveness?). The fact that these four influences all have an impact on the therapist's countertransference makes it essential for him or her to try to distinguish the sources of his or her internal experience in relation to the patient. As a rule, the sicker the patient, the more prominent is the patient's transference in generating countertransference reactions. This is because patients with more serious pathology use more primitive defense mechanisms, especially projective identification, which tends to induce elements of the patient's internal world in the therapist as part of the patient's effort to avoid feeling the full intensity of his or her inner conflict. Consequently, with borderline patients, and especially with lower-level borderline patients, much of the countertransference is determined by the patient's internalized object relations as they emerge in relation to the therapist.

The therapist's countertransference may be either concordant or complementary (Racker 1957). Concordant identification in the countertransference occurs when the therapist experiences an affective identification with the patient's current subjective affective experience (of which the patient may be more or less clearly aware). In other words, the therapist experiences empathy with the patient's current self representation. One could say that when the therapist experiences concordant countertransference, he or she learns how the patient feels through trial identification.

In contrast, complementary identification in the countertransference is identification with what the patient cannot tolerate and is projecting onto the therapist at that time; if the patient identifies with the self representation, the therapist may be identified with the object representation included in the currently active dyad. If the patient identifies with his or her object representation, the patient may be projecting his or her self representation onto the therapist, leading to the corresponding identification in the countertransference.[2]

---

[2]To speak of *self representation* and *object representation* is a shorthand that does not communicate that the patient ultimately identifies with both. In other words, at a deep level, both self representations and object representations are, in fact, self representations. In the shorthand use of these terms, self representation is the pole of the dyad with which the patient more consciously identifies and object representation is the pole of the dyad that the patient tends to see in the other or put into action without full awareness of the significance of the action.

A complementary countertransference may provide a better feel for the patient's split-off internal objects and thus for the totality of the current dyad. For example, if a patient says "I failed my test" and then remains silent, the therapist might feel sad. This would represent a concordant countertransference, in which case the therapist might say, "It may be that you're silent because you're sad and disappointed and think this is the end of the world." However, in the same situation, the therapist might feel angry and critical of the patient. This would represent a complementary countertransference, in which case the therapist might say, "It may be that you're silent because you think I might be critical of you." In this case, the therapist realizes that his or her anger is identification with the persecutory object the patient is projecting. Concordant countertransference involves the therapist's identifying with that part of the patient's psyche that the patient experiences as himself or herself; the therapist's internal experience parallels that of the patient—the self representation of which the patient is aware. Complementary countertransference involves the therapist's identifying with the object representation corresponding to the patient's current projected self representation.

The therapist's countertransference can shift between concordant and complementary within the particular relationship dyad active in the patient at any given moment. In addition, countertransference can change in accordance to shifts in the dyad that determine the patient's experience from one moment to another. The therapist's awareness of his or her countertransference and its relation to the patient's internal object world plays an essential part in following the strategies of intervention outlined above.

The therapist's countertransference can also be classified into acute and chronic countertransference reactions. *Acute countertransference reactions* are potentially very helpful in the treatment. They may shift, within each session, in relation to transference developments. *Chronic countertransference reactions* are more problematic, usually reflecting chronic, unresolved transference and countertransference developments or a treatment stalemate. The latter reactions may start insidiously, extend over many weeks or even months, and affect the therapist's position of technical neutrality by leading the therapist to blind spots in his or her perception of the patient's internal world.

In clinical practice, the therapist's clear understanding of the conditions of treatment as established in the contract helps him or her be aware of countertransference reactions. Any temptation to deviate from the established treatment frame or to accept a patient's deviation should be viewed as a sign of a countertransference reaction corresponding to some element of the patient's inner world. For example, if the therapist finds himself or herself agreeing with the patient's claim that the expectation to come to all sessions is rigid and harsh, the therapist should refrain from acting to modify that expectation and should explore the transference for a relationship dyad involving a rigid, harsh, and probably sadistic character. The therapist should include these data in his or her emerging internal formulation—for example, "I'm beginning to feel punitive and sadistic with regard to this patient. Let me observe the affect related to this relationship dyad and also be aware that the poles of the dyad may shift so I can expect to be on the receiving end of something punitive and sadistic at some deeper level or at some later point."

If the therapist is not aware of his or her countertransference and the need to explore it in object relations terms, he or she is at risk of enacting it in a way that could collude with the patient's resistance. For example, the therapist may actually decide the patient is right that he or she should not be expected to attend sessions regularly. This response would leave intact a superficial positive relationship dyad but may, in fact, represent a negative relationship on a deeper level that remained unexplored insofar as the therapist's adopting this position would in effect result in abandoning the effort necessary to help the patient. Consequently, the patient and therapist would be joined in a situation that appears friendly and supportive on the surface but that defends against a deeper level of the internal world involving irresponsible, neglectful, or even abusive relationship elements that are now being jointly enacted in the collusion to avoid exploring them.

Because countertransference reactions can originate in the therapist as well as in the patient's inner world, the therapist must be open to exploring the source of his or her reactions. This is especially important on those occasions when the patient comments on the therapist's behavior (e.g., "You seem angry" or "You looked at my cleavage").

Monitoring countertransference clearly provides key access to understanding the patient's primitive defense mechanisms of projective identification and splitting, as well as to understanding the nature of the part-object representations in the patient's internal world. In short, the therapist's reaction provides clues to the dominant question of the early phase of treatment—"How is this patient relating to me?"—to which the answer is often to be found in considering the question "How am I being made to feel?"

Further Comments on Countertransference Reactions

In conjunction with allying with the patient's observing ego, it is important that the therapist find some likeable, authentic human aspect of the patient, a potential area of ego growth that will constitute the initially small yet essential base for an authentic communication from the therapist to the patient. In other words, the therapist's position of technical neutrality implies an authentic commitment to what he or she expects or hopes constitutes an available core of interpersonal investment, of ordinary humanity within the patient—a core that suggests a capacity for authentic dependency and the establishment of a therapeutic relationship in spite of the problems that bring the patient to therapy.

The therapist's comments start from an implicit alliance between the therapist in role and the relationship-seeking aspect of the patient's personality that is the foundation for the consistent interpretation of those aspects of the patient's internal life and external behavior that reflect split-off part-representations of self and others of a purely sadistic or idealized nature. At the beginning, the therapist may have to only assume the existence of a somewhat normal self representation imprisoned in the middle of the patient's nightmarish world, and this assumption permits the therapist to systematically confront the patient's imprisonment in this world without equating the interpretations of the primitive parts with an attack on what the patient is himself or herself. This means that in spite of the patient's projection of, for example, harsh superego precursors onto the therapist and the consequent perception of any critical comment from the therapist as a savage attack to be fended off, it is important that the therapist maintain both 1) a moral stance without becoming moralistic and 2) a critical, analytic attitude without letting himself or herself be seduced into an identification with projected sadistic images or letting himself or herself be tempted into a defensive style of communication that reinforces the denial of the severe aggression rooted in the patient's internal world.

The patient's provocative behavior can pressure the therapist to move from the position of technical neutrality and authentic human concern into one of the following roles: a sadistic persecutor of the patient, a victim who submits to the patient's denial of aggression, or an indifferent other who withdraws emotionally from the patient. Sometimes, a therapist's pseudo-investment in the treatment—a friendly surface that denies the aggression in the transference-countertransference—may bring about a superficially positive therapy but without the possibility of resolving the denial and splitting processes that keep the patient in the paranoid-schizoid position and make in-depth relationships impossible.

Because the therapist is exposed to strong emotional forces in the therapy, the protection of an honest investment in the process on the therapist's part requires the objective safety of the therapist. Whenever the therapist feels threatened, the first step has to be for the therapist to assure his or her own physical, emotional, and legal safety. Safety must take precedence over any other consideration because it is the very precondition for an authentic investment in the psychotherapeutic endeavor and is therefore a basic guarantee for the survival and effectiveness of the therapy. The proper therapeutic investment requires maintaining at all times a realistic sense of what is possible. In contrast, adopting a messianic attitude of helping and saving impossible cases—going overboard to provide such patients with a "corrective emotional experience" of total dedication in the face of their provocative behavior—may create the risk that the therapist will deny the negative aspects of the countertransference, a denial that, in turn, could lead to the gradual unconscious, and eventually conscious, accumulation and possible acting out of negative feelings in the countertransference in a way that could cause the therapist to precipitously end the treatment. The tolerance of strong negative countertransference reactions to patients whose transferences may include intense projected hatred is essential to understanding the role of the hatred in the patient's dynamics.

CASE EXAMPLE

A senior female therapist felt completely paralyzed in the presence of a female borderline patient whose chronic sadomasochistic interactions with men, violent physical outbursts, instability at work, and bulimia were creating havoc in her daily life. The patient would slouch in her chair in sessions and complain angrily about a host of things going wrong in her life, shifting from one subject to the next and talking in a monotone without ever looking at the psychotherapist. The psychotherapist felt incapacitated by these endless and shifting complaints and felt intuitively resentful of the patient's despondent, passive, implicitly cavalier and arrogant behavior in the sessions.

The patient had described her mother as a grandiose, self-centered, arrogant, and neglectful person, and the patient's complaints implied that insofar as the therapist was not doing anything to change the patient's daily suffering, the therapist was behaving like the patient's mother. It was only the therapist's internal exploration of her consistent, intense countertransference that brought about the therapist's awareness that the patient was behaving toward her like the patient's own mother had behaved toward the patient, and that permitted the therapist to analyze the dominant transference situation. In this way the therapist transformed the patient's endless stream of complaints and despondent internal responses into an active exploration of the relationship between a grandiose, arrogant, neglectful mother and her helpless, paralyzed victim as the patient enacted alternatively both roles in the transference.

A strict and consistent frame of the psychotherapeutic treatment should provide the therapist with realistic security that should permit his or her exploration of the countertransference without undue pressure toward immediate action. Nevertheless, there will be times when the patient's provocative behavior will induce the therapist to some degree of countertransference acting out (i.e., the therapist's interventions being contaminated by his or her own emotional reaction). Hateful patients may triumphantly point to the fact that the therapist spoke with a clipped, angry tone; the therapist should acknowledge that behavior without either denying it or reacting with excessive guilt. In fact, the occasional loss of the position of technical neutrality as the therapist reacts may convey both his or her humanity and the expected consequence of extremely sadistic or provocative behavior on the patient's part.

It is important for the therapist to set limits on the extent to which his or her own time, space, and life situation may be affected by the patient and to adhere consistently to such limits without going out of his or her way in response to a particular transference appeal. The consistency of the therapist's behavior will permit him or her to diagnose the temptation of countertransference acting out and to trace this reaction back to the analysis of the total transference-countertransference situation. It is essential that the therapist protect the integrity of the therapeutic setting, the physical integrity and space of his or her environment, and the privacy of his or her own life outside the therapeutic relationship with the patient. Aggressive and libidinal parts within the patient will naturally be directed at the boundaries of the therapist-patient relationship, challenging those boundaries as an attempt to shift the therapist from a position of technical neutrality to enacting a part of one of the patient's internal conflicts.

CHARACTERISTICS OF SKILLFUL INTERPRETATION

The skillfulness of interpretations—the level of competence in formulating and communicating them—depends on four additional criteria: 1) clarity, 2) speed, 3) pertinence, and 4) depth.

CLARITY OF INTERPRETATION

Clarity of interpretation refers to the therapist's precise and direct communication. Even though an interpretation is a hypothesis regarding the patient's intrapsychic functioning, it is best to state interpretations directly and clearly. Although the degree of certainty about the interpretation may vary in the therapist's mind and the tone and emphasis may reflect these different degrees, to state interpretations tentatively would usually reflect an enactment of the countertransference. If the interpretation is not correct, its inaccuracy will become apparent. The hesitant, tentative communication of interpretations usually slows the pace of therapy.

EXAMPLE OF LACK OF CLARITY

At a point in therapy when a patient reported feeling increasingly depressed and experiencing a return of suicidal thoughts, the therapist had recommended that the patient consult with the psychiatrist responsible for her medication. In the therapy session following that consultation, the patient spoke of the psychopharmacologist as an idiot whose recommendations were worthless.

The therapist commented, "I think that what you're saying about Dr. Sutton has something to do with me. You know he and I work as a team. You seem to be reacting negatively to him, so I'm assuming you're having some negative feelings toward me. This could have something to do with your depressed mood and suicidal ideation too. Sometimes people envy the people who can help them. Maybe that's why you're responding negatively. And then you could get upset because part of you really does want help."

SAME INTERPRETATION MADE WITH CLARITY

"You are responding to Dr. Sutton's efforts to help you with contempt. It could be that your renewed suicidal ideation is an expression of contempt for my efforts to help you as well. Your depression may be a realistic response to that conflict that is going on within you right now between a side of you that desperately wants help and a side of you that is suspicious, envious, and angry and attacks those who may offer help. That, indeed, is quite a dilemma."

SPEED OF INTERPRETATION

For the interpretive process to have maximum impact, the interpretation must be delivered in a timely fashion. A major reason for inappropriate speed is the fragmented nature of borderline patients' verbal communications. This fragmentation may reflect a defensive avoidance of traumatic experiences ("the central phobic position" described by Green [2002] or an aggressive "attack on linking" [Bion 1967] and rejection of thinking). Our observation in supervision has revealed that some therapists tend to wait too long before interpreting. The therapist's usual explanation for waiting is the need to gather more data to ensure the accuracy of the interpretation. However, it is our impression that many therapists postpone interpretations repeatedly, sometimes over a period of weeks, because of anxiety about the patient's response. This tendency reflects the general reluctance of many therapists to accept that they are an important object in the patient's life and that the process of therapy requires that the patient's most intense emotions unfold in sessions.

With the above caveat about the risk of delay, interpretations should be used only when 1) the therapist feels clear enough to formulate a hypothesis on the basis of what the patient has communicated and/or on what the therapist has observed in the interaction; 2) the therapist is reasonably certain that this hypothesis, if shared with the patient, may increase the range of self-knowledge or, if proven wrong, will contribute to further understanding on the part of the therapist; and 3) it is unlikely that the patient would easily arrive at this hypothesis without interpretive help. Unless these three conditions are met, the therapist should either remain silent or use the techniques of clarification and confrontation (unless an early deep interpretation is required, as discussed in the "Depth of Interpretation" subsection below).

Once the three conditions apply, the interpretation should be made as soon as possible because, in addition to its therapeutic value, it offers an opportunity to evaluate the patient's response, which may indicate 1) whether the patient is ready to listen; 2) whether the patient can do something with the interpretation, such as enlarge on it or make additional associations to it; and 3) how the patient experiences the interpretation in the context of the relationship with the therapist—as a fruitful expansion of understanding, as evidence of the therapist's magical powers, as a narcissistic wound, as a gift, as worthless, and so on. This latter consideration—how the patient experiences the interpretation—provides ongoing information concerning the patient's transference.

PERTINENCE OF INTERPRETATION

The pertinence of interpretation refers to the appropriate focus on the part of the material in the session that has the most affect (the economic principle of interpretation), with the therapist addressing that dominant issue.

EXAMPLE OF A NONPERTINENT INTERPRETATION

A patient begins a session by angrily "spitting out" a dream to the therapist. The therapist responds by focusing on the content of the dream and providing an interpretation of the dream that does not relate to the patient's angry affect. A pertinent interpretation would address the patient's affect toward the therapist and may or may not refer to the content of the dream.

EXAMPLE OF A PARTIALLY PERTINENT INTERPRETATION

A therapist who has been working with a withdrawn and inhibited borderline patient for a number of months remarks on the patient's indifferent affect toward her: "You relate to me as though you have no feelings toward me. I think this is a sign that you may be afraid of feelings you actually do have for me."

EXAMPLE OF A MORE FULLY PERTINENT INTERPRETATION

A therapist reacts to a patient's seeming indifference toward him by saying, "You relate to me as though you have no feelings toward me. I believe this apparent indifference may be covering over, and protecting you from feeling, a deep concern you have about me and a profound wish that I would take care of you. I base this hypothesis on a number of things. For instance, you always arrive early for your session and look like you are waiting anxiously for me. Also, whenever I tell you that I will be away for a period of time, you say it doesn't make any difference, but your nonverbal expression communicates concern and uneasiness. If what I am saying is right, the next step would be to understand why it is so hard for you to be aware of and acknowledge feelings you may be having in relation to me."

Criteria Determining What and How to Interpret

The economic principle, the dynamic principle, and the structural principle also guide the focus and content of an interpretation (see also Chapter 7, "Tactics of Treatment and Clinical Challenges," section "Tactic 3: Choosing and Pursuing the Priority Theme"). The *economic principle* is that interpretation should be linked to the affect that is dominant in the session; this is because the patient's affect state is a marker of which of the patient's unconscious object relations is being stimulated. The object relation associated with the dominant affect in the session typically coincides with the object relation dominant in the transference. However, there are times when the affectively dominant dyad is in relation to a person or situation outside the transference and does not have a direct connection with the transference at that time. In this case, the therapist is advised to explore the area in which the affect is the strongest, even if this means not attending to material in the transference at that moment. Having said this, we have seen that affectively laden material that appears to be outside the transference almost inevitably links up with the transference at some later point.

The *dynamic principle* focuses interpretations on the forces in conflict within the psyche. This principle guides the therapist to work from surface to depth and from defense through motivation to impulse (Figure 6–1). The therapist should generally start with the data that are most immediately accessible to the patient and provide an understanding for the patient of the unconscious meaning of his or her communication in the here and now in a relatively ahistorical way. For example, the therapist might say, "Your behavior here is as if an angry child were relating to an angry and punitive parent," rather than assume that the object relationship being enacted is historically accurate and say something like "You continue to experience anger because of the harsh and punitive treatment you received from your parents." In addition to possibly being inaccurate, this latter intervention removes the patient's affect from the immediate situation with the therapist.

In general, the material closer to consciousness should be interpreted first, with exceptions to be discussed later in this chapter (see subsection "Complications in Proceeding From Surface to Depth"). In the early stages of therapy, interpretations principally address the defensive nature of the material provided by the patient. Patients tend to instinctively avoid the painful awareness of the primitive affects and internal fragmentation that are kept from consciousness but are manifested in behaviors and interpersonal relations. Much early work involves helping patients see how their behaviors, both in and outside of sessions, constitute an avoidance of looking at the material that is the most important to see and understand. This reality of the clinical work is one of the factors that underlies the hierarchy of priorities that should be addressed in treatment, as discussed in Chapter 7, subsection "Adhering to the Hierarchy of Priorities Regarding Content." Patient behaviors that are resistances to the work of exploratory therapy must be addressed before the exploratory work can be accomplished.

The *structural principle* focuses interpretations on the intrapsychic structure involved in the defense and/or impulse—that is, on the level of the tripartite structure (id, ego, and superego) in neurotic patients—and on the level of the predominant object relations dyads in patients with borderline personality organization. With the latter, the goal is to understand and interpret the object relations dyad that is serving a defensive role and to gain awareness of the deeper dyad that is being defended against and that is associated with the impulse. Pertinence of interpretation involves the therapist's making his or her interventions in accordance with the economic, dynamic, and structural principles.

DEPTH OF INTERPRETATION

Depth of interpretation refers to the progression of the interpretive process from the conscious, behavioral experience of the patient to the description of the underlying psychic structure, as well as the conflicts within it, that motivates the patient's behavior. All intrapsychic conflicts involve not only one layer of defense and impulse but rather a successive layering of impulse-defense configurations (see Figure 6–1).

Ideally, the therapist should interpret neither too superficially (that is, material that is too close to the surface and may already be evident to the patient) nor too deeply (that is, material that is not yet able to be assimilated

Defense on the surface:	The patient is silent with an angry look

Impulse that is defended against: (motivation for the defense)	Intense aggression

The therapist suggests this by saying: "You appear afraid to talk, perhaps from fear that you might 'blow up'" The patient agrees with this hypothesis.

Next level of defense:	The aggression as defense against dependency

The therapist suggests this: "Your fear of blowing up keeps you from interacting with me."

Next level of impulse:	Dependency longings

The therapist suggests: "Perhaps the urge to blow up is serving the purpose of avoiding an interaction that might bring up feelings of dependency."

As the work proceeds, the therapist and patient might find that dependency wishes in turn defend against competitive oedipal strivings. The work can go on through different levels. In addition, in BPO patients, dissociative defenses create the possibility that any defended *against* level may shift to be on the surface at a given point in time, now serving a defensive purpose. What is constant is that the parts of the conflict remain dissociated from one another until interpretive working through.

FIGURE 6–1.   Working from surface to depth

by the patient). However, the optimal level of interpretation has to be found by trial and error, and the criterion of depth of interpretation refers to the therapist's efforts to deepen interpretation as much as possible, testing the level at which the patient can understand and incorporate it.

Each defense has a motivation—that is, a reason why the corresponding impulse cannot be accepted consciously by the patient. Depth of the interpretation requires a complete spelling out of the defensive behavior, of its motivation against an opposite impulsive one, and of that impulse per se.

INTERPRETATIONS AT THREE LEVELS

An interpretation can be made at one of three levels: 1) interpreting how acting out or primitive defenses are serving to avoid awareness of internal experience, 2) interpreting a currently active object relation (describing the self and object representations in the dyad and the reversals of roles within the dyad), and 3) interpreting the object relation that the currently active object relation is defending against.

Level 1: Interpreting Primitive Defenses

Because interpretation generally proceeds from surface to depth, we first address the approach to interpreting primitive defenses. In general, defenses are mechanisms for avoiding intolerable conflicts—that is, conflicts between different parts of the psyche and between parts of the psyche and elements of external reality. Primitive defenses, as opposed to more mature ones, attempt to avoid conflict by maintaining a sharp and unrealistic intrapsychic separation between loving and hateful aspects of one's self and others so that the conflicting parts do not meet in the arena of the patient's psychological awareness. Even if these contradictory states appear in consciousness, they do so at different times and in total separation (although one state may be experienced consciously while an opposing state is simultaneously acted out in behavior but is not present in the patient's consciousness). This extreme separation of incompatible states leads to the patient's experiencing as *external to him or her* parts of his or her inner world that cannot be tolerated at the same time as the part he or she is consciously experiencing.

Splitting, the central mechanism of primitive defenses, isolates extreme, caricatured representations of the self and others in the patient's internal world, protecting loved "good" internal images from the hate associated with "bad" images. The price the patient pays for this segregation of internal representations is the ability to deal with people and situations with the flexibility and complexity characteristic of the real world. In terms of the patient's subjective experience, splitting usually leads to an erratic discontinuity in his or her experience of self, of others, and of the world. In some instances, splitting results in a fixed and rigid, but brittle, semblance of stability based on the consistent projection of bad internal objects on the external world; this is most typical of patients with narcissistic personality disorder whose internal world is structured around the pathological grandiose self (D. Diamond, F.E. Yeomans, and B.L. Stem, A Clinical Guide for Treating Narcissistic Pathology: A Transference Focused Psychotherapy, in preparation). In general, the primitive defensive operations, such as omnipotent control, projective identification, idealization, devaluation, and primitive denial, make it possible to sustain splitting through the belief that unacceptable aspects of the self are present in others instead of in the self, that bad objects are at other times good ones, and that the contradictions are of no emotional consequence.

To bring the part-self and part-object representations to the patient's awareness, the therapist often must retrieve them from their projected locations by demonstrating the use of defenses such as projection, projective identification, and omnipotent control. The patient's use of primitive idealization, devaluation, and denial is also interpreted to aid the patient in recognizing a more accurate assessment (good, bad, or mixed) of the self and object images. Once the therapist has demonstrated the repertoire of caricatured images that influence the patient's relationships (treatment strategy 1, discussed in Chapter 3), the next task is to bring together the self and object fragments. This is when the interpretation of primitive defenses is most useful. These defenses are described in the following list:

1. *Splitting:* The clearest manifestation of splitting is seen in the patient's perception of the therapist or the self as all good or all bad, with the concomitant possibility of a complete, abrupt reversal. Primitive idealization, devaluation, omnipotent control, and projective identification all derive from the split psychological structure.

   Therapist: Right now you're telling me I'm benevolent and you are totally relaxed with me.
   Patient: Sure, what's wrong with that?
   Therapist: Nothing, but I'm not sure how that fits with what you said 10 minutes ago—that you thought I could hurt you and you had to "watch me like a hawk."
   Patient: But I can *see* you're okay; I just feel it. Maybe I was wrong before.
   Therapist: But earlier you were convinced I was dangerous. How can we make sense out of my apparently changing so quickly? It's as if you know what to do with me only when you see me as at one extreme or the other. This way of experiencing me may be a way of avoiding the anxiety you might experience if I didn't fit one of those extremes.

2. *Primitive idealization and devaluation:* These two primitive defenses build on the tendency to see external objects as either totally good or totally bad by artificially and pathologically increasing their goodness or worthlessness (in extreme cases, devalued objects go beyond worthlessness to evil). Primitive idealization creates unrealistic all-good and powerful images, as reflected in the patient's treating the therapist, someone else, or himself or herself as an ideal, omnipotent, or godly figure on whom he or she can depend unquestioningly. The therapist may be seen as a potential ally against equally powerful (and equally unrealistic) all-bad objects. Alternatively, the therapist, another person, or the patient may at times be experienced as completely devalued, worthless, and/or evil.

3. *Omnipotent control:* This defense attempts to protect the patient from the threat of the aggressive affects that are projected onto external objects. It logically follows that if an individual projects and perceives aggression in the other, it is necessary to control the other to protect the self from the aggression. Thus, the only way to maintain a relation is to maintain control (Kernberg 1995). Tragically, it is often precisely this controlling atti-

tude that leads others to turn away from the patient. One form of omnipotent control can be in the patient's style of speech: a rapid-fire pressured speech—sometimes with abrupt changes from one topic to another—can be used defensively to keep the therapist from intervening in a meaningful way; this type of pressured speech must be distinguished from that of a manic episode.

4. *Projective identification:* In contrast to higher levels of projection, which are characterized by attributing to another an impulse repressed in oneself, primitive forms of projection, particularly projective identification, are characterized by 1) the fact that the patient may enact and even intermittently experience the impulse that is being projected onto the other person; 2) the experience of fear of the other person, who is now seen under the influence of that projected impulse or affect; 3) the need, therefore, to control the other person (a link with omnipotent control); and 4) the unconscious arousal of the feared and projected affect in the other person. Projective identification, therefore, implies interactions, and this may be reflected dramatically in the transference and can provide important information to the therapist through the countertransference.

Projective identification may emerge in the therapy in two ways. First, the patient who is attempting to defend against an aspect of his or her internal world by unconsciously inducing an unacceptable affect in the therapist may accuse the therapist of having that affect or reaction. For example, the patient accuses the therapist of being hateful while treating the therapist in a cold, controlling, derogatory way and simultaneously feeling the need to protect himself or herself from the therapist. Second, the therapist may begin to experience an affect that seems atypical to his or her usual response to patients and may then question where this countertransferential element is coming from. The affect, which may not appear to be directly related to the manifest level of material coming from the patient, may be evidence of an underlying process of projective identification in which the patient deals with a part of himself that he cannot tolerate in himself by inducing it in the therapist. The countertransference may be the principal means of accessing this aspect of the patient's internal experience.

A common example of projective identification involves the initial conflict between internal aggressive forces that push for destruction and libidinal forces that support the effort for life and healthy relations. In the early phase of therapy, patients often take the position that their only wish is to be dead and that the therapist and the treatment oppose this wish—a projection of the internal libidinally invested part onto the therapist. This projection is an attempt to free the patient from the internal conflict, and it puts the patient and the therapy at risk. The therapist should interpret this conflict:

> You say that you are totally in support of your wish to die, and you see me as a frustrating obstacle to that. This is a dangerous situation, and it is one that I think is not so simple. I believe there is a conflict in you and that you are not totally identified with the wish to die. For instance, there is the simple fact that you have started to come here for therapy. Also, the fact that your suicide attempts have failed suggests that you are in conflict about this wish. However, you prefer to avoid the conflict in yourself and to see it as a struggle between you and others, including me. This is a dangerous game because it could result in your being dead. It is important to acknowledge the conflict within you and to work with that side of you—no matter how weak it seems now—that wants to live your life.

A more complete vignette of working with this type of projection of one part of an internal conflict is found in Chapter 7 (see the subsection "Hospitalization").

5. *Projection:* This defense mechanism is not limited to borderline personality organization but can play an active role in borderline pathology. Most often, the patient—who cannot tolerate simultaneous awareness of both sides of an intrapsychic conflict—experiences one side of the conflict consciously while repressing and projecting the other side (embodied in a particular object representation) onto the therapist. Projection is a more advanced defense mechanism than projective identification. Because projection is based on the predominance of repression, in contrast to the dominance of splitting mechanisms in the borderline patient, its manifestations are more subtle. In projection, in contrast to projective identification, the patient does not unconsciously induce what is projected in the therapist and does not exert effort at control of the therapist under the effect of this projection.

6. *Primitive denial:* This defense in borderline patients reinforces the splitting process. The denial is generally of emotions related to thoughts or memories. These patients can remember perceptions, thoughts, and feelings about themselves or other people completely opposite to those experienced at the moment, but the memory has no emotional component and cannot influence the way they feel now. Primitive denial may also be manifested by the lack of an appropriate emotional reaction to an immediate, serious, and pressing need, conflict, or danger. The patient calmly conveys cognitive awareness of the situation while denying

its emotional implications or shuts out an entire area from awareness, thus "protecting" against a potential area of conflict.

Systematic interpretation of the primitive defenses leads to shifts in the object relations activated in the session. Such shifts are valuable in confirming the accuracy of the therapist's interpretations. The patient gradually becomes aware of contradictory internalized object images. When whole, three-dimensional internalized self and object representations have been formed, the patient has entered the more advanced phase of treatment discussed in Chapter 10, "Advanced Phase of Treatment and Termination."

Level 2: Interpreting a Currently Active Object Relation

The second level of interpretation is the most consistent application of treatment strategy 1 discussed in Chapter 3. Interpretation at this level may involve a preparatory step in which the therapist explicitly describes the patient's self and other representations that are not obvious on the surface. This step is especially helpful in situations in which either the roles being enacted in the transference are somewhat disguised (i.e., when superficial appearances belie the underlying roles being enacted) or the patient has difficulty seeing that his or her inner world is shaping his or her experience of the interaction in situations in which the patient builds on a grain of truth to claim that his or her perception and experience of the situation are strictly in line with objective reality. Interpretation at this level begins by describing the current interaction and moves a step deeper when the therapist suggests *why* the patient experiences the interaction according to these roles.

The following is an example of preparation for this level of interpretation:

> **Therapist:** To most observers you would look like a helpless child right now. In fact, I had that impression myself. However, in a subtle but consistent way, you are very strong. You represent yourself as beyond help; you reject all my attempts to further our understanding; you seem not to listen to or hear much of what I say. These things could be understood simply as evidence of your helplessness, but in my experience a helpless person usually shows some openness to the offer of help. Your tenacity in maintaining your helplessness, combined with your rejection of everything I say, creates an interesting situation in which you are coming across as the strong one and I seem weak and ineffective, even helpless. It might be worth our while to look at this situation.

Another example of preparation for this level of interpretation is the following:

Therapist: I checked with my secretary, and it's true that she asked if you could call back because she was very busy at the moment. However, I think we should look at your response to this incident because you are saying that you can't continue therapy with me unless I fire her.

Patient: How could I continue therapy with someone I don't trust? I've told you your secretary is irresponsible, and if you don't do something about it, that makes you just as irresponsible.

Therapist: Whether my secretary's action was irresponsible or not is one thing, but what you are doing with this incident is important for us to look at. You're taking this as proof in your mind that I am the irresponsible and negligent creature you've accused me of being on other occasions. You've called me a monster who doesn't care if you're dead or alive. So, we both agree about what my secretary said, but you are using that to defend a view of me that seems to come from elsewhere, and that's what we should be looking at and trying to understand right now.

The therapist in this example then began a level 2 interpretation:

Therapist: In an interesting way, you seem more relaxed when you are accusing me of being a monster. This is in contrast to how awkward you seemed in the last session when I was able to make the schedule changes you requested. For some reason, which we have yet to understand, you seem more comfortable when you feel you are dealing with a clear-cut monster that you mistrust at every step than when you are dealing with someone who might be nice to you. It seems as if you feel you know the territory when you see me as a monster. You may not be happy with thinking of me as a monster, but you don't seem to be anxious about it. Your deeply held belief that I am here to use or exploit you rather than help you may explain this lack of anxiety. If I appear to be nice, it may not fit into your expectations, and you may experience it as a setup for later mistreatment. Or, it could be that if I am nice to you, you feel guilty because of the rage and mistreatment you have directed toward me.

When dealing with the typical paranoid transference of the early phase of therapy, the therapist may propose an interpretation linking the patient's projection with their theory of mind. For example, the therapist might say, "I wonder if your anxiety that I'll 'throw you out' if you 'say the wrong thing' could come from the idea that my mind works in the same way that yours does. You've told me many examples of going from liking someone to being totally disgusted with them because of one thing they said or did."

Level 3: Interpreting the Object Relation Being Defended Against

The third level of interpretation is the most complete level because it is directed at the split psychological structure. The therapist proposes an interpretation at this level when he or she feels that enough information is available to understand what type of relationship the patient is defending against, which may not be directly visible on the surface level (see Figure 3–1 in Chapter 3). The following exemplifies such an interpretation by a therapist:

> I've noticed that every time you leave a session with any kind of a good feeling—a feeling that there may have been a positive connection with me, no matter how subtle—one of two things follows: either you leave me a phone message saying that you don't want to continue the treatment—that it is useless and that you want to end it—or you come into the next session with an angry, defiant look and state that you have nothing to say. The interesting question is what it is in you that precipitates these reactions. You have said that it's "reality"—the fact that you can't trust me and that I can't help you. However, my impression is that what sets off these repeated negative responses is that you momentarily are in touch with a part of you that is very scary to you—a part of you that wants very much to trust someone and look to someone for help, which is me in this case. At those moments you do not seem angry but instead seem to demonstrate a tentative, nervous yearning for a sincere connection—like the relation with a nurturing and caring parent. This disappears when that more familiar angry and contemptuous part returns, which may destroy the possibility of a true connection with someone but which you believe leaves you safe.

Working With the Levels of Interpretation

In working at any of the three levels of interpretation, the therapist is constantly monitoring the three channels of communication to have the necessary data to formulate interpretations. Interpretations at any level are usually preceded by the use of clarification and confrontation. Sometimes, a well-placed confrontation makes an interpretation unnecessary if the patient is able to use the confrontation, which is essentially an invitation to reflect—that is, to achieve insight on his or her own. The therapist should not make an interpretation until it is clear that the patient cannot do it unaided. The patient should first be asked how the information presented might be put together:

Therapist: Can you make anything out of the fact that you came late to the last two sessions while telling me that you've been preoccupied with how everyone is "blowing you off"?

Patient: Are you thinking that maybe I can dish out what I'm always complaining about? [The patient shows evidence of some new insight regarding the reversal of roles within the dyad.]

Interventions should stimulate the patient to integrate a step beyond current awareness. If a confrontation does not suffice to help the patient take the step, then the therapist should proceed to an interpretation.

COMPLICATIONS IN PROCEEDING FROM SURFACE TO DEPTH

The therapist working with borderline patients faces a particular problem with regard to the issue of depth of interpretation. The general principle of interpreting defensive aspects of the patient's material before content (surface before depth) is complicated by the problem of accurately differentiating what is on the surface from what lies below. The process is complicated because of the nature of splitting. With splitting, not only might one relationship dyad be closer to the surface and defending against its corresponding opposite dyad but the dyads might switch places so that the deeper one might become the one closer to the surface and the one that initially had been on the surface might become the one now defended against, as in the following example.

CASE EXAMPLE

A patient has been interacting with the therapist in an angry, hateful way, which is being communicated through two channels: mostly through her words but also through some nonverbal behavior. However, the therapist senses other aspects of nonverbal communication that indicate a longing for closeness to the therapist. He also senses a countertransference response that includes both wanting to rid himself of an angry, attacking person (a concordant countertransference) and wanting to protect a vulnerable, child-like individual (a complementary countertransference). Putting together all the data available to him, the therapist might conclude that the dyad closer to the surface—involving an angry individual experiencing hatred toward a person who has mistreated her—is defending against the experience of a dyad present at a deeper level. That dyad would involve a fragile, insecure self representation longing to love and be cared for by a nurturing individual. The therapist could make an interpretation to that effect.

However, the dyad closer to the surface and the dyad being defended against might change places. In response to some internal or external stimulus, the patient might abruptly begin to communicate a neediness and longing to be cared for by a nurturing other. In this situation, the nonverbal communication and the therapist's countertransference might provide data relating to the now-deeper dyad involving a mistrustful and hateful self in relation to a dangerous other. The countertransference might now include anxiety or wariness.

What might be confusing to the therapist is that the defense and the deeper content might alternate—that is, the "surface" and the "depth" can be interchangeable. This is the nature of splitting. The therapist working with borderline patients must be comfortable with the fact that there is no fixed defense-impulse constellation in the patient's psyche but rather a shifting situation in which the key is to observe all the parts so that the significance of their being split off from each other can be pointed out to the patient. A simple corollary of this is that the patient is not *either* a helpless child longing for nurturance *or* an angry accuser but is *both* a helpless child *and* an angry accuser. In the case example above, after having observed the alternation of the two opposed dyads, the therapist might make the following interpretation:

> At times you treat me as the enemy who must be avoided or destroyed. At other times you reveal a side of you that wants nothing more than to be totally cared for by me. The coexistence of these two parts of you makes it impossible for you to move ahead. If you begin to feel the longing to be cared for by me, your suspicious side tells you I'm the enemy who can't be trusted. If you are experiencing the hatred and wish to destroy me, you lose the possibility of being cared for. You can't win. You can't move ahead. And both sides keep you from experiencing me in a realistic way where you could appreciate my concern for you without feeling you were becoming totally and helplessly dependent on someone who is untrustworthy because he or she is not perfect.

FURTHER ELEMENTS IN THE PROCESS OF INTERPRETATION

MAKING AN EARLY DEEP INTERPRETATION OF THE TRANSFERENCE

Inasmuch as primitive transference dispositions imply a rapid shift to a deep level of experience, the therapist working with borderline patients must be prepared to shift the focus from the realistic here and now to the more unrealistic, fantasized object relation activated in the transference—one that often includes extreme and primitive characteristics that the therapist has to make explicit as far as his or her understanding permits. Such interpretations are made early in the treatment when there is a threat that the patient's internal experience will be acted out in a way that would put the patient, someone else, or the treatment at risk. For example, the therapist might say the following:

> It is just the second session since we completed our contract and agreed to work together, and you have spent the first half of this session in silence except to say that you are thinking of ending this treatment. Although I do not have a lot to go on, the first thing that strikes me is your facial expression. You are looking at me with your head cocked to one side, with a defiant air. It suggests that you experience your silence as a triumph over me, and that to speak would be to submit to me rather than to work with me. It is as though the only possibility here is a power struggle in which one of us will dominate the other. This impression, based on your expression, is supported by what you have told me about your relations with boyfriends and

employers. If I am right, it is essential that we talk about this power struggle you experience here. The alternative would be for you to end the treatment, which would leave you feeling triumphant for a moment but would leave you without the help you need.

There are certain risks to early deep interpretation. One risk is that because the therapist is basing his or her intervention on a minimal amount of data, the patient may feel that the accuracy of the therapist's observation supports the patient's primitive belief that others are capable of magic and that he or she can be magically cured without making an effort in the treatment. The patient may therefore take the interpretation as evidence that his or her primitive belief in an omniscient other is a realistic expectation.

CASE EXAMPLE

After the therapist made an interpretation that the patient felt murderous rage toward her in order to retaliate for severe injustices he had experienced in the past, the patient responded by indicating that he felt as if that meant that the therapist now knew him in a special way that no one before had ever been able to demonstrate. The therapist might say, "I notice that you focus more on your belief that I have special powers than on any effort at understanding your angry feelings toward me and why they might be present. Every time I say something to you, you act as if I have given you a tremendous gift. At the same time, by your responses I can see that you never pay any attention to what I am saying. All that seems to count is that I give you something, yet what I give you seems to get lost immediately. In fact, when I told you about your wish to 'blow me away' and why, it was only a speculation based on what you have told me so far. The truth is that I can't read your mind; only you can confirm or deny the truth of what I have said. It could be that, underneath the themes we are discussing here, there is another level of a very intense wish to find the person who could magically 'understand everything and make it all better.'"

There are other risks to early deep interpretation. The interpretation might be rejected because the patient is still too strongly defended to consider it, or the interpretation might be incorporated in an intellectualized fashion and used as resistance against true emotional understanding. Generally, focusing on the patient's reaction to the interpretation will make it possible to correct such potential misfirings, as in the case example above.

Whenever the therapist interprets the deeper aspect of the patient's psyche, the patient's motivation for his or her defensive position must be included in the interpretive statement. By providing the patient with an explanation about why it might be necessary to hold such a position, the therapist increases the probability that the patient can listen to the statement and consider it. The interpretation therefore needs to include the recognition that the patient erects defenses because of the need to protect against impulses, thoughts, or feelings that seem intolerable, dangerous, or forbidden.

DESCRIBING THE CONFLICT

The interpretation should point out that the patient is in conflict. Because splitting is an attempt to avoid intrapsychic conflict that leads to its expression in behavior, the therapist's interventions should bring the patient's attention to the conflict that is being defended against. The therapist generally interprets the defense before interpreting what is being defended against. The surface manifestation is usually more ego-syntonic, whereas what is being defended against is less acceptable to the patient and therefore arouses more anxiety. These two principles are illustrated by the following intervention:

> The therapist notes that the patient is silent and, because of the patient's clenched fists and facial expression, believes that her silence is a defense against rage toward the therapist. He says, "I wonder if you are silent and sitting with clenched fists because you are afraid that if you talk, your anger may emerge and hurt one or both of us?" First, the therapist is drawing the patient's attention to what she is doing. In this instance he describes her behavior: he notes that she is sitting silently, with clenched fists. Second, the therapist makes a hypothesis about why the patient is not talking: that she fears her own aggression (and perhaps the therapist's retaliation).

This process of describing the conflict depends on the use of clarification, confrontation, and interpretation, often addressed at discrepancies between the different channels of communication.

EXAMINING WHAT IT MEANS TO THE PATIENT TO BE GIVEN AN INTERPRETATION

In the early phase of treatment, borderline patients tend to experience the therapist's actions as powerful, concrete acts of reward and punishment. Because the therapist's most powerful act is usually that of making an interpretation (although confrontation can be a powerful intervention as well), it can be perceived as the vehicle through which the therapist dispenses magic or administers rebukes. Experiencing the interpretation as a wonderful gift is an expression of idealization, whereas seeing it as worthless signifies devaluation. In either case, the patient is responding to the intervention in accordance with his or her character structure and internal world of representations at the expense of attending to the content, which is to be expected in the early phases of therapy and which is why the therapist must also focus more on process—the way things are done—than on content in the early phases (Reich 1972).

An example of the interpretation being experienced as a gift is presented in the following dialogue. The therapist observed the patient making frequent notations on a pad during her session.

Therapist: I notice that you're taking notes whenever I speak.
Patient: Yes. I'm counting how many times you talk.
Therapist: Why do you do that?
Patient: It helps me know if you care about me. I count up the number of times you speak, and when I go home I compare that number to the last session. That's how I tell how much you're giving me.
Therapist: Does it matter what I say?
Patient: Not so much. What really counts is how many times you tell me why you think I'm doing what I'm doing. Then I know you're really listening to me and concerned about me.
Therapist: So it's very important that I care about you, and you've devised a scheme to answer that question for yourself. However, you seem to be disregarding what I actually say. So, in a paradoxical way, your effort to reassure yourself that I'm concerned about you leaves me out of the picture. It might help to think more explicitly about your difficulty imagining that I'm concerned about you.

The therapist's last comment serves at least three purposes. First, it addresses the fact that the experience of the interaction is more important to the patient than the content of the communication. Both patient and therapist should be aware of this, because it is so frequently the case and because exclusive attention to the content usually results in a mutual avoidance of the most important issues early on in the therapy. (The reader should note that this vignette began with the therapist referring to the patient's actions rather than words.) Second, this comment focuses attention on the underlying paranoid transference: the patient's belief that the therapist is not concerned about her. Finally, in pointing out that the patient is disregarding the therapist's words, the therapist refers to an underlying reversal of the paranoid dyad—an underlying devaluation by the patient of the therapist that, although it may not be present consciously at this point, is being earmarked for future exploration.

Another possible response to interpretations is that the patient may treat the interpretation as an effort to control, as seen in the following exchange:

Patient: I purposely wore this short skirt today to be sexy. I thought it would turn you on.
Therapist: And what would happen then?
Patient: Then you couldn't concentrate on your work.
Therapist: Could it be that your being "sexy" in this instance is a way of expressing anger about what we talked about last time and trying to distract me from my work?

Patient: I knew you'd say that. All you want to do is to take away my interest in sex. You're trying to impose your values on me and turn me into whoever you want.

Therapist: So your sexy outfit today is meant to counter what you see as my efforts to control you? If you see that as my goal, that would explain why it's so hard for you to think about what I say. And if you're experiencing our interaction as a struggle to see who can control the other, then I wonder what good you think could come out of our working together. But I guess that's our topic now.

ASSESSING SUPERFICIAL COMPLIANCE

In the initial phase of treatment, borderline patients—who may often fear the therapist's imagined intent to control, criticize and reject, or expose them—may be quite suspicious of the therapist and attempt to ward off the therapist's efforts by superficially seeming to comply. This is another reason why it is important for the therapist to assess the effect an interpretation has had on the patient. A productive interpretation produces further spontaneous elaboration on the patient's part. When this does not occur, such as when the patient blandly appears to agree with the interpretation and then remains silent or changes the subject, the therapist might say, "Although you say you agree, you don't seem to go further with what we are talking about."

ACTIVE ROLE OF THE THERAPIST

We include a section on the active role of the therapist because although TFP is rooted in psychoanalytic theory and technique, the level of the therapist's activity in TFP surprises some psychoanalytically trained therapists.

FEELING FREE TO CLARIFY AND CONFRONT

With regard to clarification, whenever the therapist is uncertain about what the patient is saying, he or she should not hesitate to request further clarification: "What you're saying isn't clear to me. Could you give me an example?" In addition to advancing the work of understanding by requesting clarification, the therapist indicates that he or she is not omniscient (thus confronting through action a frequent object representation), reestablishes the patient's responsibility for providing data, and helps to maintain an atmosphere of exploration and inquiry.

Our understanding of confrontation may sometimes seem to run counter to the central instruction in most psychoanalytic psychotherapy: to follow the patient's associations wherever they lead. This principle of free association applies to our model of therapy with borderline patients but with the following considerations:

1. The patient's associations may reflect a self or object representation that is split off from other representations. In this case, to follow the elaboration of that split-off part may be useful to a point, but it may become necessary for the therapist to confront the patient with material representing other split-off parts that are not present in the current associations in order to advance the process and avoid having the patient perpetuate a situation in which the fragmented internal representations remain segregated from each other.
2. The patient's free associations may serve a defensive purpose and be in the service of resistance (see the discussion on tactics, the hierarchy of priorities to address, and trivialization in Chapter 7). When this occurs, the therapist may have to confront the resistance with a comment such as the following:

> What does it mean that in this session, you are discussing at great length and without visible affect your annoyance with your sister, when two nights ago you left a message for me that you might not be at this session because you might have to go to the hospital? There seem to be feelings in you that you are not discussing in this session, and it would be important to hear about them. If you don't discuss them here, you may return home and feel just as you did the other night without having used this opportunity to try to understand what it's about.

USING FLEXIBILITY IN MAKING INTERPRETATIONS

Because of their use of splitting, borderline patients often assume that others are as rigid as they are about seeing things in black-and-white terms. This assumption of rigidity reflects the patients' difficulty separating their sense of self from their sense of the therapist. This issue can be thought of in terms of theory of mind: they assume the other's mind functions in the same way as theirs. Therefore, flexibility serves to differentiate the therapist from the patient and to provide a model for an alternative way of perceiving and thinking. By demonstrating the ability to hold alternative views of the same person or event, the therapist provides the patient with a model for tolerating ambiguity and appreciating complexity. If, for example, a therapist is considering two different explanations for the patient's behavior, the therapist might well present the patient with both and acknowledge his or her uncertainty about which is the more valid interpretation: "It could be that your difficulty getting here today was a result of your fear that I would be angry with you, but there is also evidence that it might be a message to me to not go into certain areas we were exploring in the last session. I'm not sure, at this point, which view is correct, and perhaps we can come to understand why you did this."

Careful phrasing is important to reinforce the patient's responsibility as being the final validator of any hypothesis the therapist might offer. The therapist also indicates a willingness to change an interpretation on the basis of the patient's subsequent input: "As you're showing me, my original idea no longer seems correct. It's more likely, given what you just said, that...."

SEQUENCING OF SPECIFIC INTERVENTIONS

Just as there is a priority for the focus on a theme, there is also a preferred sequence in the use of specific techniques. In general, interpretation is seen as the key technique for effecting change in TFP. Therefore, the techniques of clarification and confrontation are introduced first to prepare for the interpretations that are eventually offered. However, as discussed earlier in this chapter (see "Making an Early Deep Interpretation of the Transference"), if the patient's actions are jeopardizing the treatment, the therapist should deepen the level of interpretations more rapidly. If such interventions do not forestall acting out, or if there is no time for such a sequence, the therapist moves to set limits, using the least restrictive intervention sufficient to contain the behavior.

TECHNIQUES NOT USED IN TFP

TFP can also be characterized by describing the techniques of near-neighbor treatments (such as psychodynamically oriented supportive therapy for borderline patients) that are not generally used. Unlike supportive treatment, exploratory psychodynamic treatment strives for structural change, focuses on access to deeper levels of the patient's psyche, and does not use overt supportive techniques such as providing reassurance, giving suggestions and advice, educating the patient about life issues, and making environmental interventions (Rockland 1992).

The reason for not using directly supportive techniques (cognitive support, affective support, reeducational measures, direct interventions in the patient's environment) is that such interventions move the therapist away from a position of technical neutrality, tend to suck him or her into a reinforcement of the positive transference, or provoke him or her into an adversarial stance by the patient's eliciting support and then rejecting it. For all these reasons, supportive techniques make interpretation of the transference more difficult.

It is important to distinguish the name of the technique (i.e., exploratory or supportive) from the result or effect of the technique. Specifically, even though "exploratory" or "expressive" psychodynamic treatment does not use "supportive" techniques, the result of exploratory or expressive techniques (i.e., clarification, confrontation, and interpretation) is often that the patient feels supported in his or her efforts toward better understanding, modulation of affects, more satisfying relationships, and greater autonomy in life. Some critics consider expressive psychodynamic treatment to be nonsupportive. We feel this is a misunderstanding based on confusing the avoidance of directly *supportive techniques* with a lack of *supportive effect* of the interventions. Our avoidance of supportive techniques is not because we do not want to support the patient but rather because we believe that using such techniques undermines working within the transference-countertransference paradigm and often leads to enactments of the countertransference.

At its extreme, psychodynamic treatment has been falsely characterized as not only nonsupportive (in technique) but also harsh in its use of the techniques such as confrontation. However, as defined earlier in the chapter in the discussion of confrontation on p. 156, confrontation is not an attack on the patient but rather is a carefully worded presentation to the patient of contradictory aspects of the patient's behavior and presentation and an invitation to reflect on them. The effect of the use of confrontation—an expressive technique—can be that the patient begins to perceive and integrate disparate aspects of self and thus feels profoundly understood and supported by the psychodynamic therapist.

Interpretation is often considered risky with borderline patients because of the erroneous assumption that the patient is bombarded with explanations of his or her behavior that are beyond his or her capacity to comprehend. In TFP, we start out from the surface—that is, from a point at which patient and therapist share a common view of the immediate reality—to then help the patient become curious about a deeper aspect of what is going on and reasons why deeper aspects of his or her psychological life seem frightening or unacceptable. Interpretations, therefore, always imply a starting point of a shared view of what the patient experiences, how the patient experiences the therapist, and how the therapist helps the patient understand the factors contributing to this.

In ending this discussion of interpretation, transference analysis, technical neutrality, and the use of countertransference, we emphasize that in the therapist's mind there is a constant interplay of the techniques and their relation to the treatment frame. Clarification, confrontation, and interpretation are at the core of the work, but this set of techniques can be used in a relatively sterile way if they are not combined with transference analysis, technical neutrality, and countertransference utilization. Therapists may understand internal object relations and manage to discuss issues such as the fear of the persecutory or abandoning object, the longing for the ideal object with anger and disappointment when it is not found, and so on. However, interventions remain intellectualized if they do not connect at times with the patient's affect "in the room." The interplay of techniques consists of the therapist's listening to the patient's material and reacting internally (countertransference). The internal reaction must be experienced and appraised: Is this reaction realistic, or is it a "pull" from the patient's internal world to enact an object from that realm? Is the therapist remaining neutral in his or her response to the patient or deviating from a neutral position? If there is such deviation, what information does it provide? The answers can be unclear, and it is often only by referring to the markers of objective reality provided by the treatment frame that the therapist can ground himself or herself. This interplay of the techniques is crucial to advancing the therapy.

COMMENTARY ON VIDEOS THAT ILLUSTRATE TECHNIQUES

VIDEO 1: TECHNICAL NEUTRALITY AND TACTFUL CONFRONTATION

At this point, we suggest that the reader view Videos 1–2 and 1–3 from a session carried out by Dr. Kernberg with an individual named Albert. As with all cases in the book, "Albert" is a composite case based on elements of real cases disguised in terms of details of information. We comment on selected parts of the video below.

▶ **Video 1–2: Technical Neutrality and Tactful Confrontation Part 1 (9:15)**

Albert came to therapy in a depressed state after his girlfriend, Saskia, left him. They had come to the therapy center 5 months ago at Saskia's urging, and, according to Albert, the two therapists there talked her into leaving him abruptly. In the early part of the session, Dr. Kernberg accepts this but tries to clarify Albert's understanding of the situation as fully as possible. Albert seems perplexed by the situation, alternating between the idea that the two therapists were unfairly prejudiced against him and the vaguer idea that he must be doing something wrong because two previous relationships also ended.

It emerges on clarification that, toward the end of the relationship, Saskia complained that Albert was intrusive and controlling. Dr. Kernberg further clarifies the events leading up to Saskia's insistence that they seek counseling. At this point in the interview, it seems clear that Albert perceives that the problem is Saskia's and that it has little or nothing to do with him. In seeking further clarification about why Saskia would behave this way, Albert reluctantly tells of an incident in which Saskia "broke her finger." As Dr. Kernberg tactfully pursues clarification, it emerges that Albert broke Saskia's finger. At his point, Dr. Kernberg begins to have a fuller picture of an aggressive part of Albert that he denies but is capable of acting out.

Albert has described himself as a very loving person, leaving out any mention of his angry outbursts that have come to light in the course of the session. Dr. Kernberg brings Albert's attention to this in the form of a confrontation, inviting him to reflect on how he can be *both* loving and at times angry at the other. Albert's response is a demonstration of his split internal structure. Rather than talk about a mix or range of emotions, he falls into the opposite side of the split view of himself: "Perhaps I'm not so much a loving person" (1:45).

At this point, Dr. Kernberg turns to another confusing part of Albert's narrative: the idea that Saskia left him solely on the advice of two therapists she had just met. Albert explained he had a feeling the therapists were biased against him, especially the woman therapist. On the basis of the information obtained during the session, Dr. Kernberg describes an alternative narrative: that Saskia might have been resentful of Albert but that it would be painful for him to consider this possibility. Dr. Kernberg offers this alternative explanation without taking sides.

In this manner, Dr. Kernberg has followed a sequence of clarifications leading to an invitation to reflect in the form of a confrontation pointing to the discrepancies in Albert's perception of events. This sequence is followed by a trial interpretation: that Albert's clinging to his inconsistent narrative may be motivated by the pain it would cause to consider the alternative. This interpretation is a hypothesis about why Albert might intensely need to split off his perception of himself as all loving from his anger and why he needs to protect the picture of Saskia as desiring to come back to him from the possibility that she might have wanted to get away from him because of something negative in him.

Albert's reaction is consistent with a split internal world and inability to conceptualize complex emotional states. He cannot imagine Saskia leaving him of her own accord because "you only do that to persons you hate" (5:48). Dr. Kernberg then brings up the possibility of transference reactions within the session.

Dr. Kernberg: Could it be that perhaps you are afraid that I, in saying what I'm saying, am really taking the side of those two therapists and that again you are in the presence of a therapist who might be biased against you?

Albert: When you're saying...I had the feeling you are accusing me. I did it all wrong, it was all my fault, and it was very right of Saskia for leaving me.

Dr. Kernberg: So, you are saying that really I have reached the conclusion that you treated her badly and that she should have left you?

Albert: That is what I hear.

Dr. Kernberg: Is that what I've said? (8:10–9:15) [End of Video 1–2]

Video 1–3: Technical Neutrality and Tactful Confrontation Part 2 (10:08)

It is at this point that Dr. Kernberg's having maintained a position of neutrality throughout the interview reaps its clinical benefit. Because he has presented two possibilities *without* siding with either one, he is now in a position to examine as fully as possible Albert's perception of the therapist's attitude toward him and his situation. Dr. Kernberg can help Albert reflect more carefully on what comes from the other person's mind and what might exist in his own mind. Although it is true that Dr. Kernberg introduced an alternative explanation of events, he left both possibilities open. His assumption is that Albert is intelligent enough to consider the possibility that negative feelings had emerged in his relation with Saskia but his internal splitting has kept him from conscious awareness of this possibility. In Albert's system, if there are negative emotions there are *only* negative emotions. Specifically, if the negative emotions exist within him, he becomes *all* bad.

Dr. Kernberg's work at this point represents the most challenging and subtle aspect of TFP: helping the patient gain awareness of the segment of his internal world that he splits off and projects. This awareness can be very painful but is necessary for the patient to become whole. Dr. Kernberg summarizes Albert's situation, reflecting empathy with his internal conflict.

Dr. Kernberg: So, you are really in a dilemma at this point, if you think of it, because there are two possibilities here.

Albert: Yes.

Dr. Kernberg: One, that all of this is a terrible mistake, that really it's not your problem that she left but it's the problem of the therapists who were kind of stirring her up against you and that the problem is really, if you want to, the two therapists and Saskia who lets herself be dominated by them. And that it's not you who should be here, but she. The other possibility is that you have a problem in being controlling, suspicious, occasionally violent, frightening the women with whom you lived without being aware of it, and then suddenly faced with their leaving you because of the aspects of this violence in you that you cannot accept and cannot tolerate, and that's what you need help with. And if that was so, that here you act suspiciously with me, seeing in me the hostility that you are trying to get away from in yourself. So that's one possibility. And the other is that, yes, there's a conspiracy of the therapists and me, and you're the victim and it's not your problem at all. It's Saskia's problem for having left you. I can see these two alternatives. Do you understand what I'm saying?....

Albert: Yes, I understand what you were saying. When I try to realize it, if Saskia had left me on her own, for her own reasons, it makes me feel very...when I see that as a possibility, then I feel very strange. When I try to look at it that way, the next moment I can't think anymore (4:55–8:17).

At this point Albert's reflective process reaches its limit, but he has at least begun to reflect. Although it is just a small step, it is a beginning: Albert has heard a formulation that is not familiar to him about the split way in which he experiences life, and he has not rejected it outright. He has thought about it up to the point when the emotional pain caused by his thinking about it made him stop. Dr. Kernberg's empathy with this pain will help Albert continue this reflective path in future work.

Dr. Kernberg's empathy is crystallized in a simple phrase when he says, "It's more assuring to see me as biased against you because then *the world is in order*" (8:26). This statement demonstrates two things:

1. Naming the possibility of the negative transference ("to see me as biased against you") brings it out into the open where it can be observed and reflected on. The therapist's acknowledging this possibility can be reassuring to a paranoid patient and communicates the therapist's understanding of the patient's internal experience.
2. The therapist can empathize with the simple order that the patient's split structure imposes on his or her experience of the world as the therapist begins to invite the patient to question that structure.

VIDEO 2: PREVACATION SESSION

The reader can next view Video 2, which shows the first 15 minutes of a session that took place 6 months into therapy. The session took place the day before the therapist, Dr. Em, was going away for a week. The patient, Betty, begins by referring to Bob, her boss. As a quirk of fate, she and Bob had developed a friendship discussing their depressive states with each other.

 Video 2–1: Prevacation Session Part 1 (9:24)

This session illustrates the intertwining of the elements of TFP—transference, countertransference, treatment frame, nonverbal communication, and interpretation—discussed in this chapter. Following the first strategy of treatment, Dr. Em's first effort is to understand which dyad is being enacted in the material Betty brings in. He internally notes a discrepancy between the content of Betty's initial comment about suicide and a provocative attitude that suggests that the comment may be meant to have an impact on him or to see what his reaction would be.

As Betty talks about Bob recommending group therapy, Dr. Em wonders if this may be a way of devaluing his own work with her: "Why are you thinking of going to a therapy when you have a therapy right here?" (1:19). Her response, "I'm not getting anything out of this therapy," confirms his hypothesis. To add more data to his impression that Betty is feeling negative about therapy, he refers to her nonverbal communication in the waiting room: "You were sitting out there in the waiting room and you were looking like you were falling asleep" (1:33).

Betty's nonchalant response about taking 30 pills (1:42) provokes an anxious response from Dr. Em. His initial reaction is to follow the hierarchy of priorities: focusing on Betty's taking of the pills as a possible threat to her life and to the treatment. In this way he is attending to the frame of treatment: he checks to see if the frame (conditions of safety) is in place—in which case he can continue exploratory work—or if he has to deviate from neutrality to take action (to get Betty to the emergency room). It is important to note that even at this point when Dr. Em switches to a more practical discourse, dynamic issues continue to evolve between the two of them. Betty seems to be deriving a certain pleasure out of Dr. Em's confusion and anxiety, suggesting a sadomasochistic dynamic. The irony, and evidence of the power of the internal world over external reality, is that although she is the one whose health—and perhaps life—is at stake, he is the one who is concerned and anxious. Dr. Em takes in this countertransference data—that he is being made to suffer—to add to his understanding of the patient and to use in future interventions.

After establishing that Betty is not at medical risk, Dr. Em returns to his neutral exploratory role. Partly on the basis of the intense anxious countertransference he experienced, Dr. Em addresses the connection between the patient-therapist relationship and Betty's affects, thoughts, and behaviors: "Everything you're saying today is geared to have an impact on this relationship between you and me" (3:59). When Betty says, "Maybe this is what suicide feels like—you take an overdose and then you don't feel anything, you just feel good," Dr. Em chooses to focus on the centrality of the relation as Betty is experiencing it with him rather than pursue what could be an informative theme in the verbal communication. Although it would be helpful to know what is so painful in Betty that sedation and suicide seem preferable to awareness, Dr. Em believes the most important understanding will be gained by exploring the underlying object relationship that is motivating her experience and behavior in the moment.

Betty's response to Dr. Em's drawing attention to their relationship is typical of a person who is anxious—insecure and preoccupied—in her relations with others: she moves away from the here and now that Dr. Em directed their attention to by returning to the question of the group therapy (4:21). Dr. Em tries to understand internally what seems like an abrupt shift in Betty's discourse and has the hypothesis that his drawing attention to the relationship between them provoked anxiety in her and a consequent defensive avoidance of looking at and thinking about elements of the relation together. One could say that his comment activated her attachment system, leading to her anxiety. We would accept that formulation, and we believe that when the attachment system is activated, the therapist can then engage the patient in reflecting on his or her internal experience of the attachment.

In an effort to help Betty understand her experience of the current moment in a broader context, Dr. Em refers to a change from how she related to him at some other times. The therapist must act as the "historian" of the pair because, by virtue of dissociative defenses, the patient's entire sense of reality is determined by what he or she is feeling in the moment. Thinking about earlier sessions in which Betty had related to him in a more positive way, Dr. Em says, "You seem to be pushing me away in the past couple of sessions" (5:28). He then expresses curiosity about the internal motivation for that behavior: "I'd like to try to understand why you've escalated this behavior so much in the past two sessions."

Betty's reaction is a classic example of denial: "It's not related to your going away" (5:45), indicating her discomfort with and attempt to reject attachment/libidinal issues. Dr. Em's initial attempt at interpreting what is motivating Betty's devaluing rejection of him is a somewhat intellectualized interpretation of her affect: "I think it's a combination of anger at me—that I'm not providing the kind of perfect caretaking you wish for, and my going away just probably underlines that" (6:13). This interpretation is based on his object relations theory view of her internal world as being organized at the paranoid schizoid level, with the belief in and wish for the "ideal object" who can provide perfect care. However, this interpretation is a bit intellectualized and too close to the theory rather than to the experience of the moment. Seeing that this initial interpretation—which is an interpretation of the motivation of the negative dyad on the surface—is met with resistance, Dr. Em then makes an interpretation that is both simpler and more related to the affect he feels is being defended against: "I think what's going on right now is a really dramatic example of what happens when you begin to get attached to someone" (7:19). This is a more affect-based interpretation of the motivation for defensively staying in the negative transference and avoiding the positive underlying dyad. This brief comment is a deeper interpretation: Dr. Em allows himself to take the surface data and go slightly beyond them on the basis of information from Betty's nonverbal behavior and his countertransference that communicated that elements of positive affect were present although they were being defended against. This is not an interpretation that tries to offer an explanation at this point but rather attempts to bring a part of the patient's psychic experience—the libidinal side of her internal split—that is beyond her awareness into her awareness so that it can be observed and reflected on. The hypothesis as to why Betty reacts this way to her positive affects comes later as Dr. Em explores the internal representations behind her paranoid transference.

Betty does not accept this interpretation immediately. In fact, her response is based on her paranoid transference: "Why should I swallow everything you're saying?" (7:33) and "You say the same thing to every one of your patients" (7:56). Dr. Em is struck by the sadness of the experience Betty is communicating: the experience that a person she has been meeting with twice weekly for 6 months does not have enough care and concern about her to address her as an individual. Dr. Em responds to this with a metaphor that expresses empathy with her internal state: "It sounds like you feel like you're just an object on an assembly line here" (8:20). That understanding of her internal state seems to help Betty move momentarily beyond the paranoid transference. Her reaction is to switch into a very different state: "I don't feel I deserve to be here" (8:28), possibly reflecting some guilt as she experiences empathy from the person she has been attacking.

Dr. Em turns again to her nonverbal communication: "Why do you think it's hard for you to show your face to me right now?" (8:50). When Betty replies that she just doesn't want him to see her, he continues with interpretation of the motivation for defending against the libidinal dyad: "I think you don't want me to see you in the longing that you're feeling right now. You don't mind my seeing you in your anger and in your rejection, but it seems like you feel you have to hide the longing for fear I'd use it to humiliate you by rejecting you or turning away from you" (9:03–9:24). [End of Video 2–1]

▶ Video 2–2: Prevacation Session Part 2 (6:12)

In Video 2–2, as the session continues Betty seems a bit less defensive, but she again distances herself from Dr. Em. Rather than responding to his comment about "beginning to get attached," she removes herself from the immediate interaction and talks about her self-care. This is a typical defensive movement for someone with a paranoid transference and preoccupied attachment style. Dr. Em is patient with Betty's resistance and is willing to temporarily follow the exploration of dyads outside of the transference in her relation to her self and to others in the outside world. He interprets a form of omnipotent control: "You feel you can control the rejection that way [e.g., dressing badly].... You feel like you're in the driver's seat and maybe it hurts a little less then if you feel that" (1:02). As stated above, this is a temporary movement away from transference analysis but an opportunity to understand something about Betty's dynamics that is outside the transference for the moment.

What follows is a period (1:17–3:14) in which Betty seems to be grappling with her longing for Dr. Em and acknowledgment of positive affects in the relation while simultaneously taking a defensive distance with a return to her controlling monologue style of speech. This mix of drive and defense is typical as progress is being made in questioning a patient's defensive strategy: Betty can begin to question and reflect without fully abandoning the long-standing defensive structures. This is one reason the midphase of therapy can be long. A question the therapist must keep in mind at this stage is the degree to which the positive affect is a function of idealized internal representations that must be analyzed in contrast to being related to a more integrated and realistic positive alliance with the therapist. In most cases, the idealized representations still hold sway and must be analyzed.

Dr. Em again turns attention to the nonverbal, expressing curiosity about Betty's capacity to observe herself: "Your whole tone changed a few minutes ago; did you notice that?" (3:14). Betty acknowledges the change of tone and begins to describe a fantasy. Although the fantasy represents a return to the negative transference ("Well, my fantasy in the waiting room was to humiliate you" [3:30]), the affects are now being *discussed* rather than acted out. At the beginning of the session, Betty was acting out without any apparent awareness or reflection, but now she is able to reflect on the negative transference rather than simply enact it: she can discuss it as a fantasy, making it more accessible to thought and understanding.

As an overarching comment on this session, we would argue that Dr. Em's attention to the interaction and his ability to help Betty find and accept words for previously inchoate affect states helped move Betty from enactment to reflection. The reader will no doubt be able to discern other elements of this session that we have not discussed. It is the richness, and sometimes the frustration, of the psychoanalytic approach that there is always more to understand.

Key Clinical Concepts

- The four basic techniques of TFP include the interpretive process, transference analysis, the use of technical neutrality, and the use of countertransference.

- Because of borderline patients' lack of observing capacity, the interpretive process begins with containing powerful affects that are experienced concretely without symbolic representation and naming the experiences of self and other that seem to be related to the affect(s).

- Following initial containment, the interpretive process can proceed beyond clarification to confrontation, preparing for interpretation in the here and now.

- Transference analysis is the examination and analysis of distortions of the "real" therapist-patient relationship as it was described in the treatment contracting phase. It is observing and understanding the relationship that the patient creates on the basis of the makeup of his or her internal world.

- The TFP therapist maintains neutrality (i.e., not siding with any of the forces involved in the patient's conflicts) in order to foster the patient's awareness of internal conflict and use of self-observation and reflection to address conflicts.

- There is an intimate link between technical neutrality and countertransference. Most unintentional deviations from technical neutrality stem from countertransference reactions that are not recognized and understood by the therapist. In other words, unintended deviations from neutrality are enactments of countertransference.

- The therapist may intentionally deviate from technical neutrality if there is a threat to safety that cannot be dealt with effectively by interpretation and understanding.

SELECTED READINGS

Caligor E, Diamond D, Yeomans FE, et al: The interpretive process in the psycho-analytic psychotherapy of borderline personality pathology. J Am Psychoanal Assoc 57: 271–301, 2009

Hersoug A, Ulberg R, Høglend P: When is transference work useful in psychodynamic psychotherapy? Main results of the first experimental study of transference work (FEST). Contemporary Psychoanalysis 50:56–174, 2014

Høglend P, Bogwald KJ, Amlo S, et al: Transference interpretations in dynamic psychotherapy: Do they really yield sustained effects? Am J Psychiatry 165:763–771, 2008 [Transference interpretation as a treatment technique seems to be especially important for patients with long-standing, more severe interpersonal problems.]

Joseph B: Transference: the total situation, in Melanie Klein Today: Developments in Theory and Practice, Vol 2: Mainly Practice. Edited by Spillius EB. London, Routledge, 1988, pp 61–72

Racker H: The meanings and uses of countertransference. Psychoanal Q 26:303–357, 1957

Reich W: Character Analysis. New York, Farrar, Straus, and Giroux, 1972 [See Chapters 1–6.]

Winnicott DW: Hate in the counter-transference. Int J Psychoanal 30:69–74, 1949

TACTICS OF TREATMENT AND CLINICAL CHALLENGES

THE TACTICS OF transference-focused psychotherapy (TFP) are the maneuvers the therapist uses to set the stage for and to guide the proper use of techniques (described in Chapter 6, "Techniques of Treatment") within the individual session.

The tactics (Table 7–1) involve therapist activities that range from creating the framework for the therapy (contracting and limit setting) to guiding the therapist's choice of what material to address (determining the hierarchy of priorities) to maintaining appropriate attitudes with regard to the patient and the material. In this chapter we provide an overview of the tactics beyond contract setting, which is discussed in Chapter 5, "Establishing the Treatment Frame." We also discuss the major challenges that might arise during the treatment.

The therapist's basic attitude is alertness to what transpires between therapist and patient, especially to what is at variance from normal human interaction. "Normal" in this regard is defined as the usual form of culturally accepted verbal communication between a patient and a therapist, in

TABLE 7–1.	Tactics of treatment

1. Setting the treatment contract
2. Maintaining the frame of treatment
3. Choosing and pursuing the priority theme to address in the material that the patient is presenting (this includes monitoring the three channels of communication, following the three principles of intervention, and adhering to the hierarchy of priorities regarding types of material that come up in a session)
4. Maintaining an appropriate balance between expanding the incompatible views of reality between patient and therapist in preparation for interpretation and establishing common elements of shared reality
5. Regulating the intensity of affective involvement

particular as defined in the treatment contract at the beginning of their work together. The therapist expects the patient to communicate his or her subjective experience. If the patient does not, the therapist suspects that the patient is troubled by the activation of fantasized, primitive, irrational elements in the interaction. The therapist's awareness of and attentiveness to such unrealistic aspects is facilitated by attention to the boundaries determined by the treatment frame as well as to any deviation from the boundaries of the psychotherapeutic situation.

The therapeutic attitude is always threatened by possible acting out of transference feelings and, at times, by the temptation for the therapist to act out the countertransference. Paradoxically, the more severely ill the patient is and the more distorted the total interpersonal interaction in the psychotherapeutic relationship is, the easier it is to diagnose primitive object relations in the transference. Conversely, the healthier the patient is or the higher level the patient is at in terms of borderline organization, the more subtle the distortions in the interaction. Therefore, therapists often find it more difficult to grasp the dynamics of higher-level than of lower-level borderline patients.

TACTIC 1: ESTABLISHING THE TREATMENT CONTRACT

Establishing a mutual understanding of the goals and methods of treatment and of the frame of treatment starts with the discussion of the treatment contract that precedes therapy per se. This process is described in detail in Chapter 5.

TACTIC 2: MAINTAINING THE FRAME OF TREATMENT

Maintaining the boundaries of the treatment is generally a matter of maintaining the conditions of the treatment established in the contract and is carried out with a combination of interpretation and limit setting.

BLOCKING ACTING OUT IN THE SESSION

Certain behaviors, although they may be laden with meaning, are so distracting from the work of exploration that they must cease so that the therapy can proceed. Therefore, there may be occasions when the therapist must curb the patient's behavior. The first step in doing so is for the therapist to draw attention to the behavior and inquire as to whether the patient is aware of the behavior and has any thoughts about what motivates it. The therapist may then interpret the behavior. The patient's understanding of the motivation of a behavior may lead to the curbing of the behavior and to a more adaptive expression of what underlies it. If interpretation does not lead to an end of the disruptive behavior, the therapist can set a limit to block the behavior. Having done so, the therapist then interprets what has transpired to reestablish a position of neutrality.

CASE EXAMPLE

Halfway through a session a patient covered his ears and began yelling obscenities at the therapist. The therapist attempted to interpret the behavior, but the patient continued to yell in a way that made dialogue impossible. The therapist's next intervention was to state, "You must stop yelling before we can continue the session. Yelling and covering your ears does not permit you to hear and makes it impossible for me to be of any help to you." Once the patient stopped this behavior, the therapist interpreted it: "You're very angry at me and at the same time may have doubts about the validity of your anger. So you may make it impossible to hear what I have to say in case it might increase your doubt and make it necessary to think about your anger."

A patient may object to a therapist's interpretation, saying that the therapist had instructed the patient to express his or her most intense feelings. The therapist may then explain that the expression of thoughts and feelings is indeed essential to the process but that a limit must be set when the expression becomes an obstacle to the process. The therapist might also invoke practical reality: "I did say your role was to express all your thoughts and feelings, but your yelling interferes with my colleague's ability to do her work next door, and we have to respect the reality we're working within."

Interpreting the patient's challenges to the treatment frame often involves addressing an aggressive part of the patient attacking the health-seeking process of treatment or understanding an attempt to avoid the anxiety that arises when the patient's primitive defenses begin to fail and the patient is faced with a complex mix of feelings that do not fit the familiar "black-or-white" structure. Forms of acting out that may require limit setting include any challenge to the boundaries of treatment, whether it be a challenge to physical boundaries, time boundaries, or space boundaries. Examples are physical destructiveness to self, to the therapist, or to objects; refusal to leave the office at the end of sessions; sexual exposure or sexual gestures toward the therapist; and yelling in a way that cuts off dialogue.

The need to block acting out sometimes applies to behaviors outside the session. Although it would be unrealistic to assume that all acting-out behaviors will stop once the patient agrees to the treatment contract, certain behaviors are so dangerous or distracting that the work of therapy cannot continue until the behaviors come to an end. Setting limits around certain behaviors may require the utilization of an auxiliary therapist if the patient does not have sufficient control to stem the behavior. However, because therapists generally err on the side of underestimating the patient's capacity for control, the recommended progression is first to attempt to establish a parameter that the patient will be responsible to follow and then to engage an auxiliary therapist only if the patient is clearly unable to control the behavior.

CASE EXAMPLE

A patient with a history of anorexia initially agreed with her therapist to maintain a healthy weight. However, she began to come to sessions looking thinner and thinner. The therapist's attempts to address this by interpretation led to no change, and the patient became so thin that the therapist's anxiety about her condition made it impossible to explore the issues with peace of mind. At that point the therapist explained that therapy could not proceed in any productive way unless the patient's anorexic condition was addressed directly. He told her that in order to continue in therapy with him, the patient would have to consult with an eating disorders specialist with whom she would work out a plan to gain weight, be weighed regularly, and stay above an established minimum weight.

ELIMINATING SECONDARY GAIN

The concept of secondary gain was developed after psychoanalysis established the concept of the primary gain that an individual experiences from a symptom. Based on the idea that symptoms represent a compromise between an impulse and the prohibition against it, satisfying each to some degree, the primary gain is the decrease in anxiety achieved by this compromise, even though it means experiencing the symptom. For example, a patient's cutting may be an unconscious compromise between an aggressive impulse (or a mixed aggressive and sexual impulse) and the punishment for having that impulse. The primary gain of the symptom of cutting is the decrease in anxiety experienced as both the impulse and the prohibition against it are simultaneously satisfied to some degree. Beyond this primary gain, the patient may experience secondary gain if, for example, the cutting attracts the attention, concern, and intervention of others. Thus, secondary gain involves external benefits that accrue to the symptom and add to its value to the patient.

The external benefits of secondary gain can threaten the treatment because improvement in the patient's condition carries with it a loss of secondary gain. The most serious forms of secondary gain generally found in the borderline population are 1) the control of others that can come from self-destructive or suicidal actions (e.g., a patient saying she is suicidal because she feels her therapist is rushing her off the phone) and 2) complacency in the passive, dependent patient role involving excessive use of social services (e.g., disability benefits, financial support from the family, and possibly the treatment itself) based on the idea of a chronic disabling illness. This latter form of secondary gain is seen in patients who look to treatment not as a means of changing and developing autonomy but rather as a way of life—a substitute for having an active, independent life and other relationships. Our view is that inactivity contributes to the illness and that movement toward involvement in an active life is part of the therapeutic process.

Because of these risks, the therapist must be sure that the treatment frame does not support secondary gain. Therefore, in the contracting process, the therapist 1) makes it clear that he or she is out of the loop of the patient's self-destructive actions—that is, that these actions are in the domain of emergency or crisis services and that the therapist will not become more involved with the patient in response to his or her acting out—and 2) does not accept for treatment a patient who rejects the idea of engaging in some productive activity outside of the treatment situation. After these conditions are established in the treatment contract, they may emerge in the course of treatment at times when the patient challenges them. One pitfall we have observed in many cases is that therapists tend, imperceptibly, to develop a tolerance for the patient's pathology and behavior; this seems true especially when the pathology is expressed in passive symptoms such as inactivity. It can be appropriate for the therapist to describe secondary gain to the patient, using layman's terms, and to explain that it is incompatible with the goals of therapy:

I notice you are beginning to repeat the pattern where you seem to be very involved in therapy, but for weeks now, you have made no effort to engage in any meaningful activity outside of therapy. Although you know I think it's essential that you be involved in our therapy, I am concerned when it is the only thing you seem involved in. In my experience, there are two main reasons why people seek therapy: one is to change and get better; the other is because it feels good to be in treatment, to have someone's attention, and so on. In many cases, a person's motivation for being in treatment is some mix of the two reasons. My concern with you now is that the second reason seems to be taking over, as I believe it did in the past when you were in therapy for 4 years and didn't seem to change. We have to look at and discuss this issue because this therapy is meant to help you change and not to provide you with a substitute for other involvements in life.

The issue of secondary gain touches on the basic understanding of borderline pathology and how society responds to it. If borderline patients are viewed as having a chronic, disabling illness, then it makes sense to respond by offering long-term disability benefits. However, we view borderline personality disorder (BPD) as a condition in which 1) most patients are capable of some level of goal-directed functioning (if only a day program or volunteer job initially), even at the stage of entering treatment, and 2) most patients are capable of making substantial progress and of becoming autonomous and productive. Therefore, we believe it is damaging to the patient to be indefinitely supported by the social system. Our experience is that starting therapy while receiving disability payments is a negative prognostic factor. In cases in which the "disability payments" come from the family, the therapist can engage the family during the contracting phase in a plan to tailor support to the therapeutic goals of the treatment.

TACTIC 3: CHOOSING AND PURSUING THE PRIORITY THEME

In psychotherapy, especially with borderline patients, one of the most common problems therapists encounter is deciding which issue, among all those simultaneously present in the material, should be addressed. Sessions often appear chaotic; the activation of a number of disparate part-self and part-object representations in the patient's mind can lead to the appearance of multiple themes in the session. At times, the therapist feels flooded with information when too much seems to be going on at once, or the therapist may be at a loss because the patient may appear to be providing little of clear interest in a given session. Consequently, the therapist often feels uncertain how to proceed. A sense of clear priorities regarding what to address in the session is essential to help the therapist in this predicament. Choosing the priority theme involves 1) monitoring the three channels of communication; 2) following the economic, dynamic, and structural principles of intervention; and 3) adhering to the hierarchy of priorities regarding the types of material the patient brings up.

MONITORING THE THREE CHANNELS OF COMMUNICATION

The channels of communication are 1) the verbal content of the patient's discourse; 2) the patient's nonverbal communication, including *how* the patient says what he or she says (tone of voice, speech volume, etc.), nonverbal communication in the form of body language (posture, gestures, eye contact, etc.), and the atmosphere in the room; and 3) the therapist's countertransference. Of course, therapists who are treating nonborderline patients should also be aware of the three channels, but, as a general rule, the more primitive the pathology, the more important are the second and third channels—nonverbal communication and the countertransference—because of the split nature of the borderline patient's internal world. Patients are generally already aware of what they are saying at any given point but are unaware of the internal contradictions or of split-off parts that do not pass through awareness and are expressed only through action or somatization (Green 1993). Awareness of all three channels is especially important because when a therapist who has been trained to listen carefully to the patient's associations is not attuned to subtle observation of the patient's interaction with the therapist and of the countertransference, the patient can go on for long periods without making any progress in therapy.

ECONOMIC, DYNAMIC, AND STRUCTURAL PRINCIPLES

The economic, dynamic, and structural principles are based on psychoanalytic concepts involving the dynamic forces at work within the mind: the interaction of drives, affects, internal prohibitions, and external reality. The *economic principle* refers to the dominant investment of the patient's affect in any given material and is the principal guide in helping the therapist decide what material to focus on. The rationale for this principle is that intense affects serve as flags pointing to the dominant object relation in the transference. An issue may be considered affectively dominant either if significant affect accompanies the content or if there is a striking absence of affect appropriate to the content, which indicates that affect is being suppressed, repressed, displaced, or split off. What is affectively dominant may appear self-evident at times, such as when a patient is discussing his mother's diagnosis of cancer with intense affect. However, it could be that the patient brings up his mother's diagnosis of cancer but in the same session speaks with more affect about being late for work that day. The therapist should first inquire about and explore the affect.

If a patient's affect is discordant with what the therapist would expect it to be, then the therapist should ask for clarification. For example, a therapist might ask, "You're talking about whether you should go on living, yet you don't seem to be concerned about what you're saying." This inquiry can lead to discovering the predominant theme. When the patient's behavior and words are incongruent and his or her affective dominance is unclear, behavior is probably more important than verbal content and should be explored first. Although it may appear nothing more than a matter of common sense to follow the patient's affect, doing so can nevertheless be a very helpful guide, such as when a discrepancy exists between what might logically seem to be the priority issue (e.g., illness in a spouse) and what appears to carry the most affect (e.g., the patient's perception of the therapist's demeanor).

If the therapist has difficulty determining an area of affective dominance, he or she should next turn to any indications of transference in the content of the patient's remarks or in behaviors (transference will be further discussed next in relation to the dynamic principle) and then to the countertransference. If no significant theme has yet emerged, then the therapist should continue to evaluate the ongoing flow of material, waiting until an affectively dominant motif appears. Its absence may indicate that the patient is consciously suppressing important material. If so, the guidelines for emergency priorities, especially regarding triviality of communication (see later section "Adhering to the Hierarchy of Priorities Regarding Content"), can help focus the therapist. Absence of significant affective themes can be particularly characteristic of narcissistic patients with a dismissive style of attachment.

After the therapist has determined which material is most invested with affect, he or she then thinks in terms of the *dynamic principle*. This principle has to do with the forces in conflict in the psyche and assumes that the presence of heightened affect signals an unconscious conflict involving a defended-against impulse. Both the impulse and the defense against it are represented in the psyche by respective object relationship dyads. Because the patient's internalized relationship dyads are observed most clearly in the transference, the dynamic principle is intimately linked with a focus on the transference. The dynamic principle instructs the therapist to work from the defense, which is observable on the surface, to the impulse, which is out of awareness at a deeper level.

What the therapist observes most commonly in early sessions are transferences that serve as *resistances* to accessing deeper material. Resistances are the clinical manifestations of defensive operations. Operationally, any difficulty the patient demonstrates in participating in the treatment as agreed to in the treatment contract serves the resistance to accessing deeper material. The task of fully examining one's inner world is inevitably daunting—especially for patients whose internal world is characterized by intense, unintegrated parts—and although it is appropriate to empathize with the difficulty of that task, the therapist must always be alert to the risk of colluding with resistance. From an object relations point of view, colluding with the resistance consists of the therapist enacting the role of one of the patient's internal object representations without examining the dyad that is being enacted and the role it plays in defending against awareness of other internal dyads. An example of this is the therapist who accepts the positive transference—the role of benevolent helper—without exploring subtle suggestions of suspiciousness or wariness in the patient.

Resistances are not like walls that need to be removed but rather are a part of the psychic structure that must be appreciated for their informational value. They are defensively used dyads that should be interpreted; that is, the reason for their presence should be understood in relation to what they are defending against. The following is a simple example of such an interpretation by a therapist: "You may be experiencing me as a harsh judge, a menacing critic [defense] because it would be too frightening to experience the wish that I be available to nurture and care for you [libidinal impulse being defended against]." Interpretation from surface to depth is discussed more fully in Chapter 6. The dynamic principle is reviewed here as an aid in knowing where to intervene.

The therapist uses the dynamic principle in determining the order in which he or she addresses material in making an interpretation. In practical terms, the therapist can ask himself or herself, "What is defending against what?" and should generally choose interventions that address the defensive level first. The following is another example: "You are very insistent on seeing me as cold and depriving. Even when I offered you an alternative session because you cannot come on Monday, you harshly responded that I was only offering one alternative that was convenient for me. I've noticed that your depiction of me as cold and withholding has increased over the past weeks. Can we agree that this is the way you have been seeing me?" This intervention is describing the dyad that is serving the defensive function. If the patient agrees, the therapist could continue: "It seems this intensification of seeing me this way could be covering up other feelings you are having that you are uncomfortable with and that make you anxious. In subtle ways, such as the look in your eyes at times, you seem to be experiencing me differently. These subtle signs suggest you may be feeling something positive in regard to me, but for some reason this appears to make you anxious, resulting in a stepping up of your criticisms of me, as though to reassure yourself that nothing positive could exist between you and me." The therapist is beginning to address the affect and impulse being defended against. The final step in this process would be to understand the need to defend against these feelings (see the subsection "Interpretations at Three Levels" in Chapter 6).

Affective dominance coincides with transferential dominance most of the time, but there are occasions when the dominant affect is not centered in the transference. However, even in these situations, the transference implication is usually clear. For example, if in the first 10 minutes of the session, the patient discusses a variety of topics with consistent blandness and without paying attention to the therapist, the predominant focus might be on exploring how the patient may be experiencing and treating the therapist: "You are talking as though I were not here today." This aspect of the transference then becomes the focus of exploration.

If affect and transference diverge—that is, if there appears to be a predominant transference paradigm but some other issue is more affectively weighted—then the latter should be chosen as the focus. Usually, the connection with transference will emerge at some later point. What makes working with the transference subtle is that it is not always communicated through words—either in direct references to the therapist or indirectly through discussion of other significant individuals. The transference is often communicated through subtle behavioral gestures or an overall attitude. For example, it may be more important for the therapist to focus on the fact that the patient commented with a slight ironic laugh than to focus on the content of the comment. It may be important for the therapist first to focus on the mistrust observed in the patient's eyes and then to wonder how to link it to the content of what the patient is saying.

The *structural principle* is also helpful in guiding the therapist's interventions. This principle involves the therapist's developing understanding of the structure of the particular patient's conflicts and comes from the therapist's stepping back and getting an overview of how the specific dyads that have been activated in the transference fit together in a larger pattern. With neurotic patients, the structural analysis involves conflicts between the id, superego, ego, and external reality, or with an inconsistent element in an otherwise consolidated identity. In borderline patients, in whom the ego and superego have not become integrated, conflicts are structured around the most prominent internal relationship dyads and their relations to each other. Although the number of possible relationship dyads is immense, in clinical practice we find that each individual patient presents with a limited number of highly invested dyads that are frequently repeated in the transference. Thus, each therapy comprises a limited number of transference themes. Establishing which transference themes are prominent in a specific patient, and their relation to each other, helps the therapist guide his or her interventions. The structural principle involves determining what object relations dyads have a defensive function against specific other object relations dyads and to what extent the patient is able to look jointly at the conflict from the perspective of an "excluded other," a triadic principle that introduces the observing part of the patient's ego represented by his or her temporary identification with the analytic function of the therapist. Because in TFP we are looking at the course of developing psychological structures, thinking in terms of the structural principle also involves the therapist's thinking in terms of what the patient is becoming and can become.

In borderline patients, the most effective way of arriving at this formulation is to determine the chronic, baseline transference that underlies the shifting transferences observed from moment to moment and that represents the principal conflict at a given phase of the therapy. Although it is not always the case, most borderline patients begin therapy with a chronic paranoid transference, a self representation of a weak, vulnerable self who is on guard against any feelings of closeness that they may develop because of the belief that the object will inevitably reject, abandon, invade, hurt, or exploit him or her. (See Chapter 9, "Midphase of Treatment," for more discussion of the evolution of typical transferences.)

In summary, these three principles remind the therapist to 1) follow the patient's affect as an indicator of what the predominant object relations dyad is at a given moment, 2) look for and address first the material that seems to be serving a defensive purpose, and 3) look for the overall organization of dyads in terms of which surface dyad is defending against which underlying dyad.

ADHERING TO THE HIERARCHY OF PRIORITIES REGARDING CONTENT

Beyond the principles discussed above, there are guidelines for choosing which of the patient's issues to address. In each session, the therapist first must establish whether any *emergency priorities* are present or whether the session will involve the ordinary priorities of therapy. The therapist must give highest priority to any behaviors that threaten the safety of the patient, of the therapist, or of the treatment. The hierarchy of priorities (Table 7–2) helps the therapist determine what constitutes emergencies or threats to the treatment (Table 7–3) versus business as usual. Emergency themes (e.g., threats of suicide or self-injury, threats to discontinue treatment, withholding of information) tend to recede over the first 6 months of treatment if dealt with effectively. This allows the therapist to focus more on the themes that are listed in Table 7–2 as having lower priority because they do not threaten the treatment but that, in fact, constitute the essence of the psychotherapy—understanding the internal world of the patient.

Each theme is addressed with the appropriate technique: clarification, confrontation, interpretation, limit setting, or restoring technical neutrality. Over time, as emergency threats to the treatment diminish, the sessions should gradually become focused on the exploration of the transference themes and underlying dynamics. A therapist might consider the hierarchy of priorities as a guide to the gradual cleaning up of the interactional field of behavioral resistances so as to clear the way for a full exploration of the transference developments. The patient's resistance to addressing the relevant themes can be manifested in behaviors that threaten the ability to continue the therapy—by the patient's threatening to end the therapy outright, threatening to end his or her life, or undermining the exploratory process even though the therapy may appear to be going on. Behaviors that interfere with an ongoing channel of open verbal communication in the session must be addressed in the order of the immediacy of their threat to the communication and to the therapy itself. Table 7–2 first lists priorities that represent obstacles to exploration of the transference, going from the most direct to the more subtle. If these themes are not present or have been adequately addressed, the therapist focuses on priorities 2 and 3, transference-related material and other affect-laden material.

The Role of Information About the Patient's Life Outside of Therapy

Borderline patients often act out in their everyday lives issues that require exploration within the therapy. The therapist should be alert to clues to such acting out that may appear. Sometimes the information is only in a passing remark by the patient or in information provided by a third party. The therapist should also be alert to patients' *not* providing information about their life outside of the sessions. If a patient who has had difficulties at college or in a relationship makes no reference to that area of his or her life for an extended period, the therapist should actively inquire. Any issue that emerges in regard to the patient's external reality should alert the therapist to the possibility that it has already or will soon emerge as a transference paradigm.

TABLE 7-2.   Hierarchy of thematic priority

---

1. Obstacles to transference exploration[a]

   Suicide or homicide threats

   Overt threats to treatment continuity (e.g., financial difficulties, plans to leave town, requests to decrease session frequency)

   Dishonesty or deliberate withholding in sessions (e.g., lying to the therapist, refusing to discuss certain subjects, silences occupying most of the sessions)

   Irregular attendance or altered mental state in session

   Contract breaches (e.g., failure to meet with an auxiliary therapist when agreed on, failure to take prescribed medication)

   In-session acting out (e.g., abusing office furnishings, refusing to leave at the end of the session, shouting)

   Between-session acting out, including intrusions into the therapist's life

   Nonaffective or trivial themes

2. Overt transference manifestations

   Verbal reference to therapist

   "Acting-in" (e.g., positioning body in overtly seductive manner)

   As inferred by therapist (e.g., references to other doctors)

3. Nontransferential affect-laden material

---

[a]The obstacles to working with the overt transference manifestations are themselves infused with transference meaning in the form of resistances.

TABLE 7-3.   Examples of specific threats to treatment

Suicidal and self-destructive behaviors

Homicidal impulses or actions; threatening the therapist

Lying or withholding of information

Poor attendance at therapy sessions

Substance abuse

Coming to session in altered state of consciousness

Uncontrolled eating disorder

Excessive phone calls; other intrusions into therapist's life

Not paying the fee; creating a situation of being unable to pay (e.g., by quitting a job, discontinuing insurance)

Seeing more than one therapist simultaneously

Wasting time in session/trivialization

Problems created external to the sessions that obstruct the conduct of the therapy

A chronically passive lifestyle which, although not immediately threatening, would defeat any therapeutic effort toward change in favor of the continued secondary gain of illness

---

CASE EXAMPLE

A patient began therapy saying that she was depressed and suicidal because her husband was a tyrant. As the therapy evolved, her therapist noted at one point that she had not mentioned her husband for a month. He inquired about her relation with him. She replied, "There's nothing to discuss; I've decided to leave him." The patient had not discussed this plan with her husband or her therapist. As the therapist explored it, he learned that the patient did not have any realistic plan to provide for herself after leaving her husband and that she planned to end therapy when she left her husband. Exploration revealed that this undiscussed plan was a covert form of harming herself. Further exploration revealed that the patient was actually feeling closer to her husband, and to her therapist, in ways and that the destructive plan was based on feelings of anxiety and guilt in relation to the underlying libidinal developments.

In summary, with regard to choosing the priority theme, the therapist will be aided in determining the most important issue at the moment through analysis of what the patient says and communicates about what he or she feels, of the therapist's observations of what the patient does, and of the countertransference. This corresponds to Bion's (1962) concept of the "selected fact."

DISCUSSION OF TYPES OF OBSTACLES TO TRANSFERENCE EXPLORATION

Suicide and Homicide Threats

Threats of suicide or homicide should be addressed according to the parameters discussed in Chapter 5 on contracting and establishing the treatment frame, keeping in mind that any mention of suicidal or homicidal thoughts may have an important dynamic and interactional meaning as seen in the discussion of the beginning of Video 2, "Prevacation Session," in Chapter 6.

Threats to End the Treatment

Threats by the patient to prematurely end the treatment, whether overt or implicit, take priority over all other issues except threats to the patient's life and safety or to the lives and safety of others. The possible motives that may prompt a borderline patient to consider dropping out of treatment include the emergence of dependency needs that create anxiety in the patient, the development of a negative transference (which could be defending against an underlying positive transference that makes the patient anxious), narcissistic issues of envy of the therapist, hypomanic states or flight into health, the wish to either protect the therapist from aggressive affects or to humiliate him or her by defeating his or her efforts, and so on. The essential attitude of the therapist in these situations is to be active—for instance, to call a patient who has missed a session without having notified the therapist and to express concern and curiosity about what this represents.

The next most serious threat to the treatment is any pattern of overt or covert lack of participation in the treatment process. This lack of participation, which can take the form of dishonesty, withholding, or acting out, must be explored.

Dishonesty

The process of therapy is particularly vulnerable to dishonesty because the problem may persist for a long time before the therapist is aware of it. Obtaining a careful initial history, including history of prior treatments, can help the therapist perceive this problem. Should the therapist learn, in the course of the treatment, that the patient is being dishonest, he or she must 1) explain to the patient that a pattern of dishonest communication would effectively render the treatment ineffective and, if unresolved, bring it to an end and 2) explore with the patient the motives underlying the dishonest communication.

Lying is an expression of how the patient experiences self, others, and the therapy. Patients may lie for any of the following reasons: 1) to avoid confrontations that will result in their having to assume responsibility for their actions, 2) to avoid the therapist's disapproval or imagined retaliation, 3) to exert control over the therapist, 4) to express superiority over the therapist by duping him or her, 5) to prevent an authentic relationship from developing, and 6) to exploit the therapist. In a deeper sense, consistent lying expresses the belief that all human relationships are exploitative or persecutory and represents a chronic transference position. Because the success or failure of the therapeutic task depends on honest communication, lying must be treated as seriously as any self-destructive action. The therapist must try to interpret fully and consistently the misrepresentation or suppression of information, while acknowledging that he or she is powerless to keep the patient from communicating dishonestly if the patient chooses to do so.

Interpretive efforts focused on lying or withholding of information may take weeks or months, particularly in cases with antisocial features. However long it may take, full resolution of the implications of the patient's lying takes precedence over all other material except life-threatening acting out and danger of immediate dropout. If the patient who habitually lies also shows evidence of life-threatening or treatment-threatening acting out, the treatment should start in the hospital so as to provide the protection and accurate reporting (by hospital staff) that the patient is unable to provide.

Patients who lie habitually and give evidence of serious superego deficiencies tend to project their own lack of moral values onto the psychotherapist and to conceive of him or her as being dishonest and corrupt. The interpretive approach to this transference includes, therefore, focusing on the patient's projection of dishonesty onto the therapist: "I am not surprised that you feel that I have billed you for a session that you believe you shouldn't be charged for, because throughout our meeting today you've been making up stories instead of telling me what really happened. It's as if you can't imagine a world in which lying and exploitation aren't the common currency of communication."

Full exploration of the transference meanings of lying, like all interpretive work, proceeds from surface to depth. (See Chapter 6 for a more detailed explanation of this principle.) Transference interpretations will often focus first on lying as an expression of the patient's hostility toward self as well as toward the therapist. Deeper interpretations about the patient's despair can be made only after the aggressive and paranoid components are interpreted. The following are examples of confrontations or interpretations in circumstances in which dishonesty serves different functions:

- Lying as an expression of hostility toward the self: "You continuously change your story about what happened. This makes it impossible for me to help you and thus ends up defeating you. It's as though some part of you wants to keep you from getting the help you desperately need."
- Lying as an attack on the therapist: "You continue to tell me the same thing even after we have agreed that this is a made-up tale. You treat me, therefore, as if I'm not worthy of your respect and as if you want to render my efforts impotent."
- Lying as an expression of fear of retaliation: "You seem to fear telling me the truth about having taken my magazine from the waiting room because you think that if you told me, I would become angry and stop seeing you."
- Lying as an expression of disillusionment: "You act as if the only way you can save your skin is to create a fiction about what's happening. That means to me that you have no belief that if I really knew you anything good could come of it."

Situations arise in which the therapist has the vague sense that the patient is being dishonest without being able to pinpoint the basis for this impression. In such an instance, it is perfectly appropriate to tell the patient, "I have a sense that you're not being straight with me. Let's explore whether this is my problem or yours."

Withholding Information

Withholding, a variant of dishonesty, must be addressed as a direct threat to the treatment. In terms of the dynamics involved, dishonesty and withholding can be equally motivated by a destructive internal part of the self resisting the treatment process in order to protect itself from scrutiny and maintain the splitting that organizes the patient's experience. Evidence of withholding may come from discrepancies between what the patient reports and other sources of information, as in this example from the history-taking phase of a therapy: "You didn't tell me that your nighttime calls to Dr. Smith became an issue in your therapy with him, but when I spoke to him, he said that your increasingly frequent calls were one of the principal reasons he recommended that you seek therapy with someone else."

In addressing the lapse or failure of honest and full communication, the therapist may distinguish between occasional suppression and ongoing suppression. *Occasional suppression* is the conscious withholding of information with respect to a circumscribed area. In general, the patient will be tempted to suppress what is most conflictual, but the positive motivation of the patient will overcome this temptation. *Ongoing suppression* is the patient's systematic, conscious withholding of material over extended periods of time or the prolonged refusal to speak during most of the session over one or more sessions. Ongoing suppression may reflect efforts to control the treatment (or therapist), active competitiveness with the therapist, severe paranoid fears (as seen in psychopathic or paranoid transferences of a pervasive kind), or guilt over certain behaviors.

When the patient acknowledges that there is something difficult to talk about, the therapist should seek clarification, exploring the patient's assumptions about the consequences of revealing the secrets before dealing with the specific content being withheld. This is an example of the need to explore the defense (reason for withholding) before the content (what is being withheld). In addition to exploring the patient's fantasies, the therapist should confront and explore the conflict between the patient's agreeing to the ground rules of open communication and then withholding or lying. The meaning of the behavior toward the therapist may add a different level of understanding to the patient's assumptions about the therapist (e.g., the patient may assume that the therapist would react in an angry, critical way but, by withholding, the patient behaves in a way that is geared to provoke anger and criticism). Very often the competitiveness, fears, or guilt behind the withholding can be worked through only over an extended period of time.

Irregular Attendance

The problem of poor attendance may appear self-evident—therapy cannot happen if the two parties are not present—but this problem is not necessarily an easy one for the therapist to address. Appeals are often made by the patient on the basis of the *impossibility* of regular attendance: "In my line of work, you never know when the boss is going to spring an emergency job on you." "I have to rely on the babysitter, and you never know when she's going to get there." "My husband drives me here, and he doesn't understand the importance of being on time." "My colitis (migraines, premenstrual syndrome, etc.) acts up and I just can't leave the house." The therapist may begin to feel that the simple requirement of attending sessions is a harsh, rigid, or even sadistic demand. However, when the therapist begins to think of the basic requirements of therapy as demands, it is a sign to reflect on what is developing in the transference and countertransference. On the most real level, although the patient's getting to sessions may indeed involve considerable effort, the therapist should not forget the importance of treatment for a patient whose life may be threatened by his or her illness.

The simple fact that must be communicated to the patient at this point is that the treatment cannot happen if he or she is not there, and this reality, although obvious, should be stated to a patient who is missing sessions. One variant of the primitive defense of omnipotent control is for the patient to imagine that someone else can take care of him or her even though that person does not have the means to act effectively in any real way. If a patient who had been attending regularly begins to come late or to miss sessions, the therapist must first make it clear to the patient that those actions are a form of acting out that is disabling and could effectively end the therapy. The therapist can then go on to explore the meaning of the behavior.

Therapists in training often ask, "How many sessions can a patient miss before I end the treatment?" This way of phrasing the question suggests that two key concepts have not yet been appreciated. First, it is not the therapist who would be ending the treatment; it is the patient who, through his or her undermining actions, may make the treatment impossible and thereby end it. The therapist's responsibility is to point out that this is happening. Second, the idea that there is an absolute number of missed sessions that determines when the treatment is rendered ineffective suggests that the therapist is abdicating his or her clinical judgment in favor of an objective rule that applies to every patient in every therapy. Although such a rule might seem easier to the therapist, it is his or her responsibility to decide when missing sessions constitutes a pattern or trend that makes it pointless to continue. To choose a fixed number of missed sessions in advance may play into the patient's projection onto the therapist of a rigid and punitive person who imposes rules to which the patient must submit. This strategy may also lead to a "game of chicken" in which the patient gradually approaches the magic number of sessions, usually at a time of apparently compelling crisis, as though to dare the therapist to carry out his or her "threat" of ending the treatment.

Mental Availability in Sessions

A corollary of the requirement of attending sessions is the need for the patient to be psychologically available in them. If there is any indication that the patient may be under the influence of alcohol or drugs, the therapist should explain that this behavior would make any effective work impossible and would lead to the end of the particular session and, if it becomes a pattern, to the end of the therapy. In general, substance abuse issues are addressed in the contract setting phase. It may, however, occur that a substance abuse problem emerges in the course of treatment or that a patient does not adhere to the initial agreement and continues or returns to substance abuse. The role of the therapist in such an instance includes doing enough of an assessment to determine whether it is safe for the patient to return home or whether the patient requires hospitalization. The therapist should make it clear that when they next meet, they will explore the meaning of the patient's breach of the contract and review the parameters around substance abuse.

Contract Breaches

Many of the priorities discussed involve dealing with breaches of the universal conditions of treatment discussed in the contract. A patient can also present with breaches of any specific arrangement that has been made to address a specific problem.

CASE EXAMPLE

A patient's treatment contract included the specification that if she cut herself, she should be checked by her general practitioner to make sure that there is no need for sutures and no risk of infection before coming to the next session. At the beginning of a session, the patient mentioned that she had cut herself in a moment of anger and went on to talk about what had upset her. Her therapist interrupted to ask whether the patient had gone to her general practitioner to be checked. She had not. After establishing that no higher priority was present (e.g., suicidal threat, threat of dropping out), the therapist reminded the patient of their agreement about her cutting and told the patient that she could not continue the session as though the patient had complied with her part of the agreement. She told the patient that they could get back to the work of therapy after the patient had fulfilled her responsibility and that a first order of business would be to explore the meaning of what had happened both in terms of the patient having cut herself and in terms of her having breached their agreement. [It should be noted that not all therapists adopt this policy with regard to cutting. A specific therapist's policy is determined by his or her level of comfort—and ability to think clearly—in dealing with the issue. Some therapists are willing to discuss an episode of superficial cutting without the patient having seen the general practitioner.]

Intrusions Into the Therapist's Life

Intruding into a therapist's life is analogous to making physical threats to the therapist but differs insofar as the harm threatened is more psychological than physical and the actions involved may appear less aggressive on the surface. Intrusions may consist of calling the therapist repeatedly at home, looking up personal information on the Internet, spying on the therapist and his or her family, or appearing in public places to meet the therapist. The more aggressive forms of intrusion, such as spying, do not allow for as much flexibility as the structure around phone calls. Because spying, which often represents the behavioral manifestation of pervasive paranoid and hostile beliefs, is never justified and suggests a serious inability to contain transferential feelings within the frame of the therapy, the therapist should make a clear statement that any instance of it would call for an immediate review of the viability of the treatment.

Problems Created Outside Sessions That Impinge on the Therapy

Patients may threaten the viability of the therapy through indirect actions. Typical examples involve the patient's creating a situation in which he or she cannot pay the fee (e.g., quitting a job, discontinuing insurance, alienating parents who help fund the therapy) or one in which it is impossible for him or her to attend sessions at regular times (e.g., taking a job with an unpredictable schedule). The therapist must be alert to the implications of any actions the patient reports because the patient may bring in such news without making any connection to the implications with regard to therapy. Patients may also engage in behavior that induces strong negative reactions toward the treatment from third parties in the patient's life. For example, a patient may stimulate intense jealousy in a spouse, who then is manipulated to take action against the therapy.

Acting Out

The next priority for interpretive intervention, after life- or treatment-threatening behavior and dishonesty or other contract breaches, is that of acting out in general. Acting out is the expression of an unconscious conflict in action rather than in emotional experiencing, remembering, and verbal communication. Acting out may provide fundamental information about the patient's conflicts, but by the same token, it prevents insight or personality change by its defensive functions. Because it serves to reduce internal tension around conflict and therefore can be highly gratifying, acting out tends to perpetuate itself. Acting out should be systematically explored and, ideally, resolved by interpretation.

There are many types of acting out. Patients may act out between sessions or in sessions. Impulsive and self-destructive behaviors outside the sessions may include, in addition to self-harm, provoking aggression in others or hurling oneself impulsively into chaotic, ill-thought-out "love" affairs. Forms of in-session acting out include yelling, throwing something, coming late, or leaving early, instead of expressing oneself in words. Acting out can also take the form of very brief actions in the sessions, sometimes taking a minute or less, in which the patient does something that leaves the therapist off guard and feeling paralyzed. The patient may suddenly say something that apparently changes the entire situation—for example, "Oh, I forgot to tell you that I've been pregnant for 3 months"—and then proceed to talk about something else. This represents two forms of acting out: concealing something that has been going on for a long time outside the sessions and making a sudden statement that has a powerful effect on the session.

Interpretations must sometimes focus on how the concerns of external reality are being ignored in the service of satisfaction in the patient's internal world. The therapist might say, for example, "We've got to the idea that your sitting in silence may provide the experience of your being stronger than I am and being in control. The question is the price you pay in the real world for that inner sense of satisfaction. Because your speaking in session would help us advance our work, the sense of power may be at the expense of moving ahead."

In contrast to the ordinary types of acting out, which are relatively easy to diagnose and treat, there are more subtle forms. One type is usually expressed outside the sessions and is reflected in split-off, long-term behavior patterns that often predate the beginning of treatment; this form is seen in "living-out" rather than acting-out patterns, such as chronic morbid obesity. The therapist has to remain alert to what is going on in the patient's external life to diagnose these forms of acting out, which is sometimes difficult because they can occur subtly and may gradually increase over time.

CASE EXAMPLE

A patient in his third year of treatment announced abruptly that he could no longer see his therapist because he had lost his scholarship because of failing grades, a fact that made it impossible for him to pay for therapy. Only then did the therapist realize that for the past several months this patient had from time to time reported that he had failed to turn in assignments on time or do the required reading. As is frequently the case with such patients, he had consistently attributed (or explained away) these activities to some other force, such as a noisy roommate or an overly demanding professor. Only in retrospect did the therapist recognize that the patient's lifelong pattern of acting in passive destructive ways was reappearing in this form of threatening the treatment.

Trivial Themes

One of the most subtle challenges for the beginning TFP therapist is to determine when the material the patient is presenting amounts to trivialization and avoidance of important material. The emergence of this challenge generally takes place during the transition from the early phase to the midphase of therapy. As the patient's level of acting out diminishes and the patient's dynamics become concentrated in the frame of the treatment, he or she may begin to avoid the most affectively charged and conflictual areas of his or her pathology by falling into a general state of trivialization in the therapy. It may take a while for the therapist to become aware of this issue because the patient may at first seem to be adhering to the basic rule of free association. However, there are certain behavioral correlates to trivialization. One possibility is that the patient may appear to be working adequately in sessions (with the therapist often in a corresponding "lulled" state) but may report intense, unexplained moments of severe anxiety or dysphoria between sessions that communicate a distress not seen in the sessions.

Trivialization may also be present if a sense develops that the patient is settling into a relationship with the therapist that becomes so gratifying in itself that it begins to replace outside reality in the patient's life—a so-called "transference cure." This can appear as a flight into health where the patient seems better but, aside from a decrease in the level of acting out, there is no change in his or her life outside the sessions—no resolution of problems in interpersonal relations, level of functioning, or identity diffusion. In this state, the therapy may be principally a source of gratification, and the therapist may be experienced as an interested companion. The content of the sessions might consist of reports on the patient's daily life at the surface level, with no evidence of self-reflectiveness or ongoing consciousness of the severity of the problems that brought the patient into treatment. The therapist can be lulled into a state of forgetting the severity of the patient's problems, and effort might be necessary for the therapist to remind himself or herself of the unsatisfactory state of the patient's work, social, and love life. Therapy can become a refuge from challenges to self-esteem experienced in the outside world. The therapist's task of deciding when material represents trivialization does not counter the principle of free association but rather complements it with adequate appreciation of the power of resistance. In other words, the relevance of the patient's associations may be in demonstrating resistance to deep exploration. If that is the case, the therapist should point out the retreat into *relatively* inessential material—especially because patient histories reveal cases in which years were lost attending to trivial material in therapy while the patient's life continued to deteriorate.

TACTIC 4: EXPLORING INCOMPATIBLE VIEWS

The general approach in TFP is to have the patient elaborate his or her view of the world and, in particular, of the therapist and the patient-therapist interaction. One reason for the focus on the interaction is that it is the only setting in which the therapist can accurately assess discrepancies between the patient's *description* of his or her experience and *the experience itself.* For example, if a patient repeatedly describes his wife's callous mistreatment of him, the therapist does not usually have enough data to know if the description is accurate or includes some distortion. However, if the patient harshly criticizes the therapist for callous treatment when the latter has merely been adhering to her role, the therapist has a clearer view of the patient's tendency to perceive external real objects through the distorting lens of an internal object representation. Therefore, TFP therapists must be careful to resist the very human temptation to immediately correct a distorted image of themselves because it is precisely the exploration of this distorted image that brings essential data to the therapy.

This tactic of exploring incompatible views requires a sense of balance on the part of the therapist. On the one hand, the therapy advances by observing the patient's distortions. On the other hand, there can be no interpretation of unconscious material unless the patient agrees with the therapist on what, ultimately, the "reality" of the situation is. The only distortions of reality that can be interpreted are those that become recognized as such and become ego-dystonic. Therefore, the goal is to elaborate the patient's subjective experience or belief and then to establish whether the patient is—or can be made to be—aware of the degree to which his or her belief deviates from a commonly shared reality. This balance between elaborating and questioning the distortions on the basis of the patient's internal object world follows, to some degree, John Steiner's (1993) recommendation that in the early stages of therapy the therapist should examine the patient's image of the therapist without rejecting it and without accepting it. The internal object representation being projected onto the therapist is at first explored *without* any attempt to link it back to the patient's mind. The therapeutic expectation is that the patient's gradual exposure to and tolerance of that projected representation as it is experienced "in the room" will eventually facilitate the patient's acknowledgment of the role of that representation in his or her internal world. The therapist's consistent stance of commitment to the treatment and interest in the patient are part of what leads to the patient's questioning the image that he or she projects on the therapist. However, when the patient's distorted views threaten the advancement or the continuation of the therapy, the therapist may have to take a more active role in challenging the distortion and trying to establish common elements of shared reality (see "Case Example of Exploring Incompatible Realities" below).

Clarification, confrontation, and interpretation are the investigative tools by which the therapist assesses the patient's capacity to test reality. The process may go in several steps, as the following example illustrates.

A patient expresses the belief that her doctor is interested in having sex with her. The therapist must first clarify whether the patient is expressing an emotional experience, an intellectual speculation, a fantasy, or a delusional conviction: "Is this an idea that you have about what I might be thinking, or do you see me as actively interested in having sex with you now?" Assuming the patient indicates the latter, the therapist's next intervention is to clarify the basis for the patient's thinking: "What is there about me— either my words or action—that leads to your idea that I want to have sex with you?" The next task is to ask her to reflect on this belief in the context of the full treatment experience to date: "Is there anything in our meetings thus far that suggests to you that this might *not* be the case?"

Then the therapist should attempt to assess the degree of conviction with which the patient holds this view. It is important to remember that the amount of credibility a patient assigns to any distorted belief can vary. For example, the therapist might say, "Are you saying there's nothing I can say or do to convince you that I'm not interested in having sex with you?"

As a next step the therapist generally will interpret the defensive aspect to see if reality testing will improve: "Could it be that you hold this view of me because it expresses your deeply held belief that men are untrustworthy and interested only in taking advantage of you? Any opposite view of men that opens other alternatives would threaten your present avoidance of any intimacy with men and confront you with your self-imposed renunciation of intimacy." This interpretation is made despite there being no apparent evidence that the patient's view is ego-dystonic; the interpretation constitutes a further effort at creating a reflective space in which the patient's perception might become ego-dystonic, even though prior efforts appear to have failed.

If all the approaches described above have failed, then the therapist should still pursue efforts to find the point at which the patient's belief is ego-dystonic. To do this, it is important for the therapist to keep the inquiry internally consistent with the patient's conviction. By becoming even more logical about the patient's belief system than the patient is, the therapist may force identification of the point at which that belief system is no longer tenable for the patient. Thus, in this example, the therapist, staying within the logic of the patient's belief, might say, "Do you believe I would jeopardize my professional reputation to have sex with you?" or "If you believe this 100%, why are you staying here?" Thus, the therapist proceeds from surface to depth, first testing the limits of the patient's understanding of reality and then interpreting the inferred defense against perceiving reality accurately.

After the therapist has carried out all these steps, if it becomes evident that the patient has a delusional conviction (i.e., a false conviction that is highly idiosyncratic and motivated and that does not respond to ordinary ways of reasoning), the technique of dealing with psychotic regression in the transference should be employed.

CASE EXAMPLE

A therapist began a session 5 minutes after the scheduled time, and the patient's first words were, "It's more and more clear that you don't like me and don't want to see me. Every day there's another sign of it. Your keeping me waiting like that just shows that you wish I would go away, and I almost did. If you had kept me waiting one more minute, I would have been out of here and you wouldn't have seen me again." Many therapists would be tempted to respond with a combination of defensiveness and reassurance, intending to be supportive of the patient's efforts to change but without getting to the root of the problem. Such a therapist might say: "Let's look at your reaction here. You tend to be so rigid and demanding of yourself and others that there's no room for leeway. A 5-minute delay is not really that unusual."

A TFP therapist would rather respond in the following way: "Tell me more about how you see me right now. My opening the door 5 minutes late was evidence to you that I don't like you. Can you elaborate on how you think I feel about you and what you think the reasons for my not liking you are?" The therapist might later intervene with a comment such as, "If you are convinced that I don't like you, what is your understanding of why I am seeing you?" In many cases, the patient can achieve some insight on her own as she pursues this elaboration. She may see that her description of the therapist's attitude toward her is so extreme that it begins to "fall from its own weight" as an unrealistic caricature. The patient may see contradictions in her own reporting; she may realize that her extreme negative description of the therapist does not fit with other data available, such as the therapist at times going out of his way to reschedule sessions. This type of ability to bring together positive and negative associations represents the beginning of integration.

Nevertheless, there are also times when a patient is firmly entrenched in his or her projection and does not achieve any insight on his or her own. At these times, the therapist must take a more active role. In extreme cases, the patient's perception includes distorting objective facts. The patient from the preceding example might say, "You kept me waiting for half the session—you might as well just tell me not to come." A first order of business in a situation like this is to see to what degree the patient and therapist share a common view of the facts before exploring the meaning these facts have to the patient. The therapist might say, "When you said I kept you waiting half the session time, did you mean that literally, or was that a figure of speech?" If the patient acknowledges some exaggeration, the therapist can go on to explore the patient's view of him and the meaning of the 5-minute delay.

CASE EXAMPLE OF EXPLORING INCOMPATIBLE REALITIES

If the patient who has been kept waiting for 5 minutes says, "You kept me waiting 20 minutes, and if you don't admit it, you're a liar and I'm leaving here right now," the therapist must confront the patient with their discrepant views of reality before proceeding. For example, he might say the following:

> **Therapist:** You're saying I opened the door 20 minutes late; I'm saying I opened the door 5 minutes late. We can't both be right. We have to look at the different possibilities here. Both of us can't be right. One of us is wrong and is incapable of reconsidering his or her position. It's as if a normal person and a person not in touch with reality were in the room, and we can't decide who is who. Therefore, I suggest we agree there's an element of madness in the room and we try to figure out where this madness is coming from. The only other alternative is that one of us is lying. If you think I'm lying, please tell me so we can explore what that would mean

This method of exploring incompatible realities follows the general TFP principle of exploring the transference. The essential issue is that for the moment the therapist and patient have no common base in reality. The priority issue is then to clarify the nature of the fantasy involved in the madness. How does the patient understand the incompatible realities? Is the therapist malicious, ignorant, or crazy? Is he so inattentive or indifferent as to be unable to keep track of the time? Does he devalue the patient to the point that he would lie to her? If the patient thinks the therapist is lying, why is the therapist lying? Why does the patient come to see a therapist she believes is capable of lying?

Exploring the incompatible realities generally leads to uncovering a part of the patient's internal world being projected onto the therapist. In the case under discussion, the patient was attributing to this therapist an internal object that was highly critical and was responsible for the patient often experiencing herself as "disgusting." Her perception of herself as disgusting diminished to some degree when she was focusing on the idea that someone was rejecting her. This did not free her from the problem, but putting the source of disgust in the therapist allowed her to distance herself from it and to direct her angry disapproval toward him for being judgmental rather than direct it toward herself.

In extreme cases, a patient may firmly hold on to a view that represents a temporary loss of reality testing. In such a case the therapist must make the diagnostic distinction between an acute episode of psychosis, which can sometimes occur in the course of treatment with a borderline patient, and a transference psychosis in which the loss of reality testing occurs only in relation to the therapist and does not affect the patient's life outside the therapy.

A final comment on the balance between elaborating the distorted view and establishing common elements of reality is that in most cases the perceptions of borderline patients are based on an element of external reality—a *trigger event.* This makes it especially important for the therapist to maintain a sense of proportion and to periodically ask himself or herself a very important question: "How does the patient's reaction compare to what an expectable reaction within the normal range of thinking and behavior would be?" This question is based on a practical, operational definition of transference—that transference is any reaction of the patient to the therapist that is beyond what a normal expectable reaction might be. For example, in the case of the therapist starting the session 5 minutes late, it is true that the therapist kept the patient waiting, but it is also true that a normal expectable response would be for a person to understand that such things happen occasionally without seeing it as proof of the therapist's rejection. However, a therapist might think, "Keeping the patient waiting was very insensitive, perhaps even cruel. I should have thought about her fragility." This line of thinking confuses the patient's internal reality with external reality, suggesting a countertransference reaction that the therapist needs to reflect on. The therapist's shift to seeing himself or herself as cruel suggests that he or she has accepted the projection of an internal object: it is an example of projective identification.

The question of what part of the therapist's experience represents entering into the patient's internal world versus staying grounded in external reality is always relevant because—to stay with the affect in question in the case of the session starting 5 minutes late—therapists can in fact be insensitive or cruel, and it can require reflection to decide what is real and what is coming from the patient. In such a situation, the therapist finds his bearings in the treatment frame: the frame established by the contract sets up the *reality* of the therapeutic relationship. For example, in a session in which a patient accuses the therapist of being cruel because he will not extend the session on a day she arrived late, the therapist needs to remind himself that he is acting in accordance with the mutual initial agreement regarding session times. This helps him situate the "cruel egoist" as a persona in the patient's internal world rather than as something he has become in that moment.

Therapists' concern about patients' seeming fragility reflects concern about challenging a patient's defense system. Patients find a certain internal stability in projecting the cruel object onto others, albeit at the expense of peaceful interpersonal relations. The therapist may be concerned about the distress the patient might experience if the therapist questions the patient's projection. Therapists must remember that they need to choose either to proceed in this way, with the hope of deep change, or to offer a more "supportive" therapy that respects the patient's defensive system, leading to less distress in the moment but also less chance of deep change.

To summarize, in all interactions in therapy, it is important that the therapist remember to compare the patient's reaction to what a normal expectable reaction would be, because the power of patients' intense affects can sometimes convince others that their reading of the grain of truth is an accurate one and has nothing to do with an aspect of their inner world that needs to be analyzed. This power of conviction of the patient's way of perceiving things can be as significant in situations of idealized positive transference as it is at times of negative transference. For example, a patient might say, "It's not my imagination. I know it…you are in love with me. You wouldn't have looked at me that way if you weren't…that and the fact that I saw you smile when I said I was thinking of leaving my husband. And when you agreed that I have made progress here, I think that's your way of telling me that we can end this whole business soon, and then we'll be free to do what we both want." A seasoned therapist will not feel guilty or apologetic with regard to the fact that he had a friendly expression on his face. He will enter into exploration of the object representations activated in the patient's internal world—as simultaneously powerful and delicate as they may be—with the confidence that the frame of treatments allows for the tactful joint observation of even the most intense affects.

The need to distinguish between the patient's internal world and the external reality is an ongoing challenge. A patient stormed out of a session saying, "You're cruel. You should have told me there was going to be construction work outside your office today—you know how sensitive I am to noise." The therapist was left feeling he was indeed cruel until he reminded himself that he had had no advance notice that the work would be taking place.

Difficulty in distinguishing between internal and external reality, and some patients' ability to convince others that their internal reality *is* the objective reality, can lead to severe practical problems in the treatment of borderline patients, including charges of mistreatment or inappropriate behavior on the part of the therapist.

TACTIC 5: REGULATING THE INTENSITY OF AFFECTIVE INVOLVEMENT

It is important for the therapist to observe the patient's affect intensity and to respond appropriately in making interventions. Patients with borderline personality organization (BPO) may become absorbed in their own affect and may not attend to or hear a therapist who is extremely calm and relatively quiet during an affect storm, an intense outburst by the patient (for a clinical example, see Video 3, "Affect Storm"). In fact, a patient might experience a therapist's calm, quiet tone as dismissive. A therapist's cool, unemotional response may leave the patient feeling as if he or she is not heard or understood. The therapist may need to use a firm tone to get the attention of the patient and to emphasize a point of view different from that of the patient.

▶ Video 3–1: Affect Storm Part 1 (9:28)

▶ Video 3–2: Affect Storm Part 2 (9:26)

▶ Video 3–3: Affect Storm Part 3 (10:10)

When the patient manifests little affect concerning life-threatening or treatment-threatening behaviors (e.g., blandly smiling while telling of cutting self), the therapist should include affect, reflecting concern, in his or her discussion and interpretation of the behavior that is affectively cut off. The therapist's matching the patient's affect intensity or complementing the patient's lack of affective intensity is not a violation of technical neutrality.

THERAPIST FLEXIBILITY IN USING THE TACTICS

Although transference themes are the focus of this therapy, they are not always the highest priority. There are times when intense affect-laden experiences take place outside the direct transferential field. Under these circumstances, the therapist should be able and willing to focus on such other affect-laden material.

COMMON TREATMENT CHALLENGES

Treatment challenges occur when the acting out of an underlying conflict threatens to overwhelm the treatment and derail or end the therapeutic process. Although these moments in treatment have the potential of rendering the therapist so anxious that it is difficult to pursue exploratory therapy, they also offer important opportunities to advance the work of therapy. In managing challenges the therapist may, on a practical level, become more proactive in the sense of calling the patient at home or communicating with a family member and, on a technical level, increase the speed of interpretations or make deeper interpretations. Dealing with crises may involve reinforcing adherence to the treatment frame or may involve temporarily deviating from technical neutrality.

In the early phase of therapy, the patient's participation—that is, discussion of problem areas (interpersonal conflict, self-destructive behavior, depression, etc.)—generally consists mostly of thoughts of which the patient is already aware. The character pathology—in particular, the internal splitting—so fundamentally underlies and determines the patient's experience in the world that he or she is not aware of it; the structure of the pathology is the structure of the patient's subjective reality. This deeper level of disturbance—the disorder of psychic structure—is initially most evident in the patient's actions, creating the need to pay special attention to actions and the therapeutic interaction. When the patient's actions threaten to derail or end the treatment, the opportunity for deeper understanding goes hand in hand with the threat because it is a sign that intense affects have been activated in the treatment, usually at a time when the patient's internal splitting is less effective in keeping a disturbing self or other representation from consciousness. To a large extent, it is in dealing with treatment crises that the patient's inner world becomes available for observation and exploration.

Crises, especially in the early phase of treatment, may include a component of challenging the treatment frame to see whether the therapist will adhere to or abandon the parameters set up in the treatment contract. Adherence to the parameters by the therapist is generally reassuring to patients who at some level are aware of a need for containment. Crises may also occur after the patient has settled into the treatment frame. Crises may correspond to moments when therapy has disrupted the precarious balance of primitive defense mechanisms or when the chaos of the patient's life has calmed down enough for the patient to consciously experience the identity diffusion that leaves him or her feeling empty and lost in the world. The patient may feel less anxious in a storm of crises than in the awareness that he or she has no clear sense of self or direction in life.

Crises often represent enactments of feelings aroused in the transference, so a first question for a therapist to consider when a crisis develops is the following: "What is going on right now in the patient's experience of me and the therapy that would lead to a threat to drop out (noncompliance with contract, psychotic regression, etc.)?" It may be that in order for the patient to avoid a painful self-awareness, the projection of an undesired internal representation becomes so intense that the patient's experience of the therapist is overwhelmed by the projected negative affect.

Because these challenges in treatment tend to elicit strong reactions in the therapist (e.g., anxiety, frustration, despair, hatred), the exploration of these episodes requires careful management lest the therapist get drawn into a pathological mutual enactment with the patient, leading to abandonment of the exploratory effort or the therapy altogether. The therapist's acting out in the countertransference generally takes one of two forms. The first is that of a superficially supportive response to a patient's demands that—although it may appear to save the therapy—aborts the opportunity to understand in depth the object relations dyad being enacted. The second consists of a superficially neutral (structured) but essentially rigid and rejecting response to the patient that is not receptive to the patient's affect and is, unconsciously on the part of the therapist, geared to precipitate the end of the therapy. Exploratory therapy requires maintaining the effort to understand the dynamic meaning of the challenge to the frame rather than letting the crisis overwhelm the frame and distort the treatment.

It is not surprising that the most common crises in treatment (Table 7–4) parallel to a large extent the hierarchy of thematic priorities that we discussed earlier in the section on tactic 3, because treatment crises take priority over other material. It is also not surprising that the most common crises are areas that may have been discussed in establishing the treatment contract because the contract is meant to predict the ways in which characteristics of an individual patient may later pose a threat to the treatment and to establish contingencies to deal with these potential threats. In fact, if the potential for a specific threat to the treatment has been discussed in the contract setting, the first step in addressing a crisis is to bring up the question of why, at this point,

TABLE 7–4.   Examples of common treatment complications
Suicidal and self-destructive behavior
Threatened aggression and intrusions into privacy
Threats of discontinuing treatment
Noncompliance with adjunctive treatments
Issues related to a history of sexual abuse
Psychotic episodes
Dissociative reactions
Depressive episodes
Emergency room visits
Hospitalization
Patient telephone calls
Therapist's absence and coverage management
Patient's silence
Somatization

the patient is creating a situation that was predicted in the contract—in other words, what is the meaning of the deviation from the contract?

MANAGING SUICIDE THREATS AND ATTEMPTS DURING TREATMENT

The threat of self-destructive and suicidal behavior is the most powerful issue in the treatment of borderline patients and is the topic that most often leads therapists to deviate from their role in exploratory psychotherapy. Despite the multiplicity of meanings that suicidal ideation may represent, a few general statements may be made. If the material comes up shortly after the beginning of treatment, it is often a test on the part of the patient to see if the therapist will adhere to the role he or she defined for himself or herself in the contract. Many patients, even if they intellectually grasp and embrace the idea of exploratory work, function on the basis of intense primary longings for—alternating with fear of or rage against—closeness, merging, and caretaking. In light of this, patients may act in a way that deviates from their stated commitment to the exploratory process in an effort to see whether the therapist will deviate from his or her defined role to assume an overt caretaking role vis-à-vis the patient.

Suicidal ideation may also represent an expression of rage, an attempt to control, a means of torture, or a sign of distress. Because suicidal ideation is so full of meaning, discussion about it is an important part of the exploratory process. When the patient makes any mention of suicide, the therapist's first priority is to establish whether the suicidal ideation is in the context of a major depressive episode, which would call for other interventions, such as medication or hospitalization. Once it has been established that no major depressive episode is present, it is important to deal with suicide as both an intrapsychic issue and an interpersonal one and to try to understand the roles of aggressor and victim in the suicide scenario. The therapist should keep in mind the following questions: "Who, in the patient's internal world or external reality, is the target of aggression?" and "What function, at this point in time and in this interpersonal context, does the emergence of suicidal ideation serve?" Finally, although we know that suicidality is a multifaceted phenomenon, in some instances it plays a particular role in interpersonal interactions—a trump card.

The unpredictability of borderline patients' behavior often means that the threat of suicide can come and go unexpectedly. Especially when chronic threats of suicide have become incorporated into the patient's way of life, the therapist should make it clear before beginning the therapy—to the patient and, if indicated, to the family—that the patient is chronically at risk of suicide, indicating that the patient has a serious psychiatric illness with a risk of mortality. The therapist should express to those concerned the willingness to engage in a therapeutic effort to help the patient overcome the illness but should not guarantee protection from suicide. Realistically discussing the limits of the treatment may be the most effective way to protect the therapeutic relationship from the possibility that the patient may try to control the therapy by inducing in the therapist a countertransference characterized by guilt feelings and/or paranoid fears regarding third parties.

It is important for patients to learn that their threat of suicide has no inordinate power over the therapist (i.e., it is important to eliminate the secondary gain). The therapist should make it clear that although he or she would feel sad if the patient died, the therapist would not feel responsible and his or her life would not be significantly altered by such an event. The therapist's acceptance of the possibility of a negative outcome with a patient is a crucial element in the treatment of patients with severe suicide potential. The patient's unconscious or conscious fantasy that the therapist could not tolerate the patient's death, and that the patient therefore has power over the therapist—or that the therapist has the magical power to save the patient—needs to be explored and resolved.

Every attempted or completed suicide involves the activation of intense aggression not only within the patient but also within the immediate interpersonal field. The therapist who seems to react only with sorrow and concern for the suicidal patient is denying his or her counteraggression and other possible reactions. Openness to countertransference feelings will enable the therapist to empathize with the patient's suicide temptations, with the despair, with the longing for peace, with the excitement of self-directed aggression, with the pleasure in taking revenge against significant others, with the wish to escape from guilt, and with the exhilarating sense of power involved in suicidal urges. Only that kind of empathy on the part of the therapist may permit the patient to explore these issues openly in the treatment.

Guidelines for Decision Making Regarding Issues of Suicide

Because patients often do not completely abide by the conditions of the contract, the therapist may find himself or herself confronted with a patient who is threatening suicidal action or has already made an attempt. Broad guidelines can be offered for the decision-making process in the evaluation and management of suicide threats and suicidal behavior. The first task is to make clear whether the patient's suicidal ideation is either a manifestation of a major depressive episode with the concomitant hopelessness and giving up on life or the anxious urge to die of agitated depression. If a major depressive episode is present, the therapist must assess the severity of the depression. The severity can be gauged by the degree to which behavior and ideation are slowed down (and concentration thus affected) and sadness is replaced by an empty, frozen mood with a subjective sense of depersonalization. In addition, the presence or absence of biological symptoms of depression (reflected in eating and sleeping patterns, weight, digestive functions, daily rhythm of depressive affect, menstrual patterns, sexual desire, and muscle tone) supplies crucial information regarding the severity of the depression. In general, the more severe the clinical depression accompanying suicidal ideation and intention, the more acute the danger is. Medication and/or hospitalization may be indicated. Patients in states of severe depression vary in their ability to control the urge to act on the suicidal impulse. The therapist's judgment on this question is based on the quality of the relationship with the patient and on whether impulsive, antisocial, dishonest, paranoid, schizoid-aloof, or psychotic aspects make the patient's verbal commitments unreliable. In addition, the patient's alcohol and drug history will be highly relevant in judging whether commitments can be relied on. Patients who lose a sense of rapport with the therapist, become too depressed to communicate, or begin to make preparations for suicide must be protected. In cases of major depression, the therapist should take a proactive stance that is different from the stance with characterological suicidality. The therapist might recommend that the patient be hospitalized or that the family be engaged in monitoring the patient's condition. A patient may feel relieved by the therapist's alertness to the cues—which may increase the patient's ability to experience the therapist as helpful rather than as punitive or adversarial—and hence this may lead to the patient's becoming less endangered by suicidal impulses.

If the suicidal ideation is *not* a function of an episode of a major affective disorder, the therapist's next task is to establish the presence or absence of suicidal *intent*. If the ideation appears to be linked to intent, the therapist reminds the patient of his or her responsibility to engage emergency help as needed (by calling 911, mobilizing family members, going to an emergency room [ER], etc.). If the ideation does not include current intent, the therapist pursues exploration of the material. This exploration includes listening to the patient's associations to the suicidal material and reflecting in particular on what is going on at this precise moment in the transference that would help understand the emergence of suicidal thoughts and how they make sense at this time: what they might be indirectly communicating or what they might be defending against. Exploration frequently reveals that suicidal gestures are attempts to establish or reestablish control over the environment by evoking anxiety and guilt feelings in others. As treatment evolves, the therapist is likely to become involved in these dynamics. Therefore, talk or threats of suicide in the absence of clinical depression often call attention to transferential issues. Active measures to increase the structure of the treatment help the therapist feel more comfortable and hence more capable of managing the powerful feelings evoked by suicidal patients. The therapist who allows himself or herself to be pressed beyond reasonable limits (such as when an idealizing patient evokes an omnipotent countertransference reaction) often eventually withdraws emotionally in self-defense (e.g., by beginning to think about transferring the case), an action that is far more damaging to the treatment than the firm setting of a structure before the therapist's resources have become exhausted.

As discussed in Chapter 5, patients who feel they cannot control a suicidal urge have the responsibility of going to an ER. If the ER physician recommends hospitalization and the patient is not willing to follow that recommendation, the therapist should make it clear to the patient and the family that he or she cannot take further responsibility for the patient because doing so would mean accepting the patient back to a level of treatment not deemed adequate to his or her current condition. This fact should also be made clear to the ER physician so that the patient will not be left without treatment but will either be hospitalized involuntarily (if deemed necessary) or be referred to an appropriate clinic or therapist. It may seem illogical to refer the patient to a therapist after he or she has just refused to work within the parameters of the therapy. However, for many patients the experience of a therapist who holds to the parameters of treatment, even in the face of ending the treatment, is a powerful confrontation of the patient's omnipotent control. This action by the therapist might be the first time someone has not given in to the patient, and it may alert the patient to the fact that a therapist may mean what he or she says in a way that can be reassuring at a deep level. After this experience, the patient may be more ready to seriously engage in therapy and work within its parameters.

THREATS TO OTHERS

Patients' threats to other people occur less frequently. Such threats may be directed to the therapist or people outside the therapy, leaving the therapist to decide whether to notify a third party of a risk. If the issue of potential threat comes up in the evaluation and contract setting phase, the therapist first explains the legal obligation to inform an outside party whom he or she judges may be at risk. The therapist then discusses with the patient how such an eventuality would damage the therapy as well as the rest of the patient's life: it would take attention away from the therapist and patient's mutual endeavor of understanding. If the therapist's safety is in question, it is evident that the therapist cannot maintain a neutral, observing stance. Threats could include threats to body, reputation, family, or property and may also include threats communicated by or involving others. The therapist's stated concern for himself or herself may provide useful role modeling for patients who often have problems with self-esteem and for whom an identification with the therapist may be part of the therapeutic process. It is important to distinguish between a patient who may be elaborating a fantasy about the therapist—a perfectly valid use of therapy—and one who is expressing direct homicidal ideation.

THREATENED AGGRESSION AND INTRUSIONS

Although borderline patients direct overt aggression more often toward themselves than toward others, therapists may be the target either of more or less veiled threats of aggression from midrange borderline patients or of direct threats of aggression from patients in the malignant narcissistic to antisocial range. To begin with, patients are aware to varying degrees that aggression toward themselves is also aggression toward the therapist. This is because of the therapist's human concern for the patient, because of the therapist's investment in the outcome of his or her work, and because of the specter of malpractice litigation. We discussed earlier in this section the management of treatment crises involving threats to the self. We add some thoughts concerning the implicit threat to the therapist implied in these threats to the self.

When beginning to treat a patient with a history of serious self-destructive behavior, the therapist should directly address the fact that the patient might harm or kill himself or herself in a way that would also attack the therapist. The therapist must make it clear that he or she takes this potential very seriously and is proposing a treatment to help the patient move beyond this position in life but also that although the therapist would regret it if the patient did harm or kill herself, the therapist's life would go on as it had before. If a therapist feels that he or she could not cope with the eventuality of a patient's death, it is essential to work through that either in supervision or in the therapist's own therapy or analysis. If the therapist continues to feel that he or she could not accept the possibility of the patient's death, he or she should not treat severely ill borderline patients. If a therapist who could not accept this possibility begins to treat such a patient, the patient may sense the therapist's fear and is in a position to control the treatment (in ways that defend against integration of the split-off aggressive part) and also to act out or indulge his or her aggression by torturing the therapist with concerns about suicide. It is important to emphasize that accepting the possibility that the patient could commit suicide allows the therapist to work more effectively and therefore makes this possibility less likely.

One way a therapist might decrease his or her anxiety about the possible death of the patient in cases of life-threatening pathology is to arrange a meeting with the patient and his or her family as part of the contracting phase. The family meeting is an extension of the contract setting process and addresses the family's understanding of and expectations from the therapy and the therapist. The meeting would include the patient's parents if he or she is young or continues to be dependent on them (e.g., financially or as a major emotional connection) or a spouse or partner if indicated. Family members sometimes assume that the patient's being in therapy guarantees that he or she will be automatically "cured," or at least will be out of risk. This idealization of treatment can represent a denial of the seriousness of the patient's pathology and can quickly change to an angry attack on the therapist if the magical expectations are not met. It is important that the therapist explain to the family that the pathology is very serious and that although therapy offers the possibility of real change, there is no guarantee of a good outcome or of completely eliminating the possibility of suicide. If family members can accept this reality, the therapist will be less at risk of attack through the patient's self-destructiveness, and the patient will be safer because a possible motivation for suicide will have been defused. If the family cannot accept this position, it is better that they seek treatment from someone who feels he or she can give them the assurance they seek.

Another way of attacking the therapist is to besmirch his or her reputation in the community. A therapist who becomes aware of such behavior must address the motivation leading to the behavior, which is usually a manifestation of the patient's envy. A clinical illustration of this is provided in the case history in Kernberg's (1984) work. Because this behavior does not usually go so far as to threaten the therapist's well-being, it is normally dealt with in the context of the treatment without having to consider ending the treatment. It is also possible that a patient may create situations in which the therapist's well-being is put at risk through indirect means. Patients have been known to create such a negative reaction to the therapist in a significant other (e.g., boyfriend) that the other person becomes threatening to the therapist. The therapist must make it clear that he or she cannot work with the patient under such circumstances and that the threats must cease for the therapy to continue.

THREATS OF DISCONTINUING TREATMENT

The rate of premature treatment termination has traditionally been very high in the borderline population (Yeomans et al. 1994). Increased use of treatments designed specifically for patients with BPD has helped decrease the dropout rate, but treatment discontinuation continues to be an issue for many reasons, including resistance to exploration. The phenomenon is most common in the early phase of treatment, but threats of dropping out may also occur in the midphase. Dropout talk and behavior can create a crisis for the TFP therapist, who may wonder if a more immediately gratifying treatment would keep the patient in therapy. Although different factors may contribute to the patient's threat to drop out (Table 7–5)—and those factors must be explored to the fullest extent possible—this discussion focuses on the management of this type of crisis.

The threat of dropping out calls for a level of therapist activity that is surprising to many analytically trained therapists, who might, for instance, deal with a patient's missing a session by waiting to see if the patient comes to the next session. The TFP therapist takes a more active role—in terms of both practical interventions and the timing and depth of interpretations—when the treatment is at risk. At times the therapist must function as the observing ego because the patient may completely lose this capacity for periods of time. This situation requires the therapist to temporarily abandon the position of neutrality. When the therapist takes a more active role, his or her actions may provide a confrontation in action to a patient's conviction, by projection, that the therapist is, at best, indifferent and callous or, at worst, exploitative or malevolent.

CASE EXAMPLE

A patient began therapy with a strong paranoid transference that her therapist had no genuine concern for her and was interested in her only to the

TABLE 7–5.	Factors that may contribute to the patient's urge to drop out of treatment

Negative transference

> The patient "deposits" hated internal representations into the therapist and then attempts to separate from them by leaving.

> The patient threatens to leave therapy as a protest against the therapist, who, by not providing the ideal care the patient desires, is perceived as uncaring or even persecutory.

Narcissistic issues

> The patient experiences feelings of competitiveness and envy in relation to the therapist, feels humiliated in relation to someone he or she experiences as superior because of the therapist's capacity to help the patient, and thus flees therapy both to get away from these feelings and to "defeat" the therapist.

> The patient experiences jealousy with regard to the therapist's other patients and other interests.

Attachment and dependency issues

> The patient becomes anxious because of attachment feelings that develop in the positive transference (which may be hidden from view) and leaves therapy to avoid the anxiety associated with dependency.

Fear of hurting the therapist/wish to protect the therapist

> The patient feels that his or her intense (aggressive and/or affectionate) affects are too much for the therapist, or anyone, to bear and decides to leave before this becomes apparent. The patient may also experience a milder form of this guilt or shame over sadistic or libidinal feelings.

The patient feels pressure from his or her family to quit treatment when change in the patient is perceived as threatening the equilibrium of the family system.

---

degree that he could exploit her for his personal gain. At the beginning of the next calendar year, the therapist increased his fee by $10. He announced this increase to the patient, adding, as he did for all his patients, that this increase would not apply if the patient felt she could not afford it. The patient became enraged and proclaimed, with a note of victory in her rage, that this was proof of her conviction that his only interest in her was to exploit her. She brushed off as meaningless the reminder that the increase was dependent on her ability to pay.

The therapist attempted to discuss the patient's reaction in terms of their ongoing effort to explore her suspiciousness of others. The patient angrily shouted that he should have made an exception in her case if he cared about her at all because he could have predicted her reaction. The therapist took issue with this point of view and explained that it was precisely because he did care that he did not make an exception. To make an exception for her would be to bend to her pathology, and whereas he could do that in therapy, it was not realistic to expect that the world as a whole would treat her differently from others because of her deeply rooted suspicions. He saw his job as an effort to help her function better and find more satisfaction in her life, and he did not know how he could do this if he colluded with her to avoid addressing her pathology rather than confronting it.

The patient stated that the therapist had made an irremediable error that made it impossible for them to work together and then stormed out of the room 5 minutes before the session was over. The next day she left a vitriolic phone message stating that if he had not already understood, she was ending the therapy and would never return. The therapist called the patient at home. She said she was surprised to hear from him. He explained that he was calling because he believed the situation was very serious. He further explained that although only she could decide what to do, his opinion was that it would be a tragic error to quit treatment right now because she was in the thick of one of her most serious issues—the belief that the world offered only exploitation. This issue was right in front of them now, and the options were either to go on leaving this conviction unquestioned or to try to work on it. The patient responded with pained confusion. She believed that he was "like everyone else," but she could not understand why he was calling and seemed concerned about her. She agreed to come to the next session. In that session the patient stated she would never have come back to treatment if he had not called—that his call caused her to question her conviction. In more technical terms, his call provided an element of external reality that confronted her projection of the exploiting other onto him (the patient was of course capable of enacting the exploiting role herself). Without his call, that projection might have remained intact and left the patient comfortable in her conviction that she was escaping from a corrupt therapist.

One factor that many therapists forget in the midst of the threat of a patient's dropping out is that the negatively charged object relations dyad activated on the surface is generally defending against a deeper one based on the wish for ideal love and nurturing. Remembering that this is the other side of the coin of the intense and stormy negative transference can help therapists remain calm, steady, and available during crises in a way that can be reassuring to the patient.

NONCOMPLIANCE WITH ADJUNCTIVE TREATMENT

The therapeutic frame may include adjunctive forms of treatment, such as attending 12-step meetings or being monitored by a dietitian. A patient's noncompliance with such treatments often carries with it the issue of honest communication because often the noncompliance is not immediately reported to the therapist. When faced with such an occurrence, the therapist must explore both the quality of the patient's communication and the meaning and consequences of the noncompliance. The noncompliance may represent a number of issues: It may be a test to see if the therapist cares enough to pay attention to the parameters that the therapist and patient set up. It may be a challenge to see if the patient can control the therapist— control that may be superficially desired but is often a source of distress at a deeper level. It may also be an attack on the treatment that represents resistance to the exploratory process because that process stirs up anxiety in the patient.

TREATMENT OF PATIENTS WITH BPO AND A HISTORY OF SEXUAL ABUSE

The etiology of BPO—and, more narrowly, that of BPD—is multifaceted, and there are multiple developmental pathways to the adult condition. The precise role of early sexual and physical abuse in the pathway to adult personality pathology is not clear, but the fact of such abuse in a subgroup of borderline patients has become evident in research. The percentage of patients with BPD who have experienced physical and sexual abuse varies tremendously from sample to sample, from 26% to 71% (Perry and Herman 1993) and even as high as 91% (Zanarini et al. 1997). However, it is also reported that only 15%–20% of individuals who experience abuse go on to develop a psychiatric illness (Paris 1994). It is important to consider these findings in debates over the role of abuse in the etiology of BPD. Sexual and/or physical abuse represents a range of experiences because the perpetrators of the abuse, the duration of the abuse, and the combination of sex and aggression are all specific to the individual case. Paris's (1994) data show that although the overall rate of childhood sexual abuse in patients with BPD was on the order of 70% in a number of studies, most of these studies did not carefully consider levels of severity of abuse. Paris's own study explored the dimension of severity and found that 30% of the abused subjects with BPD had experienced severe childhood sexual abuse with penetration.

Not only are the objective events different from case to case but each individual internalizes these early experiences with his or her own cognitions and affects. Traumatic childhood experiences are both the precursors of and the contributors to personality pathology and in turn are interpreted through the lens of the current personality organization of the patient. Therefore, the integration of these experiences in a treatment process will be through the patient's level of personality organization. Patients with BPO and those with neurotic personality organization will experience and re-create early trauma during the treatment in different ways. Those with BPO are much more likely to manifest—in polarized ways—the roles of victim and aggressor.

Past sexual and physical abuse comes up in the here-and-now transference in many ways. What is important to the treatment of the patient with BPD and a history of abuse is the manner in which these abuse experiences, like other important early experiences, have been remembered and integrated into the personality structure of the adult. Fonagy et al. (1996) found an association between borderline personality and lack of resolution of loss or trauma on the Adult Attachment Interview. Unresolved early experiences may enter into the transference as situations in which the patient experiences himself or herself as a victim at the hands of the therapist or, alternatively, attacks and victimizes the therapist. The issues discussed here focus on the treatment of patients with BPO, of whom some have clearly been abused in the past and others hint that they have been or wonder if they have been. One can differentiate between patients in whom early sexual and physical abuse has inhibited or even extinguished any sexuality and those who have experienced early sexual abuse combined with aggression in a way that has led to adult sexuality involving promiscuity, often with significant sadomasochistic features.

In patients with BPO in whom sexual abuse has left pathological consequences, the following treatment implications and guidelines apply:

1. The abuse will be activated in the transference. For patients with prior sadomasochistic relations,[1] the patient identifies as both victim and perpetrator, and these experiences will appear alternately in the transference. At certain times the patient will feel himself or herself to be the victim of the therapist, experiencing the therapist as an aggressor. Alternately, the patient may idealize the therapist and see others as aggressors and look to the therapist as the rescuer. At yet other times the patient will act as the aggressor and will victimize others, often including the therapist.
2. It is the therapist's task to bring to the surface the patient's identification with *both* victim and aggressor. A gradual tolerance on the part of the patient for his or her identification as both victim and aggressor will permit the patient to gain mastery over aggressive impulses that, when split off and out of consciousness, had overwhelmed him or her. This development will facilitate the disentanglement of sex and sadomasochistic aggression, leading to the possibility of sexual satisfaction and allowing the patient to explore in depth the experience of the sexual abuse

---

[1]We refer to sadomasochistic relations in the broad sense, which includes experiencing satisfaction in conjunction with psychological or emotional pain and is not limited to the experience of pleasure in relation to physical pain.

(e.g., the sense of violent destruction, destruction of the idealized care-taker, the possible triumph of being the sexual object of the parent, guilt over such feelings). Eventually, the whole range of feelings—fear, disgust, excitement, triumph—can be integrated into adult sexuality.

If a patient appears to be entering a dissociated state in the course of a session, the therapist can make use of basic grounding techniques to reengage the patient in dialogue. Coming to terms with the past on the part of victims of abuse involves the recognition of the anxiety, pain, and terror as well as rage and hatred derived from the painful physical or sexual invasion of body boundaries. A further level involves understanding the threatening effects of the corruption of early superego structures by the sadistic and dishonest behaviors of parental figures. Coming to terms with the past also involves recognizing the sexual and sadistic satisfactions that might have been part of the traumatic experiences of the past, as well as their repetitions throughout time. Fixation on past traumatic experiences has many functions, reflected in the repetition compulsion in the treatment (Freud 1920/1958), and these functions need to be systematically explored: the endless search for an ideal object behind the persecutory one (in the case of masochistic trends); the need to take revenge on a hated object by its violent destruction; the effort to transform a traumatic, painful experience into a sexually exciting one and, at the same time, the utilization of sexual gratification for purposes of revenge; and the urge to fuse with the therapist as an omnipotent, primitive, inexhaustible provider of love and gratification.

PSYCHOTIC EPISODES

Before discussing psychotic experiences associated with the transference, we wish to emphasize that although many BPD patients can be treated without medication, low-dose neuroleptics may help patients prone to psychotic distortions to maintain better contact with reality.

Acute Psychotic Experience Within the Transference

Transference psychosis differs from simple paranoid regression in the transference in that the psychosis expands outside the transference relationship to include secondary delusions and hallucinations. This phenomenon starts in the transference and then expands to affect other aspects of the patient's life. This expansion is more likely to occur if the transference issues remain closed to discussion in the sessions. In borderline patients with no comorbid pathology (e.g., bipolar illness), episodes of psychosis that occur in the course of treatment are generally related to the transference.

CASE EXAMPLE

A patient with low-level BPD had begun to experience libidinal longings for her therapist after a long initial period of fear and mistrust in relation to him. At that point, she started a session saying that she had an experience that she knew the therapist would not believe but that was true. She said the devil had appeared in her bedroom the previous night—not a dream or a fantasy, but the devil himself. The therapist became concerned she was entering a psychotic episode. As he explored the patient's experience, she said she had left out one part of the experience: the devil was him, her therapist. This opened the experience to transference exploration and to discussion of her intense regression to paranoid fears regarding him. The emergence of feelings of closeness had activated her anxieties about attachment and provoked the idea that he was only tricking her into feeling comfortable with him so that he could hurt her more intensely. Discussion of this experience and the related internal objects helped move it from a psychotic-seeming "reality" to fantasy material that could be explored.

Transference psychosis must be distinguished from a more general psychotic experience; the test of the situation is the possibility of keeping it within the transference while working on it and resolving it. If this does not work, the therapist must consider seeking consultation, prescribing medication, or recommending hospitalization.

Drug-Induced Psychosis

A variety of substances that influence bodily perceptions, mental state, or sensitivity to external stimuli may induce psychotic experiences in some borderline patients. Drug-induced psychotic experiences include feelings of depersonalization and loss of reality, visual or auditory hallucinations, and paranoid delusions. The management of drug-induced psychoses begins with acquiring accurate data about the patient's current drug use. In addition to substances of abuse and prescription medications, over-the-counter preparations (especially those with anticholinergic effects) should be considered. Brief hospitalization may be indicated when the substance abuse cannot be controlled in the outpatient setting.

DISSOCIATIVE REACTIONS

A particular expression of severe splitting between idealized and persecutory relationships may be observed in patients with dissociative reactions. Dissociative reactions may present in the form of a patient who appears to withdraw internally and to cease responding to external stimuli, including the therapist. In such a case, the therapist may employ basic grounding techniques and should continue to address the patient with the assumption that a degree of observing ego remains active in the patient. Dissociative reactions may also present in the form of the controversial syndrome of multiple personalities—dissociative identity disorder in DSM-5 (American Psychiatric Association 2013). Management of a case with this complication is presented in Chapter 9. The therapist's interpretation of the nature of the object relationship activated during the dissociated state, and of the defensive function of its being split off from alternative object relations in the transference, facilitates the object relationship's gradual elaboration and reduction. In such situations the main dangers are the therapist's anxiety and confusion when first faced with this contingency and the temptation to be seduced by the dissociated state into treating a "different person" instead of a split-off object relation in the transference.

DEPRESSIVE EPISODES

Evaluation of a patient presenting with depression is discussed above in the subsection "Managing Suicide Threats and Attempts During Treatment."

EMERGENCY ROOM VISITS

It may be appropriate for a patient to go to the ER at times when he or she feels uncertain about his or her ability to control self-destructive impulses. Evaluation in the ER may help clarify the situation. The fact of seeking help rather than acting on an impulse may itself be a sign of positive change. In our experience, a number of patients went through a phase in which, after engaging in therapy, they had one or two brief hospitalizations after going to the ER because of concern about acting on self-destructive impulses. This differed from their earlier pattern of being hospitalized *after* having acted out in a self-destructive way. In most instances, both ER visits and hospitalizations stopped after the patient fully realized that these behaviors would not bring about the secondary gain of getting the therapist more involved in his or her life.

Nonetheless, ER visits can present a dilemma for the therapist. This is because ER staff often feel that the outpatient therapist should accept total responsibility for the patient. If this occurs, the therapist can explain to the ER staff that the therapist's taking charge in emergency situations would provide secondary gain to the patient and therefore would be counterproductive. Even though the therapist knows the patient in greater depth, it is the ER doctor who has information about the patient's immediate condition. Therefore, although the former may provide information to the latter, it is the ER doctor's decision whether or not the patient should be admitted to the hospital. The information most relevant for the therapist to provide to the ER doctor is the patient's level of engagement in therapy and ability to make a commitment, the presence of any acute stressors, the risk of substance abuse, and the presence of antisocial features. ER visits usually taper off if they are handled in this way.

HOSPITALIZATION

Hospitalization itself does not necessarily represent a crisis in treatment. A patient who seeks the protection of a hospital setting when he or she is at risk of self-destructive actions *before* carrying them out may be demonstrating good judgment and improvement in his or her condition. In such instances the role of the therapist is to work with the patient to understand what contributed to the acute sense of risk. Hospitalization might also be the appropriate intervention for an episode of major depressive illness or a psychotic regression (although these can often be managed in the context of the therapy).

Depending on the circumstances, the therapist may be able to have one or more sessions with the patient on the hospital ward. If so, the therapist might be able to make progress addressing an issue that the patient is strongly defended against (such as Amy's defending against awareness of her aggressive side in the case discussed beginning in Chapter 8, "Early Treatment Phase"). However, in this age of short hospitalizations, sometimes the only contact possible between therapist and patient during the course of the hospitalization will be over the telephone, in which case the therapist's principal task is to establish whether the outpatient treatment frame is adequate for the patient to return to therapy and to determine whether the patient is motivated to resume therapy—especially in cases where events around the hospitalization may have involved the patient's breaking the frame of treatment (e.g., resuming substance abuse, withholding important information from the therapist).

In addition to communicating with the patient about the resumption of therapy, it is essential for the therapist to communicate with the person in charge of the patient's treatment in the hospital. Under the best of circumstances, that doctor, psychologist, or social worker will have some understanding of psychodynamic therapy and will help in determining whether and how to transfer the patient back to the outpatient treatment frame. However, sometimes the hospital therapist becomes involved in enactments of the patient's dynamics. The most typical scenario occurs in situations in which the hospital staff views the patient as being incapable of taking responsibility in his or her treatment and life. Patients sometimes discuss their outpatient therapy in a way that depicts the therapist as unreasonable, demanding, and dictatorial. In this situation, the therapist should make the interpretation that the patient is externalizing his or her conflict around dependency versus autonomy and projecting the part of him or her that is interested in more independent functioning onto the therapist while seeming to be content to remain a passive recipient of a more chronic supportive treatment. The therapist should remind the patient that he or she is free to choose which path to pursue, but the therapist should predict to the patient that the conflict will continue even if the patient, for the moment, seems comfortable choosing one side of it. It is also helpful for the therapist to point out that although the choice of a more chronic patient role may seem validated by the hospital staff and may seem to make life easy for the moment, it could be tragic to abandon the potential for higher functioning over the years to come.

A patient's hospitalization sometimes brings to light the need to review and modify the treatment contract. For example, a patient who had previously concealed his use of alcohol was hospitalized after he became disinhibited when intoxicated and impulsively took a handful of pills. This brought to the therapist's attention the importance of discussing 1) the patient's need to make a commitment to open communication in therapy and 2) the need to establish a treatment parameter requiring the patient to attend Alcoholics Anonymous meetings before returning to therapy.

Hospitalization can represent different things. Especially in the early phase of treatment, it can be a protest and a message to the therapist that the patient believes that the conditions of treatment set up in the contract are too difficult to comply with. The therapist offers this interpretation to the patient and openly reviews whether the patient wishes to commit himself or herself to this type of treatment. In some cases, being hospitalized is part of an enactment of split borderline dynamics that have not been contained within the structure of the treatment and that may be dealt with by interpretation.

CASE EXAMPLE

Edie, a patient with strong narcissistic features and a history of very serious suicide attempts had been doing relatively well in therapy for 2 years. She had stopped making suicide attempts, maintained a job, and had become involved in a steady relationship with a boyfriend. However, she continued to be highly critical of herself and very devaluing of her therapist. She maintained that she was incompetent at work despite getting very good feedback from her supervisor. Her anxiety about her "incompetence" at work led to her staying home so much that she eventually lost her job. Even though she quickly found another job, this event marked the beginning of a downward spiral.

Edie reported to her therapist, Dr. Todd, one day that she had not gone to work the previous day but instead had gone to a local dam to kill herself by jumping. Dr. Todd explored the behavior and addressed the patient's commitment to adhering to the treatment contract, which included the understanding that she would go to a hospital if she felt she could not control her suicidal impulses. Edie reported that she could not be sure from one minute to the next whether she could control her impulse to kill herself and could not give a commitment to go to a hospital if she felt like giving in to the urge. After probing to assess Edie's ability to make a commitment at that time, Dr. Todd agreed that for whatever reason she was acutely at risk of serious self-destructive behavior. The therapist and patient reviewed the options: Edie could either return home and be monitored by family members or she could be hospitalized. After some initial resistance, she agreed with Dr. Todd that the hospital was the better choice.

In the hospital, the staff found Edie to be obsessed with the idea of killing herself. The hospital treatment consisted of starting mood-stabilizing medication and working on coping skills. Edie was discharged after 2 weeks with the plan to return to her job on a part-time basis and attend a hospital day program 5 afternoons a week while returning to her twice-a-week therapy. Dr. Todd reemphasized the treatment contract, in particular Edie's responsibilities with regard to managing her suicidal ideation. The second week after discharge, Edie confessed in the middle of a session that she was hiding the fact that she had not gone to her job or the day program the previous day but had returned to the dam to jump. After a discussion with regard to her suicide risk, she was rehospitalized. During her 10 days in the hospital, the treatment focused on her anxiety about work and attempted to help her develop coping skills so that she could better tolerate her work setting.

The week after discharge, Edie called Dr. Todd just when their morning session was scheduled to begin and reported that her alarm clock had not gone off and that she would not be able to get to the session that day. She added that she was fine and would see him at the next session. Dr. Todd, on the basis of his knowledge of this patient, confronted Edie with his doubt that this report was true. He said it did not ring true that 1 week out of the hospital, she could miss a session with such apparent indifference. Edie acknowledged that she planned to go to the dam that day to kill herself instead of going to her session or to work. Dr. Todd outlined the three possible outcomes of this situation: 1) she could go to the hospital for readmission, 2) she could come to the therapist's office for a session later in the morning, or 3) she could proceed with her plan to kill herself. He added that if she chose the third option, he would notify the police to look for her at the dam, but he made it clear that this would be no guarantee that she would not kill herself.

Edie said she would come to the session. In the time before the session, Dr. Todd called a colleague to seek consultation. He felt he had lost perspective on this case since the first hospitalization and that he was functioning mainly with the goal of keeping Edie alive, with a loss of the psychodynamic perspective. The colleague helped Dr. Todd regain that perspective and reviewed with him that he had an honest choice when he saw Edie that morning: he could decide to work with her on the level of interpretation within the sessions or, if he did not feel safe with that, he could recommend another hospitalization. Dr. Todd decided he would explore the possibility of working with interpretation and then, depending on his assessment of Edie's response, he would decide whether to continue this approach or to support the option of hospitalization.

When Edie came to session, Dr. Todd proposed the following interpretation of the recent events: "You are acting as though there is no conflict in you about whether you want to live or die. You say that all you want is your death and that it is only others who prevent you from killing yourself. Your actions—your repeated visits to the dam—appear, at first glance, to support this view. However, I believe you are trying to find a way out of a dramatic conflict that is taking place *within you:* while there *is* a destructive part of you that seeks your death, for reasons we have not yet fully understood, there is also a part of you that does *not* want this, a part of you that wants to live and seeks connections with others. You seem to be trying to resolve this conflict by denying this latter part of you and acting as though only others feel that way. This denial would free you to act in accordance with the destructive part in a mad fling with death. However, your actions show that you cannot get out of this conflict so easily. First, you are alive; if all you wanted was to be dead, you would be dead by now. Second, you come to therapy, which you know is on the side of your living. Third, despite your repeated trips to the dam, you do not jump—you go so far and then stop. I would like to help you resolve this conflict, but I have had difficulty doing so recently because there has been so much focus on *action*, on your apparent need to be hospitalized. It may be that you need to be hospitalized again today, but I have been reflecting on this and it seems to me that if you wanted to be dead, you would be by now. So I think there is some other issue going on and that the way to look at it is not to have you back in the hospital but to continue the therapy. But we can only do that if you stay alive. What do you think?"

Edie, who had looked interested and somewhat surprised as Dr. Todd had been talking, replied, "I think you might be right, although I hadn't thought about it that way. All I *feel* at those times is the urge to kill myself, but you're right: I don't. I go to the dam and just sit there and sit there and sit there…for hours, but I don't jump. I don't know what stops me, but maybe it's what you're talking about."

Dr. Todd replied, "It would be helpful to explore what goes on in your mind at those times—what thoughts, what images, what fantasies—and we can do that here, if we are comfortable enough to do it. But I would like to comment on another aspect of the situation. I have a hypothesis that may or may not be accurate. It seems to me that you get some pleasure from seeing me squirm when you talk about your visits to the dam—a sadistic pleasure. I don't know if you feel this, but looking back, I believe this side of you has increased since you lost your job. I wonder if it has to do with a sense of humiliation and a related envy. We know how hard you are on yourself. Losing your job may have seemed to confirm to you your sense of worthlessness. Yet there is a side of you that feels superior to others and can't tolerate feeling that anyone is better than you. It may be that since you lost your job, the only way you have found—instinctively—to feel good about yourself is to feel superior to me by becoming my torturer—a part of you that, of course, attacks yourself just as it can attack me. This may be one reason you are still alive, because of the pleasure of seeing me squirm—although I believe there is also a part of you that wishes for a more positive connection. If anything of what I say is true, then we should look at it; to have envious, aggressive, or even sadistic feelings does not mean you deserve to die—a lot of people have such feelings. But if you deny them or condemn yourself for them in a way that makes it impossible for us to explore them, then those feelings will not be under your control but rather will control you."

Edie smiled in recognition when Dr. Todd referred to the possibility of sadistic pleasure and said, "I have to admit I do get some pleasure out of seeing you squirm.... I didn't know you saw that."

Dr. Todd and Edie went on to discuss a treatment plan. Edie felt that Dr. Todd's interventions had clarified what was going on in a way that would allow her to resist the temptation to go to the dam. His interventions had also helped free her to discuss certain feelings of which she had been only partially aware. The two agreed to proceed without an additional hospitalization. The therapy progressed from that point with a deeper exploration of the dynamic issues and without further hospitalization.

Although this vignette demonstrates a number of aspects of treatment, the emphasis here is on how the patient's hospitalizations fit into an underlying dynamic and how the therapist intervened in what was becoming a crisis of repeated hospitalizations. The patient's attempts to externalize her conflict around living versus dying, as well as around establishing connections versus destroying them, resulted in hospitalizations that were part of the overall enactment of the dynamic: the fact of hospitalization and those involved in the hospitalization, including the therapist, represented the split-off healthier side of the patient. A second theme involved the patient's envy and her wish both to make the therapist squirm and to show, through repeated hospitalizations, that his therapy was no good. Until these themes were interpreted, the cycle of hospitalizations was likely to continue.

PATIENT TELEPHONE CALLS

A careful assessment reveals whether a patient has had problems in previous therapy with telephone calling, emailing, or texting a therapist. If so, the contracting therapist should present a structure for dealing with that eventuality to contain the behavior and rechannel the patient's communications to the therapist back into the framework of the sessions, where work can be done.

THERAPIST ABSENCE AND COVERAGE MANAGEMENT

Routine absences from the office by the therapist for vacations, professional meetings, and so on can be occasions for skilled management with borderline patients. In all cases the therapist must arrange for a colleague to be available during the period of absence. The therapist's absence is most likely to provoke a crisis during the first year of treatment. During that period, the therapist may arrange for the patient to have scheduled sessions with the covering therapist if indicated. Generally, in the course of the first year, therapists are able to work with the dynamic issues catalyzed by an absence so that such events cease being experienced as a crisis.

The therapist should explore the patient's difficulty in maintaining an internal image of the therapist. The patient's rage at the perceived "abandoning object" frequently attacks the internal image of the "caring object" and leaves the patient with no sense of connection to the therapist during periods of absence. Interpreting that this is likely to happen, or that it has happened on previous occasions, can help the patient avoid this destruction of the internal image. A patient who said with anxiety, "Every time you go away, I think I'll never see you again; I picture your plane blowing up as soon as it takes off," provided her therapist with evidence of her anger attacking the internal link with him.

Patients frequently talk about feeling "abandoned." It is helpful to explore why a patient experiences the interruption in treatment this way. It often turns out that the patient feels that the interruption provides proof of what the patient has "known" all along—for instance, that the therapist does not care at all about the patient or that the therapist finds the patient disgusting and wants to get away from him or her. In other words, the interruption reinforces a negative internal representation. The therapist should question whether his or her being away constitutes proof of indifference and point out that although the patient is angry and disappointed, the patient almost seems relieved to have "proof" that the therapist does not care. This relief corresponds to how much anxiety is provoked when the defense of splitting begins to break down and the patient experiences the possibility of a good relationship. The therapist can interpret the fact that his or her going away reinforces the split as follows: "You were beginning to think that I might have some genuine concern for you, even if it is not all you want. You seem to be taking the news of my upcoming absence as an opportunity to reestablish the status quo. It's a sad status quo, because in it neither I nor anyone cares about you, but it's a reassuring status quo insofar as you feel you know the score and therefore won't be vulnerable."

PATIENT SILENCE

Observing the nonverbal reaction of the silent patient to questions about what is on his or her mind, along with reflecting on the therapist's own countertransference under such conditions, facilitates the understanding of the experience of self and other behind the silence. The patient's silence may represent fear, guilt, shame, arrogance, provocation, or other affects. The therapist's observations may permit him or her to work interpretively with the activated object relation despite the patient's silence. The technique of stimulating the patient to talk, followed by an analysis of the nature of the patient's nonverbal response and the therapist's countertransference, then a tentative interpretation of the present object relationship in light of this analysis, and then renewed observation of the patient before stimulating the patient once more to talk, constitutes a nonthreatening cycle of transference analysis and interpretation that usually permits the resolution of even protracted silences. In extreme cases in which the patient remains silent despite the therapist's best interpretive efforts, the therapist may have to address the question of whether the therapy can continue when the patient is consistently failing to adhere to the treatment parameter that calls for the reporting of thoughts and feelings. A detailed example of this is provided in Yeomans et al. (1992, Chapter 7, Case Study #2).

SOMATIZATION

Along with acting out, somatization is a form of managing affects and internal conflicts that keeps the material from conscious awareness. Somatization is a particular challenge for exploratory therapy because patients often reject the idea that there is a psychological contribution to the physical problem. Indeed, therapists must ensure that adequate medical investigation has taken place to rule out, to the degree that it is possible, a biological cause of the somatic complaint. In working with somatizing patients, therapists should listen for emotional issues that the patient is trying to avoid and be attentive to countertransference developments that suggest affective material that is not present in the content of the patient's discourse. TFP considers somatization to be a presymbolic expression of affect. The therapeutic approach is to attempt to describe the underlying affect in terms of a relationship dyad related to the somatic problem.

CASE EXAMPLE

A single, middle-aged man came to therapy for help with depression and anxiety. The structural interview led to a diagnosis of high-level BPO with rigid narcissistic features. The patient suffered from years of gastrointestinal (GI) symptoms. In the course of an extensive GI workup that included a number of second opinions, the therapist, whose countertransference included the feeling of always being under scrutiny, pointed out the patient's pattern of harshly finding fault with each of the specialists he consulted with. The therapist proposed to the patient that within his mind there was a "tyrant" demanding meticulous perfection from others and probably, at a different level, from himself. As the patient reflected on this possibility, he was more aware of anger in him related to feeling neglected by caretakers who did not meet his standards. As he discussed his anger more, he began to experience a lessening of his GI symptoms, an improvement of his mood that was accompanied by an increase in a sarcastic sense of humor (a higher level of metabolizing aggressive affect), and an increased openness to dating. Although this brief example gives a flavor of the work with somatizing patients, the reader should be aware that therapy with this type of patient can be arduous and involve very strong resistances to gaining access to underlying affects.

COMMENTARY ON VIDEO 3: AFFECT STORM SESSION

The cases we have presented as illustrative of TFP are composite cases based on elements of real cases that have been disguised. The session in Video 3, which demonstrates working with the dyads underlying intense affect states, is typical of a patient with a predominant paranoid transference. This segment was based on a session that took place a year into the therapy. The patient, Carolyn, begins by referring to the taping of the session, saying "It affects how I feel in here" and asking the therapist, Dr. Hamilton, to turn off the camera. The taping was agreed on at the beginning of therapy and was part of the frame of treatment. Carolyn understood that the recordings would be used in a supervision group both for the purposes of teaching and to get colleagues' input on the case. Dr. Hamilton's first intervention is to try to clarify what Carolyn is experiencing in the moment because her position is a change from her initial agreement to the contract. He asks her to say more about her "paranoia."

 Video 3–1: Affect Storm Part 1 (9:28)

One issue that is illustrated in this session is an attempt to establish the boundary between internal and external reality. One could take the position that the camera is objectively a hostile intrusion. However, Dr. Hamilton is interested in what Carolyn is projecting at this moment on the camera and on him. The camera is not new, but Carolyn's reaction to it is. Dr. Hamilton suspects that what is threatening is a part of Carolyn's internal world that has been activated. He follows the basic strategy of understanding the object relation that underlies the affect.

Some of Carolyn's early comments suggest a libidinal element that is hard to perceive in the midst of the anger: "This is supposed to be a relationship between you and me, right? I have enough trouble even wanting to have a relationship with you, and now it has to be this?" These may be the affects the paranoia is defending against in a patient who, as Dr. Hamilton will point out toward the end of the video, seems more comfortable when the relationship is hostile than when it is positive.

Following the first strategy of TFP, Dr. Hamilton tries to focus on the object relation underlying the affect in the moment: "What's making things especially difficult right now?" (1:50). He also attempts to define the active dyad: "You seem to feel I'm treating you just by the book" (2:12) and "[You feel I'm] a cold robot" (3:24). Carolyn agrees but with the conviction that this is the simple reality as she elaborates her negative transference in the moment: "You are a New York psychoanalytic psychotherapist who does one type of therapy!" (3:31).

Dr. Hamilton continues to elaborate the dyad: "You're telling me basically that my clinical treatment of you is extremely painful and disorganizing" (4:25) in the hope that the description of what Carolyn is feeling will encourage taking the time to observe and reflect on it. Carolyn persists in the negative transference, not reflecting on Dr. Hamilton's comments. He notes a rigidity in her position that seems to embody what she is describing in him and suggests that "the only way you can react to this is to imitate me in this…, and you're doing that right now [as Carolyn starts to read her papers]—to close yourself to whatever I say" (7:40). He is describing an oscillation, a reversal of the dyad that is in Carolyn's behavior but not in her awareness: she is enacting the rigid, ungiving other that she fears and feels she is encountering in him. Dr. Hamilton goes on to name the interaction and to describe their different opinions in a way that touches on the technique of incompatible realities: "So we could say there's a lack of attention here, a lack of taking in the other—and you're convinced it's me who's doing that" (8:20).

For a moment Carolyn becomes calmer and speaks in a way that is more characteristic of a "normal" therapy session, describing her concern about how she has been feeling. However, it takes only a few seconds of Dr. Hamilton's listening in silence to reactivate the negative dyad and projection; Carolyn drops the narrative of how she was feeling and interjects "Stonewall—very good!" (9:22). [End of Video 3–1]

Video 3–2: Affect Storm Part 2 (9:26)

In Video 3–2, Dr. Hamilton again follows the strategy of naming the dyad: "So you experienced my silence as a combination of indifference and rejection?" He points out the reversal again: "Just notice what's going on right now because you experience me as not being interested in what you're saying at the moment when you're telling me the same thing" (00:30). He goes on to empathize with her internal state: "You have the feeling that I either don't listen or that I attack you—that's a very painful experience. So it's worthwhile to examine whether this is the situation or not" (1:55).

This leads to a discussion of the harsh demandingness that characterizes part of Carolyn's split internal world. First she describes this rigid quality of thinking as she sees it in Dr. Hamilton: "You want me to appreciate everything that you have to offer and say" (2:38). Dr. Hamilton describes this object, leaving open the matter as to where it originates: "It's as if there's one part of you operating either within you or that you see operating in me that's so perfectionistic and demanding that it can only either be total perfection or total devaluing" (3:46).

Carolyn agrees with the formulation but can initially say so only in an ironic and mocking tone. Dr. Hamilton notes the defensiveness of the tone: "You started out there by making fun of me, hiding the fact that you're actually acknowledging part of what I was saying" (5:04). He is pointing to her anxiety about both her sense of humiliation at having a problem and the possibility of positive affects in the relation, an anxiety that is typical in the context of a paranoid transference that cannot imagine that attachment could work out well.

Carolyn agrees that she is acknowledging that Dr. Hamilton has a point: "You do [have a point]" (5:29), which she says with what might be seen as an ironic smile. (It should be noted that the actress in the video does not quite communicate the ambiguous affect of the actual patient.) Dr. Hamilton misinterprets this as Carolyn being ironic again; he does not realize that her internal state has changed from irony to sincerity. She reacts to his lack of understanding with rage, getting up, throwing her papers on the floor, and yelling, "You are fucking full of shit!" (5:38).

The key to working with an affect storm is to carefully pursue the strategy of accurately identifying the underlying self-other dyad. Dr. Hamilton quickly recognizes his mistake and acknowledges it: "You're absolutely right—I missed something" (6:25). Although it is unfortunate that he did not follow Carolyn in her shift from one internal state to another, it is not always easy to follow the abrupt changes of state that characterize the borderline experience. He links this experience to the demanding of perfection: "That's what we were talking about that happened just now...I missed a few seconds..., and you flew into this rage" (6:35).

Dr. Hamilton puts his understanding of Carolyn's experience into words: "I think you felt betrayed by me" (7:08). This is the patient's greatest fear: to let down her guard/defense, to reveal the part of her internal world that she is defending against (the longing/wish for attachment), and to feel rejected/criticized.

As Dr. Hamilton reflects on the interaction (and it can take a while to "unpack" all that happens in the very condensed experience of an affect storm), he acknowledges Carolyn's insight (8:05). As he is acknowledging her positive input, he notes her continued, and perhaps even increasing, distress. This observation brings his thoughts back to the basic internal split and discomfort with any positive experience in a relationship. He observes, "Why are you now unhappy under the condition when I'm acknowledging that I missed your expression and, on top of that, I missed an interpretation you had...? That could be a positive experience but for some reason you're experiencing it as painful. I think at this time, when you experience me as a decent human being, you are suffering. Something in you doesn't permit you to experience me as a decent human being" (8:40). [End of Video 3–2]

Video 3–3: Affect Storm Part 3 (10:10)

At the beginning of Video 3–3, Carolyn acknowledges the dyad and sees it in herself: "It doesn't permit *me* to experience myself as a decent human being" (00:02). She calms down at this point and seems more reflective. However, she shifts back to a negative transference: "Do you know how hard it is to sit here and feel humiliated in front of somebody who looks at you like this?" (she makes a caricature of a stone face) (2:52). Dr. Hamilton replies, "We could learn a lot from how you perceive me." He acknowledges her perception of him as expressionless but decides to return to what he feels is the deeper material at this point: her discomfort with him when the affect is positive: "But if I *do* respond..., it's hard for you in a different way" (3:23). He continues this line of reflection a bit later, referring to "a moment when there was good communication between you and me—but then it blew up.... The question is why it's so fragile, this positive thing we had for a moment" (6:16).

Carolyn points to his misunderstanding: "You blew it!"

Dr. Hamilton returns to the theme of her discomfort with the positive connection: "I missed something—but it seems that when you experience yourself in a good relationship with me, maybe just for a few seconds, for some reason you get more anxious" (6:35). Carolyn has difficulty staying with this theme: "I'm not doing this!" Dr. Hamilton then points out, "You seem more comfortable fighting than talking peacefully, as sad as that might be."

Dr. Hamilton tries to be more specific about the immediate object relation underlying the affect: "What is it right now that's making the treatment unbearable? [At the beginning of the session] you said it's hard enough to have a relation—I think that's the issue.... You opened up, I missed it, and then it seemed like a disaster struck." He continues, "The problem is right in front of us again, except that we're talking about it a little bit more right now" (7:17–8:13).

Carolyn (looking sadder rather than angry) says, "I've tried too many times—it's never different.... It's like slapping an eager puppy" (8:40). Dr. Hamilton picks up on the metaphor, saying that it was hard to see the eager puppy when it turned into a raging bull (8:57)—pointing out the defensive nature of her anger. Carolyn acknowledges the defense, saying it's better to be alone than to be bruised (9:34). Dr. Hamilton agrees, "[but only] if those are the only two options."

Carolyn points out that Dr. Hamilton has a different, nonparanoid view: "I know you think people can be nice. I'm not sure you're right...maybe you're the naïve one" (9:45). Ending the session, Dr. Hamilton maintains neutrality and opens the question for exploration: "It would be good to look at those two possibilities."

Key Clinical Concepts

- The tactics of TFP set the stage for the use of the treatment techniques.

- The treatment contract serves many purposes that must be kept in mind throughout the therapy (see Chapter 5).

- It is essential to always listen to the three channels of communication: 1) the content of the patient's discourse, 2) nonverbal behaviors and attitudes, and 3) the therapist's countertransference. Therapists often pay attention to the patient's verbal content more than the other channels of communication; this can lead to a therapy that favors a cognitive focus at the expense of an appreciation of deeper affective issues.

- TFP guides therapists in their choice of what material to address by providing clear guidelines on how to choose the priority material.

- Following the patient's affect is a fundamental rule. In addition to generally providing access to deeper material, this approach provides a model for the ability to contain and reflect on affect and helps the therapist avoid colluding with the patient's defenses against intense affect.

- After being guided by attention to the patient's affect, the therapist follows the hierarchy of priorities regarding content. This hierarchy first addresses patient behaviors and attitudes that act as resistances to exploration.

SELECTED READINGS

Clarkin JF, Yeomans FE. Managing negative reactions to clients with borderline personality disorder in transference-focused psychotherapy, in Transforming Negative Reactions to Clients. Edited by Wolf A, Goldfried M, Muran JC. Washington, DC: American Psychological Association, 2012, pp 175–188

Koenigsberg H, Kernberg OF, Stone M, et al. Borderline Personality Disorder: Stretching the Limits of Treatability. New York, Basic Books, 2000

Yeomans FE, Selzer MA, Clarkin JF. Treating the Borderline Patient: A Contract-Based Approach. New York, Basic Books, 1992

CHAPTER

8

EARLY TREATMENT PHASE

Tests of the Frame, Impulse Containment, and Identifying Dyads

IN THIS and the following two chapters, we explore the major issues that arise in the different phases of transference-focused psychotherapy (TFP) and the progressive changes that occur in patients. We can generalize about the major issues that arise in the early, middle, and late phases of treatment; however, individual differences are to be expected among patients across the borderline personality organization (BPO) range as they progress through treatment. To relate the principles of TFP to individual cases, we have chosen to illustrate the interaction of principles and individual patients by following two representative cases across the phases of TFP (Table 8–1). These are composite cases with details changed to protect confidentiality. Because two cases cannot capture all the possible major variations found in patients, we also present examples of other specific clinical situations in the three chapters. Both cases meet the criteria for borderline personality disorder (BPD). Amy is a prototypical patient with low-level BPO at the beginning of treatment. In contrast, Betty, who was introduced in Chapter 4 ("Assessment Phase"), is a prototypical example of high-level

271

BPO, with prominent identity diffusion and isolation but less aggression than Amy. These differences in level of personality organization have an impact on the treatment process in the early phases of treatment, but the differences begin to fade as the goals of treatment are achieved.

The goals and related tasks of the early treatment phase (Table 8–2) reflect the nature of borderline pathology and the manner in which psychodynamic treatment begins to shape the interaction. The therapist begins to apply the treatment strategies (see Chapter 3, "Strategies of Transference-Focused Psychotherapy"). However, the goal of beginning to identify the internal object representations can take place only in a context that is not excessively disrupted by the patient's acting out. Therefore, paying attention to adherence to the treatment contract, as well as focusing attention on deviations from it, is especially important in this phase of therapy. Acting out in this phase often takes the form of challenging or testing the frame of treatment that was established in the contracting phase. Another common early type of acting out comes in the form of the patient's impulses to leave the therapy as attention to the patient's intense affects and internal world provoke anxiety.

If the early phase of treatment goes well, the patient begins to demonstrate increased control over impulsive and self-destructive behaviors in conjunction with an increased ability to experience intense affects. This progression is also in response to the elimination of secondary gain from acting out, as established in the treatment contract. As the patient's impulse control is strengthened, his or her chaotic and socially inappropriate behavior is reduced—although not necessarily eliminated—outside the treatment setting. Limit setting tends to shift the experience of affect into the therapeutic relationship, where the underlying object relations dyads are activated in the transference. Limit setting and the decrease in acting out allow the therapist to begin to use the analytic techniques of TFP.

Intense affects tend to become concentrated in the treatment situation, which has been defined as a space where all affects can be tolerated. The therapist has the opportunity to link the patient's impulses to act and symptoms such as anxiety, rage, emptiness, or depressed mood to vicissitudes in the relationship with the therapist that reflect the dominant, underlying object relations in the patient's inner world as they are activated in the transference. As the patient becomes more confident in the possibility of expressing intense affects in the treatment setting, the therapeutic alliance increases even as the therapeutic relation may be stormy at times; the ability of the patient to experience and express intense affects in relation to the therapist *and* to come back to the next session reflects a strong alliance. Even so, the patient's urges to drop out may occur in response to a number of possible developments: 1) the anxiety of reflecting on uncomfortable as-

TABLE 8–1. Two continuous cases across phases of treatment

	Amy	Betty
Patient characteristics	Low-level borderline personality organization; 23-year-old married female; unemployed; in treatment for 7 years prior for anxiety, depression, and self-destructive behavior; multiple hospitalizations	High-level borderline personality organization; 33-year-old single female; unemployed with no friends; in treatment since age 16 for depression and superficial wrist cutting
Early treatment phase (Chapter 8)	Patient cuts both wrists in emergency room with subsequent hospitalization. Exploration of this leads to initiating interpretation of her pleasure in aggression.	Patient makes use of omnipotent control in early sessions. Her defenses against libidinal longings become clear.
Midphase of treatment (Chapter 9)	Patient ends aggressive attacks on self. Her paranoid orientation decreases but remains evident in more subtle ways. She takes up college studies and decides to have a child. She experiences a shift in her mistrust of those in her expanding environment.	Patient takes volunteer job and goes to college but experiences mistrust of people in these environments. She experiences ambivalence about her success and demonstrates competitive strivings with classmates and therapist.
Advanced treatment phase (Chapter 10)	Patient and therapist examine her perception of therapist as condescending. Patient begins to recognize that attitude in herself. She has a phase of idealized erotic transference. She undergoes an evolving perception of therapist as benevolent and collaborating.	Patient is making new friends but continues to be sensitive to rejection. Her awareness of her own critical and judgmental side is increasing. She is becoming better able to contextualize the immediate emotional response and balance it with awareness of the broader reality. She develops an intimate relationship and gets married.

TABLE 8–2. Areas of focus and change in the early treatment phase

The patient's capacity to maintain the relationship with the therapist with all its intensely fluctuating affect states increases, and there is a reduction in the risk of premature dropout from treatment. The therapist's capacity to be open to and contain the range and intensity of the patient's affect states helps the patient "sit with" them without acting out, increasing the possibility of reflecting on them and exploring the conflicts related to them.

There is a reduction in suicidal, self-destructive behavior and other chaotic behavior outside the sessions by maintaining the treatment frame, reducing secondary gain, and transforming action into observation of the dominant object relations in the treatment relationship.

Intense affects and affect storms become concentrated in the treatment situation, and symptoms such as anxiety, rage, emptiness, or depressed mood are linked to the vicissitudes in the relationship with the therapist and others and understood in terms of the object relations dyad that underlies the affect. This work reflects the clinical observation that in many instances, the patient's affect is the reflection of an underlying object relation—an internal sense of self in relation to other—that the patient experiences but of which he or she is not consciously aware and in relation to which he or she can take no observing distance. His or her experience *is* the reality of the situation rather than an experience on which to reflect. The techniques of clarification, confrontation, and interpretation will begin to introduce an observing distance.

The patient begins to accept a work or study role in everyday life. This follows from discussion in the contracting phase. The patient's reports of experiences in the world outside therapy provide important information to complement the transference analysis.

The patient's basic lack of a stable concept of self and/or others is not expected to change yet. The increased engagement in life tasks reflects the impact of the frame of treatment and not a change in identity integration at this point. It is assumed that the patient's problematic internal representations and use of primitive defense mechanisms will lead to a repetition of earlier difficulties in life experiences, but the patient will be encouraged to use the safe haven of the therapy to understand those difficulties in a way that will allow for a decrease in misunderstandings and conflicts with others and an increase in engagement in activities and with others.

pects of the patient's internal world, 2) increasing attachment to the therapist that may be threatened by the anxiety of attachment itself and by related fears of abandonment, and 3) initial glimpses of awareness of dissociated or projected aggression, with paradoxical increases in paranoid reactions in the transference.

CAPACITY TO MAINTAIN THE RELATIONSHIP WITH THE THERAPIST

THERAPEUTIC ALLIANCE

In the early phase of treatment, the relatively high dropout rate by borderline patients compared with other patients is a serious consideration. A review of treatment completion by patients with BPD (Barnicot et al. 2011) indicated that the following were important factors in dropping out: high impulsivity, anger, anxiety, lack of commitment to treatment, low motivation to change, higher experiential avoidance, and poor therapeutic alliance. In a large study comparing dialectical behavior therapy and general psychiatric management, the strongest predictor of dropout was poor therapeutic alliance (Wnuk et al. 2013). One of the most robust findings in all of psychotherapy research is the importance of the early therapeutic alliance in relation to treatment process and outcome (Crits-Christoph et al. 2013). This literature makes little distinction between patients in terms of diagnosis and in terms of levels of personality organization (e.g., neurotic vs. borderline). Our knowledge of the attachment difficulties of borderline patients suggests that forming a treatment alliance with them is more complicated and more difficult than forming one with neurotic patients. In addition, most of the literature indicating the importance of the early alliance refers to treatments of brief duration.

TFP, by definition, focuses on the relationship between patient and therapist. The relationship is complex in that on one level it is real and on another level it is a creation of the patient, based on how the patient's internal representations of self and other determine his or her perception of the therapist. Ultimately, it is the therapist's exploration of these latter perceptions that helps the patient advance to a more stable psychological structure. The more reality-based aspects of the relationship with the therapist constitute the therapeutic alliance (Gill 1982)—the awareness that both parties are joining together in an attempt to help the patient. In successful therapies, this relationship becomes a very important part of the patient's life, and the patient's wish to maintain it becomes one of his or her motivations to work within the treatment frame.

Questions about the therapeutic alliance inevitably arise: What is the importance of the early treatment alliance in the long-term treatment of borderline patients in terms of process and outcome? What is the nature or character of the therapeutic alliance in TFP compared with that in supportive treatment or cognitive-behavioral treatment? How are threats to the alliance handled in TFP? In the psychoanalytic literature the working relationship or therapeutic alliance is described as the relationship between the therapist in role and the patient's observing ego. The working alliance is therefore the collaboration between the therapist and the healthy part of the patient—the part that can join the therapist in observing and reflecting. At the start of therapy, this part of the patient's psychological makeup may be small and fragile in contrast to the floods of affect the patient experiences. Therefore, our interpretive approach begins with attention to the experience shared between patient and therapist. Use of this interactive process depends on the capacity of the patient to trust someone without excessive idealization, which is a particular challenge for borderline patients. The working alliance must be distinguished from an idealization that leads the patient to see the therapist as a magic healer and the derivatives of this in early manifestations of a positive transference; as therapy proceeds, the alliance overlaps more and more with a positive transference.

Certain personality characteristics complicate the patient's ability to engage in a working treatment alliance. First, the working alliance is limited by antisocial and severely narcissistic personality structures. Antisocial patients experience others as objects to use and exploit, and severely narcissistic patients may respond to others with such intense envy that they tend to attack the envied object rather than engage cooperatively. Second, and more positively, the treatment alliance is promoted by the ability of the patient and the therapist to maintain the relationship even under the stress of aggression, and often in later phases idealized love, from the patient in the transference. Finally, the capacity of the therapist to provide authentic interest in the patient, despite the patient's aggression and possible disagreeableness, is essential to the process. Successful therapists must find something likable in a difficult patient, even if it is based largely on being able to *imagine* the patient better in the future. Nonetheless, often the main contribution to the establishment and strengthening of the therapeutic alliance with these patients depends on the analysis of the manifest and latent negative transference. Because negative assumptions regarding others— such as suspicion, fear, or envy—tend to color borderline patients' experiences of relationships, the most authentic relationship with such a patient will be one that can accept and include those feelings.

The nature of the therapeutic alliance in a specific case is indicated or manifested in seven ways.

1. *The nature of the patient's and the therapist's understanding of the patient's difficulties.* The assessment phase leads to a discussion of the therapist's impression of the nature of the patient's difficulties. Taking into consideration that BPD is a complex phenomenon and often comes with other comorbid conditions, the therapist and patient need to agree that the patient

would benefit from psychological exploration as the focus. What is needed is a minimum joint agreement on the reason for and objectives of the treatment.

2. *The achievement of a relative consensus as to the conditions of treatment.* The contracting process is evidence of the therapist's attention to and interest in the patient. The process is a bid to engage the patient in joint reflection on how to address problem areas. Achieving an adequate degree of consensus is a step in building the alliance.

3. *The nature of both the patient's and the therapist's expectations of the treatment.* These include both the expectation regarding the outcome from treatment and the expectation of what the process of the treatment will be. Questions to consider include these: Does the patient expect the focus of the treatment to be on getting advice and guidance or medication, or do patient and therapist agree that the focus will be on the patient's learning about himself or herself in conjunction with the therapist? Can the therapist visualize this particular patient advancing to a better experience of self and others and a better level of functioning and satisfaction in life?

4. *The affective investment of the therapist in the patient.* The ability of the therapist to engage affectively with the patient may depend on the therapist's ability to imagine that the patient's initially small healthy part can join in the effort to change from internal conflict and chaos to successful integration. The affective investment is largely in what the patient might develop into, in the therapist's realistic hopefulness.

5. *The tolerance of intense affects by both therapist and patient.* Aggressive affects are often more prominent in the initial phase of therapy. The therapeutic relationship must be such that the duo can accept and work with these affects, being open to the expression and experience of intense affects without subtly or overtly backing away from them or acting them out.

6. *The ability of both patient and therapist to meaningfully participate in the dialogue.* This is manifested in the ability of the patient to consider and build on the therapist's interventions. Early in therapy, participation by the patient might be a matter of considering the therapist's way of describing the current interaction and the affect linked to it. In later stages, it involves considering the therapist's interpretations. In a symmetric way, the therapist manifests the ability to listen effectively to the patient, to immerse himself or herself in the affect of the session, and then to coherently elaborate these experiences.

7. *The early approach to diagnosing and resolving manifest negative transference.* Clarifying and tolerating negative affective reactions in the transference may be a dominant way to permit the emergence of whatever potential the patient has for a more trusting relationship.

In-depth exploratory therapy, by its nature, challenges the therapeutic alliance. This is because such therapy questions the patient's current defensive functioning in the process of helping him or her change to a psychological structure—a way of relating to self and the world—that is more adaptive and satisfying. The challenge comes from the fact that patients' initial defensive structure—their way of trying to balance the interface among competing emotions, internal rules, and the pressures of external reality—is the only one they know. Even if this structure is not adaptive in the long run, it provides some relief from anxiety in the short run. For example, splitting *does* provide an order to a person's experience, but it does not fit well with the complexity of the world. New ways of processing one's experience may be more adaptive but will initially be unfamiliar and thus a source of anxiety and subject to doubt. When this general truth about exploratory therapy is combined with the intensity of affects that borderline patients bring to the transference, it is clear that maintaining the therapeutic alliance might require active interpretive intervention from early on.

TESTS OF THE TREATMENT AND FRAME

Patients frequently but not always begin treatment by testing the frame established by the contract, which reflects certain typical dynamics. On one level, this behavior stems from borderline patients' difficulty trusting others. Because they tend not to trust the other to be there for them, they often feel they have to control the other—to take charge—to avoid abandonment and hurt. In more narcissistic and antisocial patients, this might be combined with a pleasure in power. A test of the contract may be a test to see if the patient can control the therapist. A variant of this pattern is the patient who believes that all relationships are based on one person controlling the other, leading to a belief that "If I do not control him, he will control me."

On another level, testing the frame may be the manifestation of a deep-seated, and hidden, wish for the therapist to be strong enough to confront and contain the patient's challenge—that is, for the therapist to care enough to be firm. In the most extreme form, this wish is a manifestation of the primitive desire to find the imagined omnipotent other. It is therefore important for the therapist to make clear that although he or she can do what is possible to maintain the treatment, he or she is not all-powerful and may not be able to successfully fend off all challenges the patient may pose to it.

As an example of testing the treatment frame, we discuss the case of Amy, a patient with low-level BPO, whom we will follow through different phases of treatment (Chapters 8–10).

CLINICAL ILLUSTRATION: AMY

Amy began TFP at age 23, after 7 years of prior treatment for depression, anxiety, and self-destructive and suicidal behaviors. Her diagnoses had included bipolar illness, recurrent major depression, and BPD. At the time of referral, BPD was the primary diagnosis. Prior treatments included supportive psychotherapies, medication (antidepressants, mood stabilizers, anxiolytics, and low-dose neuroleptics), and a number of hospitalizations.

Amy was married and unemployed at the beginning of treatment. She did not work or attend classes because of her fear that others would be critical and rejecting of her. Her prior therapist considered Amy the victim of neglectful parents and offered her extra contact outside of sessions in an attempt to soothe her feelings of loneliness and emptiness. This strategy did not help because Amy's symptoms continued and she was hospitalized after yet another suicide attempt. She was discharged from the hospital to TFP with Dr. Jones. At that point her medications were an SSRI antidepressant, a benzodiazepine, and diphenhydramine for sleep, all at higher than recommended doses. Her medication regimen was reduced over the first months of therapy.

In the discussion of the treatment contract, Amy agreed with some reluctance to the stipulation that she would go to an emergency room (ER) if she could not control her suicidal impulses. A corollary was that if psychiatric hospitalization were recommended, she would accept the recommendation. Dr. Jones was aware of her ambivalence but judged her agreement to be good enough to begin the therapy. Because Dr. Jones considered Amy to be at high risk for suicide, he had included her husband in one of the contracting sessions so that the conditions and realistic expectations of treatment would be clear to him as well.

Two weeks after beginning therapy, Amy took an overdose and was taken by her husband to the local hospital, where she was admitted to a medical floor for observation. The next day, after medical clearance, the hospital's consulting psychiatrist recommended transfer to a psychiatric unit. Amy refused and asked to be discharged. The hospital psychiatrist called Dr. Jones to report that the patient was being discharged against medical advice. Dr. Jones quickly made it clear that he could not accept Amy back into treatment under those conditions because the hospital psychiatrist assessed her as needing a higher level of care. He explained that Amy knew that it was her responsibility within their treatment agreement to accept a recommendation for hospitalization.

The hospital psychiatrist communicated Dr. Jones's comments to Amy, explaining that it would be necessary to arrange a new outpatient treatment. Dr. Jones then received a call from Amy's husband accusing him of unprofessional behavior and of abandoning Amy in her moment of need. The therapist reminded Amy's husband of the understanding in the contract and repeated that his response was based on treatment principles that involved his wife's best interests. The husband, who was calling from Amy's room on the medical ward, put her on the phone.

She proceeded to address Dr. Jones with a combination of entreaty and accusation: "You have to understand—I'm better now. I got it out of my system. You don't know what it's like to be on a psychiatric unit. It's horrible! That will make me want to kill myself.... I knew you would do this to me. You enjoy torturing patients. Just when I was beginning to trust you, you throw me to the wolves!"

The discussion provoked anxiety in Dr. Jones. Although he believed he was taking the correct therapeutic position, he began to feel that he was being harsh, unreasonable, and even sadistic in refusing Amy's pleas to get back into treatment with him without the recommended admission to the psychiatric hospital. However, a quick reflection on his part—a check of his countertransference—reminded him that he was not refusing treatment but rather was offering treatment on the proper terms. He understood that Amy was evoking in him a sense of being harsh and rejecting. He assumed this corresponded to an object representation in Amy's mind that would be important to explore and interpret if she returned to treatment. For now, however, he was attending to the frame.

Dr. Jones repeated his position. Amy repeated her entreaties and accusations. When it was apparent that the discussion was not advancing, Dr. Jones stated that they had both made their positions clear and that it was up to Amy to decide what she would do and then let him know. Internally, he accepted the possibility that she might choose to end the therapy. Later that day he received a message that she had agreed to be transferred to the psychiatric unit and would be returning to therapy with him at discharge.

This was not Amy's last challenge to the frame of treatment, but it did establish that the therapist was capable of maintaining the frame. After such events, it is always important to address the meaning of the challenge to see what can be learned from it. In this case Dr. Jones and Amy went on to explore her intense need to "get her way." Over time, and after observing related material, they came to understand that this need was based, on one level, on the fear that if she did not control the other, then the other would hurt her and, on another level, on the hidden wish to find someone strong enough and concerned enough not to give in to her unhealthy demands and thereby neglect her.

This example is one of many ways that a patient might test the newly established treatment frame. Other typical ways of doing this include frequently missing sessions, not following up on commitments to engage in work or studies, and not complying with attendance at 12-step meetings.

MISSING SESSIONS EARLY IN THE TREATMENT

Some patients agree to the treatment contract but then begin to attend sessions on an irregular basis. This behavior requires the therapist to be active. The therapist generally calls the patient, asking about the absence and reminding him or her of the need for regular sessions for the treatment to have a chance. If the patient expresses reluctance or ambivalence about attending therapy, the therapist makes it clear that the decision is up to the patient but lets the patient know, in a way that offers a bit of psychoeducation and encourages the expression of affect, that sessions are often the most productive when the patient finds them difficult to attend.

BRINGING IMPULSIVE AND SELF-DESTRUCTIVE BEHAVIOR UNDER CONTROL

THREATS OF SUICIDE AND SELF-DESTRUCTIVE BEHAVIOR

The treatment contract describes the responsibilities of patient and therapist with regard to suicidal impulses. The limits of the therapist's responsibility, the extent of the patient's responsibility, and, if relevant, the role of the patient's family with regard to the risk of suicide should have been discussed during the contract setting. If suicidal thoughts or behaviors emerge in the course of the treatment, the therapist should address them as the first priority (see section "Adhering to the Hierarchy of Priorities Regarding Content" in Chapter 7, "Tactics of Treatment and Clinical Challenges"). This may seem obvious, but it should be made clear because a patient may approach his or her suicidal impulses with a dismissive attitude. The therapist must address the issue of self-destructiveness 1) to establish that the patient is dealing with this issue in accordance with the agreement established in the contract and 2) to explore the meaning of the emergence of the issue at this particular point in time.

Even while adhering to the hierarchy of priorities, the therapist must always use his or her best clinical judgment in individual situations. An exception to the rule of always addressing suicidal or self-destructive material first is made when the therapist senses that the patient has realized that bringing up such material can distract the therapist from other material that the patient finds more difficult to deal with. In such an instance, the therapist might say, "I've noticed that whenever the topic of your sense of humiliation regarding your body comes up, you immediately go on to mention suicidal ideation. Could it be that your awareness that I always explore suicidal material as a priority is leading you—consciously or unconsciously—to bring up this topic as a way to avoid dealing with a topic that is more painful to you?"

SETTING PARAMETERS IN THE COURSE OF TREATMENT AND MEDICOLEGAL CONCERNS

If, in the course of treatment, suicidal thoughts and impulses or any other major issue emerges as a new issue in a case, the therapist must take time to add to the treatment contract an understanding of how these matters will be dealt with. In addition to clinical considerations, medicolegal concerns—such as the threat that the patient or the patient's family will sue the therapist if the patient injures or kills himself or herself—add to the complexity of dealing with suicidal patients. The therapist should not hesitate to address these concerns directly, because they are part of the real context of the treatment and touch on the central principle of working in a context where the therapist can maintain a position of feeling safe to be able to think clearly. Not only does the therapist have a right to be concerned about the risk of legal action but the treatment requires that this risk be addressed so that the therapist does not feel constrained or blackmailed in carrying out his or her role. If it is not addressed, anxiety about potential legal action can lead the therapist to attempt to deflect the negative transference away from himself or herself or can otherwise lead to abandonment of the exploratory task. Once the issue has been addressed, the therapist can then proceed to explore the transference meaning of the sense of threat to the therapist that has emerged.

The position described here vis-à-vis suicidality differs from a medical model approach to issues of responsibility in the treatment in which a professional who has accepted a patient into his or her care takes responsibility to save that person, while the patient is seen as the passive recipient of treatment.[1] The TFP position differs from this model for two reasons:

1. The medical model does not take into account the fact that patients with BPD may put themselves at risk to provoke the therapist to become more involved in their lives—to extend himself or herself beyond the frame of the therapy in terms of both time and emotional involvement (the issue of secondary gain). A more informed point of view with regard to the responsibility of the therapist in the psychodynamic treatment of a borderline patient takes into account both the need for the therapist to define his or her role as one of reflection rather than action and the need for treatment arrangements that do not feed into a cycle whereby the therapist's response to acting-out behaviors provides gratifications that lead to perpetuating or escalating the acting out.
2. The medical model fosters ongoing dependency of the patient on the therapist (therapy as a crutch), whereas TFP fosters the development of autonomy in the patient.

---

[1]Even this medical model, as described here, does not apply in most medical interactions—short of a patient's being unconscious or under anesthesia—because the patient's active cooperation with treatment recommendations is important in most treatment situations.

The TFP therapist would not be shirking his or her legal and ethical responsibilities by adhering to the contract. The treatment has built-in safeguards in the form of 1) advance planning for how both therapist and patient will respond to the patient's suicidal impulses, 2) emphasis on the quality of communication between patient and therapist, and 3) placing a high priority on addressing suicidality when it is an issue.

NONLETHAL SELF-DESTRUCTIVENESS

Patients with BPD often present with parasuicidal behaviors that are self-destructive without being lethal, such as superficial cutting or "mini" over-doses. Therapists often are uncertain of how to consider these behaviors: From a dynamic point of view, are they the same as suicidal behaviors? From a practical point of view, should the same conditions of therapy hold for these behaviors as for behaviors with a clear lethal potential? The following is a typical reaction from a therapist struggling with appropriate limit setting: "I can understand the need for the patient to go to an ER if she is at risk of killing herself, but is that necessary if she is dealing with an urge to inflict a superficial cut?"

It is helpful to remember that a principal rationale of limit setting is to keep the patient's affects within the treatment setting rather than permitting them to be discharged through acting out. Therefore, the main question is "What will the impact of the nonlethal self-destructive behaviors be on the work of the therapy?" Exploratory therapy is based on the principle of allowing the patient to communicate, to discover, and to examine his or her own story, with the help of the therapist, to move beyond defensive obstacles to understanding. The therapy leads to new understanding and a more coherent narrative of the self. Yet this process can threaten a patient's current psychological equilibrium, as maladaptive as that equilibrium may be. Consequently, patients may act in ways that take attention away from the mutual effort to understand—acting out as a form of resistance to exploration. It is unreasonable to expect that a therapist will discern in advance all the possible resistances that a particular patient may bring into the treatment. It is also possible that a patient may develop new behaviors as resistances to exploration in the course of therapy. Therefore, the therapist should continue to watch for such developments and be prepared to introduce new parameters as needed at any point in the treatment. With regard to self-harm, it may take time for the therapist to know whether the patient cuts because it is a learned behavior for coping with anger, an enactment of an internalized object relationship involving trauma and including an identification with both perpetrator and victim, an attempt to influence the therapist or make him squirm, or some combination of all of these.

With regard to nonlethal self-destructive behaviors in general, the main consideration is the degree to which these behaviors are likely to undermine the exploratory therapy. Some cases, such as the following, are relatively straightforward.

CASE EXAMPLE

A young woman's prior therapy of 3 years had been characterized by her repeatedly cutting and burning herself to the extent that her therapist's role was largely confined to monitoring the degree of these behaviors and evaluating her condition to determine whether it was necessary for her to seek medical treatment or be admitted to a hospital. In this case the new therapist outlined her position:

Therapist: Your prior therapy was rendered ineffective by your cutting and burning, which became the focus of the work and made it impossible to use the sessions to explore your feelings and conflicts and to advance. Your behaviors led your therapist on an endless chase after your self-destructive actions. These behaviors may have inhibited your therapist from actively pursuing the work of exploration because it sounds as if she was afraid that you would hurt yourself if she said the wrong thing. I would like to emphasize that as your therapist I am interested in your actions and symptoms primarily to the extent that looking at them will help us understand more about you and will help you get beyond them. If you continue to engage in self-destructive behaviors without any improvement while in therapy, I would wonder if this was your way of communicating that you are not interested in this type of exploration and of effectively ending the treatment. If so, case management would be more appropriate because that type of treatment would focus on these symptomatic actions and behaviors themselves—and we can arrange for that, if you think it would be best. However, the fact that you are here for an evaluation is a sign that part of you is interested in exploring your actions and getting beyond them. To think about and explore them, we need to be free of the preoccupation that you might be inflicting tissue damage and might be inhibiting the exploratory work here, as happened before. Therefore, I would recommend that you take some time to think about the kind of treatment you are interested in before signing on here.

In this discussion the therapist appeals to the patient's interest in changing from engaging in self-destructive behaviors to attempting to understand what lies behind them. Many patients protest, claiming that they have no control over self-destructive behaviors. However, extensive clinical experience shows that most patients are able to control urges to some degree when encouraged to do so.

In some cases, this discussion and the patient's efforts suffice to put an end to the self-destructive behaviors. However, in many cases, the patient's acting out reappears at some point in early treatment. Any such instance is explored in terms of the patient's affects, relation to self, and relation to others, such as the therapist. Moments of acting out do not in themselves signal stalemate or failure if there is a pattern of decreased frequency and intensity over time. However, if there is no decrease during the first 3–6 months, the therapist should discuss with the patient whether a more behaviorally or pharmacologically oriented treatment would be preferable at that point or, if the patient continues to express motivation for exploratory therapy, what additional parameters might help the patient engage better in the treatment.

In some extreme situations, therapists might find themselves working with a patient who seems to create a situation of brinksmanship in the form of continuing to act out until the therapist questions the viability of the treatment and then exhibiting control for a period of time only to return to the acting out. In patients with strong aggression, this could represent the chronic enactment of a sadomasochistic relationship that can be interpreted. Some patients act in a way that pushes the therapist to be tempted to set an ultimatum (e.g., "If you burn yourself one more time, it will mean the end of the therapy"). In such cases, it is important to make it clear to the patient that the therapist's thinking is informed by a *pattern* over time and that the patient's provoking an ultimatum likely represents an aggression to both himself or herself and the therapist in combination with an effort to have a sense of control that would be concordant with a paranoid or antisocial transference.

Some forms of minor self-harming behavior may be controlled by setting a parameter in the contract specifying that each time the patient cuts or hurts himself or herself, he or she needs to be examined by an internist or general practitioner to check for the need for wound care before returning to outpatient therapy. The objectives are to make it clear that self-injurious behavior is outside the realm of TFP, to ensure the patient's safety, and to provide the time and space to interpret the meaning of the behavior as well as the meaning in the transference of having to establish a parameter. The question of whether to adopt this position depends mostly on the underlying principle that the therapist should establish conditions that allow him or her to think and reflect. Therapists who are more disturbed by minor cutting or other nonlethal forms of acting out may wish to adopt this parameter.

AFFECT STORMS AND THEIR TRANSFORMATION INTO DOMINANT OBJECT RELATIONS

OVERT AFFECT STORMS

Affect storms are bursts of intense affect. Two types occur in the treatment of patients with BPO (Kernberg 2004). First, there are open, blatant affect explosions in the session, as seen in Video 3. These affect storms usually have an intensely aggressive and demanding quality, but they can also contain a sexualized quality. The patient seems driven to action under the power of intense affective experience that is difficult to reflect on. In fact, the capacity for self-reflection and communication of internal states appears to be all but eliminated in these storms.

▶ **Video 3–1: Affect Storm Part 1 (9:28)**

▶ **Video 3–2: Affect Storm Part 2 (9:26)**

▶ **Video 3–3: Affect Storm Part 3 (10:10)**

SILENT AFFECT STORMS

The second type of affect storm involves patients who demonstrate rigid, repetitive behavior characterized by a flat, monotonous affective tone that serves to stifle affect. It is as if the patient is only partially alive, and the therapist can feel bored or indifferent or even become enraged by the futility of the situation. Recognizing the monotonous affective tone and tedious content of the communication from the patient as the communication of a certain dominant relationship theme, the therapist may interpret the situation and find that the patient responds with an intense affect that the monotonous control had defended against and masked.

INTERVENTION IN AFFECT STORMS

During affect storms the patient may not be able to accept any interpretation from the therapist, perceiving any such intervention as an assault, which results in inflammation of the situation. What is called for here is first an emphasis on the therapist's ability to contain the affect—to sit with it without avoiding it—and then what Steiner (1993) described as an *object-centered* interpretation. This involves the therapist's describing in detail the patient's apparent perception of the therapist without either accepting that perception or rejecting it (e.g., "I see how it can be frustrating coming back again and again to someone who seems totally lacking in empathy"; "So right now I'm being harshly critical of you?"). This careful articulation of the patient's experience of the therapist without yet suggesting that what is being discussed is an element of the patient's internal world allows the patient to gradually tolerate what is being projected, to consider it, and to accept it as "in the room," clarifying the nature of what is projected and eventually linking it to the patient and interpreting the reason for its being projected.

During the patient's intense affective arousal and outburst, the therapist's affective state—not only the content of his or her statements—is an important part of interventions. Interventions made with a wooden, flat, unresponsive tone usually inflame an ongoing affect storm. Such an affective demeanor on the therapist's part could convey that he or she does not understand the patient, is detached and contemptuous of the patient's loss of affective control, or is terrified and paralyzed by the patient's feelings and behavior. As described in Chapter 7, the therapist must engage the patient at an affective level that communicates affective involvement in the situation with the patient yet manages to contain the affect of the patient.

With an appropriate affective response, the therapist can gradually interpret the dominant object relations from surface to depth, starting with the patient's conscious experience and proceeding to the unconscious, dissociated, repressed, or projected aspects of the patient's experience and the motivations for defending against it. This process of affective engagement and gradual interpretation transforms the affect storm, characterized by a flood of affective intensity, into a reflective experience in which the patient's affect and cognition become connected by the clarification of the object relations dyad that underlay the storm.

LIFE OUTSIDE THE THERAPY HOURS

Many patients come to treatment both in a state of chronic symptomatic distress and without any structured involvement in study or work in their daily lives. Clinical experience has shown that participating in therapy without engaging in any meaningful life activity is generally a fruitless process. The therapist should explain to the patient that gradually assuming a study or work role in daily life is an essential part of treatment (see Chapter 5, "Establishing the Treatment Frame"). Some patients have not worked for a long time, if ever, and have received little professional or vocational training. Others, however, have extensive professional training but have not worked because of their symptoms and difficulties with interpersonal relations. Therefore, the level of engagement in structured activity can vary from attending a day hospital for the most impaired patients to starting a paid job for the more skilled. In the early phase of therapy, it is important to discuss the anxieties and problems that arise in the work setting along with exploring transference issues; the two often overlap. The therapist should periodically inquire as to the state of the patient's activities outside of therapy if the patient does not bring up that material. In some cases, the patient may be compliant in sessions but act out aspects of his or her pathology in the workplace. An example is a patient with combined BPD and narcissistic personality disorder who appeared reflective about issues in his sessions but who continued to act in a haughty and arrogant way at work. It was only after the patient lost his job that the therapist learned about the latter problem. The therapist then understood that she had been lulled into listening to the patient in an attentive and even admiring way—thus gratifying some aspects of the patient's narcissism—while the patient continued to act out narcissistic dynamics in a way that was destructive to his career.

PROGRESSION OF A SESSION IN THE EARLY TREATMENT PHASE

TFP is a principle-driven treatment, based on the concept that the patient's dominant internal object relations will unfold in an appropriately defined treatment setting. In contrast to treatments that describe the therapist's agenda for each session, in TFP the therapist is silent at the beginning of the session and waits for the patient to start with what is on his or her mind. The initial treatment contract includes the instruction for the patient to talk about current problems and preoccupations and, if none are pressing, to say whatever comes to mind. Once this instruction, which defines the reality of the treatment relationship, has been given, the therapist assesses the extent to which the patient carries it out. Patients will follow the instruction to varying degrees; any deviation from this basic rule of therapy can be explored in terms of transference analysis—understanding the patient's experience of himself or herself in relation to the therapist that is motivating the deviation (e.g., expecting that the therapist will be sharply critical of anything the patient says or waiting for the therapist to dispense magic).

The following example provides an illustration of an early treatment session and is an example of the principle that an affect is a manifestation of an underlying object relation.

CASE EXAMPLE

Greg entered therapy with a diagnosis of high-level BPD at age 35 after a suicide attempt. He held a steady job and had a set of friends. However, he was chronically depressed and could not establish a love relationship. After the evaluation and contracting sessions, Greg began the first therapy session almost mute. After long silences, he repeated phrases such as "My life is miserable." His therapist, Ms. Ot, entered into the process of clarification with questions such as "What's making your life miserable right now?" After a number of minutes, Greg responded, "What I haven't achieved" and fell silent again. Although this statement may appear minor, it signaled the introduction of internal conflict into the dialogue. Greg's earlier statements ("My life is miserable") described a state. The comment about not achieving implies two parties: a judge of what should be achieved and the recipient of the judgment. Ms. Ot continued with the clarification process, inquiring about what Greg felt he should have achieved. He said he liked to paint but felt a failure at that. With further inquiry, Ms. Ot learned that Greg was very interested in a specific type of painting, nineteenth-century academic style, a type of painting that requires training in technique. However, Greg had never taken any courses in technique in the 15 years that he attempted to paint in that style. Ms. Ot saw this as a contradiction and wondered if it represented a way Greg related to himself: that he neglected or even frustrated his own desires, a relation to self that might well lead to depressed affect. She verbalized this thought to him with a combination of confrontation, asking him to reflect on the apparent contradiction of having an interest and not attending to it, and an early step of interpretation, verbalizing the relation to self she thought that the contradiction implied.

At that point in the session, Greg became visibly anxious; he had difficulty speaking but managed to say, in a halting way, that he was having trouble breathing. Ms. Ot asked if this happened often. Greg shook his head "no," saying he was feeling very anxious. Ms. Ot pointed out that anxiety is generally related to fear and asked Greg if he were afraid of something in the moment. He again shook his head "no." Ms. Ot then formulated a hypothesis about their interaction and began an interpretive process: "I wonder if something in the interaction with me might have affected how you feel. I asked you a number of questions over the past 10 minutes and you may have experienced them as criticism." Greg said "No," but he started to become less anxious. Ms. Ot pointed out that while he was disagreeing, his state appeared to be changing for the better. She then elaborated the transference interpretation corresponding to the first strategy with some advance to the second strategy:[2] "It could be that as you heard my questions, you felt you were being subjected to criticism. In addition, my comments speculated that you treat yourself badly. So your anxious reaction may have reflected not only an experience of criticism from me but also a moment of awareness that you have a harsh part in yourself that treats you badly. That awareness could be very disturbing—and it is interesting that your anxiety has gone away as you've listened to me discuss these possibilities." Greg went on to consider the hypothesis.

---

[2]This example does not present the second strategy (a reversal of roles within the dyad) but does show a description of the patient's identification with both poles of the dyad.

This example illustrates the early emphasis on clarification of internal states and how it can lead to employing the first treatment strategy. Even though this was a good start to the therapy, the case continued for a number of years. The second year of treatment was characterized by an important reversal within the dyad during which Greg became harshly critical of everything about Ms. Ot. During that phase, Ms. Ot was then able to see the grandiose narcissistic structure behind Greg's chronic depressed affect. He harbored harsh primitive superego elements that condemned himself but, when turned outward, provided him a solace in positioning him as superior to a world he devalued.

In a certain sense, then, the patient sets the agenda. However, although the initiation of the session and the content of the session are introduced by the patient, the therapist then begins to address resistance, if present, and to focus on the most central theme(s) that have emerged as affectively dominant. The therapist's chosen theme(s) may or may not be what the patient is directly discussing because often the most important information is communicated through nonverbal channels, especially at the beginning of treatment. For example, a patient may be talking at length about a problem at work, but rather than comment on the content of the patient's discourse, the therapist might say, "I hear what you are saying, but you seem to be talking about the work issue in a monotonous way without a great deal of affect. On the other hand, there seems to be a lot of feeling in the intense way you are looking at me, as though you are scrutinizing me for any hint of how I may be reacting to what you are saying. It might be helpful to think about that."

Although the general rule is that the therapist should not initiate the first topic, he or she may have an idea of things that must be discussed in the course of the session according to affective dominance and urgent priorities (see Chapter 7)—for example, if a patient left a message between sessions suggesting that she was unable to control herself and needed to go to the ER, or if the patient ended the prior session with a statement about something that, if left unexamined, would threaten the continuation of the therapy. Even under these circumstances the therapist waits to see what material the patient will introduce at the beginning of the session. If a patient begins the session with no mention of the important material she had previously introduced and left unresolved, the therapist should seek clarification and confront the patient about the meaning of her behavior: "Last time, just as you were leaving, you mentioned that you had lost your job and didn't know how you were going to be able to continue to pay for therapy. Today, you've begun the session with no reference to that. This affects whether we can continue to work together, so I'd like to hear more about it. I'm also curious about the fact that you introduced this and yet are continuing as if nothing happened, and about what *that* means."

Another reason to let the patient speak first even when the therapist intends to bring up material is because the patient may have a more urgent issue to present. Even though we follow the customary practice in psychodynamic therapy of letting the patient speak first, many psychodynamic therapists are surprised to see both 1) how quickly the TFP therapist may begin to intervene in the session and 2) how much the TFP therapist contributes to the dialogue. The reason for participating more actively than is usual for psychodynamic therapists treating nonborderline patients is that in the early phase of treatment of borderline patients, the most important material is not as much what the patient says as the discrepancies between the channels of communication; splitting keeps the various aspects of the patient's personality apart. The therapist's effort is to link what is being communicated verbally with parts of the personality that are being communicated through the other channels. In addition, patients often tend to discuss relatively trivial material because the more important material can be very disturbing. A principal task of the therapist in the early and middle phases of treatment is to refocus discussion on the most important issues: "Your conflicts with your sister are important, but just last week you were experiencing strong suicidal urges again, and we have not yet understood what was underlying them. It may be that what you're saying now is related to that issue, but I'm bringing this question up because I have the impression you might be more comfortable not thinking about the suicidal urges until they take you by surprise again."

ENDING A SESSION

In general, it is advisable not to bring up new material at the end of a session or to offer interpretations when time does not permit the therapist to follow them up with exploration of the patient's reactions to them or to their accuracy or appropriate level of depth. Moreover, the patient needs time at the end of a session to integrate what has already been presented. The end of a session will often provide important clues about the patient's attitudes toward leaving the therapist and, more broadly, toward handling issues of separation and loss.

Whenever possible, the therapist should end a session at the agreed-on time. However, the exquisite sensitivity to loss experienced by patients with BPD often expresses itself in efforts to extend sessions, with behavior ranging from bringing up new material to literally refusing to leave. For example, a patient may wait until the end of a session to announce a particularly potent issue, one that might threaten the continuity of the treatment. The therapist may then feel that there is no choice but to deal with the matter at the moment.

CASE EXAMPLE

A patient announced at the end of the session that she had decided to take a 3-week trip with an old boyfriend with whom she used to use drugs. The therapist, feeling that this would be a threat to the patient's well-being and to the treatment, said, "Because you've waited until the end of the session to tell me this, we weren't able to discuss it during our regular time. Taking 3 weeks off with this man, without prior discussion, threatens your sobriety and our work together. I suggest that we continue this session long enough to understand something about this. We can discuss later how to handle the arrangements related to the additional time at the end of this session."

The therapist then explored 1) whether the patient waited until the end of the session because she was trying to avoid the awareness, which would inevitably come with discussion, that this was a dangerous plan and 2) whether she waited until the end to see how the therapist would react, especially to see if he would seem indifferent and end the session at the appointed time or take action in response to what she said.

This example illustrates the complexity of therapy. On the basis of a statement by the patient at the end of the session, the therapist's reaction included a countertransference reaction ("This is destructive, and she should not do it"), attention to the hierarchy of priorities (threat to self and to the treatment), the decision to deviate from the frame by extending the session, and the decision (which followed as the discussion went on) about whether or not to deviate from neutrality and state a position about the patient's plan.

CLINICAL ILLUSTRATIONS OF EARLY SESSIONS

In the following illustration, we return to the case of Amy, the patient with low-level BPO who was introduced earlier in this chapter (see "Tests of the Treatment and Frame").

CLINICAL ILLUSTRATION: AMY

Amy's initial response/transference to her new therapist was to experience him as a cold, uncaring robot. The trigger for this was the therapist's beginning the treatment with more emphasis on the treatment frame than had existed in Amy's prior therapy. One element of this frame was that phone contact between sessions was limited to calling about practical arrangements or true emergencies (which referred to unusual stressful events, in contrast to Amy's chronic distress, chaos, and wish for immediate but fleeting support). Dr. Jones attempted to work on helping Amy see that her negative perception of and response to the treatment frame might provide valuable information about her tendency to experience herself as the object of the uncaring neglect of others and to use this observation of her automatic negative perception to more accurately appraise her encounters with others, including considering the possibility that she may perceive in others dissociated aspects of herself. However, as can happen, the patient's affective experience temporarily took precedence over her ability to understand, appreciate, and apply the ideas being discussed. The negative images from her internal world flooded the treatment situation, as is common: the patient's projection became *her* reality. The first step in working with this requires that the therapist calmly contain the affects evoked. In sessions Amy began to report thoughts about dangerous acting out. Dr. Jones experienced anxiety and discomfort as he listened to these reports, but Amy maintained a calm, almost indifferent, tone.

Dr. Jones hypothesized that this part of their interaction might be an expression in action of another set of internal representations of self and other: in addition to the neglected-neglector dyad, the patient's internal world seemed to be populated by a persecutor-victim dyad, and the therapist experienced himself as the victim of Amy's cool but frightening discourse. He attempted to engage her attention in considering the possible impact on him of her apparently carefree urges to hurt herself. He wondered whether, in addition to the internal relief that she reported from harming herself, there might be an interpersonal element, such as 1) trying to engage more active involvement from him, 2) trying to show that she was stronger than he, 3) getting some gratification from the discomfort her destructiveness could evoke in him, or 4) some combination of these three.

However, Amy's reports of urges to hurt herself increased to the point that she went to the ER one evening. Because the ER staff was familiar with her capacity for self-destructive behavior, they placed her on "one-to-one observation" with a security guard. In that setting, she took a razor blade she had hidden and cut both wrists without the guard's immediate notice. She was then hospitalized.

Dr. Jones arranged a session with Amy in the hospital. His focus in that session was on understanding Amy's experience rather than more directly changing her behavior. As she narrated the events leading to the hospitalization, Amy described her being able to cut herself in the presence of the guard with a visible pleasure, seeming to enjoy the fact that she could outwit him and make him look incompetent and foolish. Dr. Jones stopped Amy at that point in her narrative and inquired what she thought about her affect. She seemed confused and asked what he meant. He asked if she might agree that she expressed some pleasure in her telling of the story. Amy responded with indignation, accusing him of labeling her a sadist and angrily denouncing him for cruelty for suggesting such a thing. Dr. Jones observed Amy's discomfort with the term *sadist*, which she had introduced, and observed that she seemed to find it difficult to consider that she might experience some pleasure in aggressive impulses. He pointed out that she had used the term *sadist*—a noun that would define her—and suggested that this all-or-nothing way of thinking might make it difficult to consider that within a more complex self, she might experience a measure of sadistic feelings, as many people do. This way of portraying Amy's experience spoke to BPD patients' tendency to experience whatever part of them that is active in the moment as the totality of who they are. This inability to situate one or another element of who they are in a broader context of sense of self stems from the dissociative defensive system. Dr. Jones's comments were an attempt to engage awareness of the broader whole.

Amy remained angry and said she was not sure she wanted to continue the therapy. Dr. Jones suggested she reflect on the issue. Amy told him in the next session that she had decided to continue. In the therapy sessions after discharge, the focus continued to be an exploration of her relationship to her aggressive side—often an essential part of the change process in therapy. She came to understand that those aggressive emotions constituted a part of her that she had always been very uncomfortable acknowledging. She had typically dealt with them in one of two ways. Most often, she confused the source of the aggressive affect in a relationship and experienced it as present in others rather than in herself, as she had done in accusing Dr. Jones of cruelty in talking about the gratification she could get from being aggressive. This type of projection of aggressive affects was behind her anxiety in relation to working, studying, or otherwise interacting with others whom she tended automatically to see as aggressive. The second way Amy dealt with aggressive affects was to put them into action without a conscious awareness of the aggression involved; for instance, although she was very sensitive to and objected to any display of aggression on the part of others (e.g., boys "roughhousing" in the park), she did not consider that there was any aggression—either to herself or to those who cared about her—in her cutting or otherwise harming herself.

This discussion of Amy's relation to her aggressive affects appeared to help her acknowledge and begin to integrate this part of herself that she had typically experienced as part of a relationship rather than part of her. In other words, one aspect of her experience of self had traditionally been that of the victim of others' judgments, criticisms, and aggression. This view of self and other existed *within* her and guided her perception of herself in relation to others in the world and also guided her behavior in relation to others. She was wary and avoidant, anticipating negative responses. Nevertheless, she also identified with the persecutor side of the victim-persecutor relationship dyad, enacting the persecutor 1) in relation to herself by means of judgments, criticisms, and at times self-destructive actions, and 2) in her relation to others as seen in the example in the ER and in her tendency to cause pain in others through her attacks on herself.

Dr. Jones's interventions succeeded in getting Amy to begin to know and symbolically represent and reflect on her aggressive affects and had a positive impact in reducing her self-destructive acting out in that she stopped self-cutting and overdosing, her two most dramatic symptoms for many years. However, even without those dramatic problems, she continued to experience difficulties in her life, especially in the form of anxiety in relation to others. In accordance with the treatment contract, Amy began to attend college courses to complete her undergraduate degree. At this stage, the most common theme in sessions became her conviction that the other students disliked and disapproved of her. She also had associated symptoms of anxiety and depressive affect. Amy was diagnosed as low-level BPO because of her level of aggression. We will continue with this example in Chapter 9, "Midphase of Treatment."

The following case illustrates an early session with Betty, a high-level BPO patient whose history is presented in Chapter 4. (A modified session can be seen in Video 2.)

 Video 2–1: Prevacation Session Part 1 (9:24)

 Video 2–2: Prevacation Session Part 2 (6:12)

CLINICAL ILLUSTRATION: BETTY

Betty started therapy in a dramatic fashion. She walked into the first consultation session complaining vociferously about a woman on the subway before she even sat down or gave her therapist, Dr. Em, the chance to introduce himself: "That woman was looking right at me—I could tell she hated me, so I looked right back and showed her I hated her too."

Dr. Em had to talk over Betty to remind her that this was a consultation session and that he could not address a specific problem with her because he had not discussed the nature of her condition or agreed on an approach to treatment. Betty's level of animated discussion and her lack of meaningful contact with Dr. Em helped him understand why Betty had been diagnosed with bipolar disorder for many years. She was 33 years old and had been in treatment since age 16. In addition to bipolar disorder, she had been treated for major depressive disorder. She had been hospitalized twice for overdoses. One hospitalization included a course of electroconvulsive therapy. Her therapies had been supportive in nature—a combination of medication and help with interpersonal difficulties and life decisions. Her medications had included alprazolam, sertraline, clonazepam, risperidone, paroxetine, and lithium. She was taking a mood stabilizer when she began TFP. By the end of the first year of TFP, she was taking only an as-needed dose of risperidone 0.25 mg, up to twice daily, which helped her when she became agitated because of her paranoid fears.

In spite of her years of treatment, Betty's condition and situation in life had worsened over time. Although she was trained in a technical field, she had been unemployed for the past year after having been fired from a string of jobs over a number of years. She blamed her firings on prejudice against her because she was not as cute as the "perky blondes," as she described them, who she felt were always treated better than she was.

It was difficult for Dr. Em to conduct the usual structural interview because of Betty's communication style. His efforts were severely limited by her ignoring his questions and engaging in a pressured monologue. After completing the evaluation the best he could, Dr. Em presented his understanding that her main problem was BPD with narcissistic features (see Chapter 5 for a review of discussing the diagnosis with the patient). The contracting included parameters regarding suicidal risk, self-destructive behaviors, and the need to find a structured activity. After initially protesting against the latter idea, Betty reported the next week that she had found a half-time volunteer position in a social service center. When therapy per se began, Betty continued as she had started, flooding Dr. Em with a torrent of discourse. Her main theme was that she was constantly neglected and mistreated because blondes got all the attention. She provided one example after another and continually made the point that she could never succeed in life because of the animosity others held toward her. This continued for the first 2 months of therapy.

Dr. Em noted Betty's tendency to control every interaction between them. Although the "basic rule" is for free association, there was the risk that Betty would continue indefinitely with a controlling discourse (channel 1 of communication, as described in Chapter 7) if Dr. Em did not address the style of interaction itself (channel 2 of communication) and the representations of self and other that he perceived behind it and include information from his countertransference (channel 3). His thoughts centered on three things: 1) She was flooding him with material. Was this an implicit request or a demand that he fix or take care of her? 2) However, every time he spoke up, she disregarded him and spoke over him, which suggested that her need to be in control predominated over dependency issues, at least for the moment. 3) His experience was of being mistreated, of being treated rudely and with no consideration, just as Betty complained she was treated by others.

Following the first TFP strategy (described in Chapter 3, "Strategies of Transference-Focused Psychotherapy"), Dr. Em began to name the actors in the interaction. He wondered if she might consider that she was treating him in a devaluing, inconsiderate way. However, she gave no indication of reflecting on what he said. Her typical response was to escalate her examples of how people treated her badly and to suggest that he was just like everyone else because he was not listening to her. As she kept talking over him, Dr. Em felt more sure that, rather than address the content of what Betty was saying, he should focus on her style of interacting (channel 2 of communication) and the defense it represented.

Dr. Em: Would you agree that you are speaking in a way that makes it difficult for me to participate in the dialogue?

Betty: You told me to say everything that's on my mind—are you contradicting yourself now?

Dr. Em: That's correct; I did say that. However, I also mentioned that part of my role in therapy would be to contribute any ideas I might have, and it's been difficult to do that.

Betty: What have you got to say?

Dr. Em: Sometimes the most important thing to think about is how a person is communicating, how the person is saying things—how the person is interacting. Your way of talking without stopping may reflect something important in terms of how you feel in relation to me.

Betty: Like what?

Dr. Em: Not leaving me room to talk may serve the purpose of "pinning me down," of keeping me in a particular place that you control.

Betty (*with an abrupt change of affect, bursting into tears*): If I didn't control you, you'd leave me, like everyone else.

This exchange began to shed light on Betty's use of omnipotent control. This defense is a logical extension of the splitting at the base of the paranoid schizoid position. If a person unconsciously splits off and projects the negative and aggressive segment of his or her internal world, it follows that others carry those affects and present a danger; therefore, they must be controlled for the person to feel safe. The attempts at control can take various forms. Betty's version was to attempt control through a never-ending discourse.

Dr. Em pointed out that Betty's way of interacting did not allow her the possibility to know anything but her preexisting conviction; her assumption determined her experience. By attempting to control the interaction in order to keep Dr. Em, Betty perpetuated the conviction that his own wish was to leave. (Dr. Em deferred discussion of the fact that her controlling behavior contributed to people turning away from her.) This was the first time in therapy that the discussion shifted from Betty's repeated stories of mistreatment. For the first time she appeared interested in Dr. Em's comments. Therefore, he went on to point out that because she was relating to him as she believed him to be, she was remaining indifferent to him as an independent and separate person; her monopolizing the interaction did not allow him to be in the room as anything but the person she imagined. He existed there like a two-dimensional cardboard cutout that she controlled. He wondered if this attitude toward him, an attitude that may well apply to others in her life, interfered with establishing relations. At that point there seemed to be a dialogue in the room. Betty became calmer and could reflect on her way of not allowing him to exist in the room because of her fear that he would leave if she left him to his own devices. As the discussion continued, it became clear that this strategy of hers left her alone, a condition for which she had blamed others.

After this productive session, Betty returned to treatment with much the same style of interaction that she had presented from the beginning. Dr. Em had to return repeatedly to the interpretation of her omnipotent control and the fear it represented. It was only after discussing this interpretation many times, in the context of the therapeutic relationship where Betty allowed herself to sense Dr. Em's interest in her—a feeling that evoked anxiety in her, as we will see later—that Betty's behavior began to change. Her capacity to "let Dr. Em exist" and to listen to him increased. We will return to this case in Chapter 9.

Key Clinical Concepts

- The therapeutic alliance between the borderline patient and therapist in a long-term treatment involves a developing working relationship in the context of positive and negative transference and the patient's ability to maintain the relationship despite intense affects that emerge in relation to the therapist.

- The therapist's capacity to contain intense affects—to reflect on them without either distancing himself or herself emotionally or reacting or retaliating defensively—is the first essential step in treatment as the therapy begins.

- A goal of the early treatment phase is to bring impulsive and self-destructive behavior under control, including impulses to end the treatment. The parameters established in the treatment contract minimize the secondary gain of acting out and encourage verbal expression over acting out.

- Affect storms, both affect explosions and rigidly controlled affect, must be managed by the therapist in a way that encourages transformation of unmetabolized affect into language through elaborating the patient's experience of self and other that underlie the affect.

- Early treatment often includes a challenge to the treatment contract. Should this occur, the therapist's management of it can provide insight into the patient's dynamics and point the therapy in a productive direction or set the stage for repeated breaks of the frame.

SELECTED READING

LaFarge L: Interpretation and containment. Int J Psychoanal 81:67–84, 2000

9

MIDPHASE OF TREATMENT

Movement Toward Integration With Episodes of Regression

THE PATIENT enters the midphase of treatment when some equilibrium is established, characterized by increased acceptance of the treatment frame and a corresponding decrease in the chaos in the patient's life and intensification of affects in the sessions. The overt behavioral manifestations of conflict and turmoil that may characterize the beginning phase are contained for the most part. Affects, both positive and negative but usually extreme, become more intense in the sessions. The work of deepening the exploration of the transference themes can progress with a diminished threat of treatment dropout or acting-out behavior (although these may recur at times of regression). Time in the sessions alternates between reexperiencing intense conflicts in the relationship with the therapist and mutual exploration of these conflicts, with the goal of increasing the patient's capacity to reflect on his or her internal experience and on its impact on his or her relationship with others outside the sessions.

The intensification of affects in the session may not occur if the patient maintains an idealized and consequently superficial transference, keeping negative affects stably split off and chronically projected on a "bad" object or objects outside the treatment setting. This issue occurs more frequently with more novice therapists who are not comfortable with the negative transference and may enact their countertransference anxiety about this in ways in which the therapist attempts to keep peace and remain "the good guy." However, it is also possible that the negative transference is predominant and that the patient defends against positive affect in the transference. This situation, in fact, is more common because the majority of patients with borderline personality disorder (BPD) are anxious about positive, libidinal affects that do not fit with the insecure internal model of attachment that characterizes almost all patients with this diagnosis. However, a negative transference early in the treatment does not often have the superficial quality of an idealizing transference. In addition to the latter, another stable, but static, scenario that may occur as treatment enters the midphase is that low-grade acting out may continue on a chronic basis, creating a situation in which the patient experiences secondary gain (i.e., a sense of gratification) from being in treatment and wishes to perpetuate it rather than work toward changing.

PRIMARY TASKS OF THE MIDPHASE OF TREATMENT

The primary tasks in the midphase (Table 9–1) begin with deepening the understanding of the split-off representations of self and other that have been named in the dominant transference themes. Therapists must distinguish between two levels of gaining awareness. The first has to do with the interchange of the roles of self and other within a particular dyad (i.e., the oscillation within the dyad that we described in Chapter 3, "Strategies of Transference-Focused Psychotherapy"). The therapist helps the patient observe and reflect on elements of himself or herself that the patient has had difficulty seeing. The second level of gaining awareness has to do with the fundamental split between dyads that are imbued with totally negative and aggressive affects and those imbued with idealized libidinal affects. The eventual integration of these two extreme segments of the patient's internal experience helps increase affect regulation as the extreme and discontinuous parts of the self that contribute to ongoing conflict become mutually toned down and modulated in a more complex whole.

TABLE 9–1. Primary tasks in the midphase of treatment

The patient experiences a deepening awareness and understanding of the self and object representations present in the dominant transference themes, with shorter repetitions of the activation of these dyads in the interaction with the therapist. Repetitious working-through of the dominant transference themes is needed.

The patient begins a gradual and transient integration of the extreme, discontinuous (idealized and persecutory) parts of the self. The patient becomes aware of the split and contradictory nature of experience and aware of the shifts between idealized and persecutory experiences. Therapy brings special attention to one dyad chronically defending against another dyad. There are periodic regressions from the developing integrated structure back to a more split structure.

The patient is better able to observe his or her own mental experience. There are moments of increasing capacity for triangulation of thought and the capacity to appreciate the symbolic nature of thought. This leads to further containment of affect and reduces the overwhelming nature of affective experience.

The further integration of representations and affects of internal object relations enacted in the treatment leads to increasing capacity for taking responsibility for aggression, increasing capacity for repression of object relations that remain more highly charged, consolidation of self representations and object representations with gradual resolution of identity diffusion, and partial working-through of depressive anxieties.

New ways of conceptualizing self and others and behaving in other relationships begin to be applied beyond the transference.

DEEPENING UNDERSTANDING OF THE MAJOR TRANSFERENCE PATTERNS

In Chapter 3 (Table 3–2) we describe typical transference role pairs that are enacted between therapist and patient. Here we describe the way the therapist achieves an overview of how these transference themes appear, are understood, and are interpreted in the midphase. There are times when the themes are obvious and emerge in a way clear to any observer (e.g., the patient may announce the negative transference loud and clear, as in "I don't think you're trying your hardest with me; in fact, I think you intentionally slow things down so I'll keep coming and paying you"). On other occasions, however, the transference themes—the patient's current experience of the therapist or the relationship that he or she may unconsciously be trying to create—are much more subtle and difficult to perceive. However, the therapist's ability to perceive the current transference theme amidst the multiple subjects the patient brings up and the intense affects in sessions is crucial to the practice of transference-focused psychotherapy (TFP). An example of a more subtle transference manifestation is a patient who speaks freely and appears to listen attentively whenever the therapist comments but who then returns to his or her associations with no evidence of having considered what the therapist said. This could be a devaluing or dismissing transference and may be reflective of a grandiosity and avoidance of dependency in the patient. Another example of the patient trying to create a particular relationship with the therapist is a patient who repeatedly describes an urgent problem in his or her life and then falls silent. This could be an attempt to provoke the therapist to become like a hovering parent who swoops in to solve the dependent child's every problem.

There are four basic chronic transference paradigms in the treatment of patients with borderline personality organization (BPO): narcissistic, antisocial, paranoid, and depressive. Any of these basic transference paradigms may be colored by pervasive narcissistic defenses, giving the underlying transference a narcissistic flavor.

Narcissistic transferences are characterized by an incapacity to depend on the therapist, unconscious dismissal of him or her, and more or less overt devaluation of the therapist in an effort to eliminate him or her as an important object who would otherwise be feared and envied. Narcissistic transferences are generally defenses against the deepening of an underlying paranoid or depressive transference. An extreme narcissistic transference may be in the form of either intense devaluing of the therapist or, less frequently, a superficial idealization of the therapist. In the former, the patient treats the therapist with such pervasive devaluation and indifference that it may appear on the surface that there is no transference—that the therapist does not matter enough for the patient to care about. However, this devaluation may, for example, hide the underlying fear and anxiety of a paranoid transference that would emerge if the patient acknowledged any feelings of or wish for dependency. In these cases, narcissistic defenses can be interpreted to reveal the underlying transference. In some cases, the narcissistic defenses remain in place over months. This occurs in narcissistic personality disorder proper, which can range in functioning from higher level to antisocial. In these cases, the priority issue is the continued analysis of the narcissistic defenses. TFP for narcissistic personality disorder is described in detail elsewhere (Diamond et al. 2011; Stern et al. 2013).

Antisocial transferences characterize the lowest levels of personality pathology and appear as frank dishonesty in the patient combined with the expectation, by projection, that the therapist is dishonest and interested only in exploiting the patient. Antisocial transferences are generally dominant in patients with antisocial personality disorder (ASPD). Our structural system of diagnosis reserves the diagnosis of ASPD for patients who have no interest in others except to use and exploit them; these patients are psychopathic. There seems to be no internal split or conflict in them because of the combination of a pathological grandiose self—the underlying structure in common with the narcissistic personality disorder—and a severe or total deterioration or absence of internalized libidinal relationships. Patients with ASPD rarely present for treatment except when they are forced to do so by their family or the legal system. Patients with other severe personality disorders can have antisocial *traits* without an antisocial *transference* because antisocial behaviors—active (assault, theft) or passive (the using of others or the system)—can exist in individuals who do desire relations with others and who thus experience internal conflict. ASPD is usually untreatable. In some cases, however, there is the possibility of working with the antisocial, or psychopathic, transference by attempting to transform it into a paranoid transference, a transference type against which the antisocial transference may defend (Jacobson 1971).

CASE EXAMPLE: ANTISOCIAL TRANSFERENCE

The parents of a 22-year-old man sent him to therapy because his substance abuse, gambling, and writing of bad checks would have led to criminal charges if they had not bailed him out. The patient missed sessions regularly and responded to his therapist's attempts to explore this behavior by saying, "What does it matter to you? My father pays you anyway, and you can spend the time reading the paper." The patient's antisocial transference assumed that the therapist is as corrupt as he is. The therapist responded, "So there are two possibilities. The first [describing the antisocial transference] is that I am as dishonest as you and have no concern about you but only about my income—even though I pretend to hide that. The second possibility is that I keep bringing up your missing sessions because I am concerned about you; this possibility does not seem to cross your mind." This discussion led the patient from his usual calm, untroubled state to a feeling of unease. The world, as he imagined it, consisted only of two groups of people: those who were out to "con" others and their gullible victims. Genuine concern for another did not fit into his system—it was unknown and foreign to him and, therefore, threatening. The patient began to experience a paranoid transference as he became uncomfortable trying to grapple with what the therapist's motives might be if they were not the same as his own.

Paranoid transferences may manifest either as direct paranoid features with fear of harm from the therapist or as chronic masochistic or sadomasochistic transferences. The majority of patients with BPO begin treatment with a predominantly paranoid transference, with the expectation that the patient will be rejected or hurt by the therapist. Paranoid transferences defend both against idealized libidinal transferences, which represent the other side of the split internal world, and against the depressive transferences that therapists hope to see emerge as the process of integrating the split internal structure helps the patient move from the paranoid-schizoid position (projecting aggression) to the depressive position within which the patient is able to recognize the internal origin of the aggressive impulses that previously were projected, to tolerate ambivalent reactions toward objects, and to experience guilt feelings, concerns, and impulses to repair previously damaged relationships. In most cases, the arc of the work in TFP involves helping a patient to evolve from a predominantly paranoid transference to a depressive one and then resolving the latter.

Depressive transferences are characterized by intense guilt over the aggressive impulses that are no longer projected and include the possibility of a negative therapeutic reaction based on guilt and feelings that one is too demanding and not worthy of being helped.

The evolution from paranoid to depressive transference is the major change in TFP. It is accompanied by resolution of the structural characteristics of BPO—that is, identity diffusion and predominant use of primitive defenses. This evolution involves two overall steps. The first step in the transformation, which occurs as the reversals within dyads are observed and discussed, is the gradual acceptance by the patient of his or her identification with the persecutory as well as the persecuted objects within him or her, along with the corresponding hateful and yearning impulses. The second step is the gradual change from split internal representations of persecutory and ideal experiences to integration into a more complex whole as the alternation between opposing dyads is worked through.

STEPS IN INTEGRATING NEGATIVE AFFECT

The treatment of negative affect—including anger, scorn, rage, and hatred—in the transference first involves the patient's gaining awareness and tolerating the experience of the affect. Tolerating negative affects as part of his or her internal world involves the patient's accepting both that these affects are part of the range of human emotions and that these affects not only are experienced as reactions to being treated badly but also exist innately and can be a source of satisfaction in themselves (especially in lower-level BPO). The patient's tolerating negative affects and understanding his or her motivation for having projected them facilitates the integration of these affects with the set of idealized internal self and object representations. Acknowledging what has been projected may be the single most difficult step of the therapeutic process; it can be almost intolerable for some patients to see that these affects are a part of who they are. When this integration takes place, the patient moves toward the depressive position, characterized by concern and guilt with regard to aggressive feelings toward objects who were previously perceived as all bad and who now are seen as a realistic mixture of good and bad qualities.

Therapists who are inexperienced with severe borderline patients often have trouble accepting that patients who behave in angry, spiteful, aggressive, and even hateful ways may not consciously experience the affect of hatred but rather experience their behavior as a natural reaction to present or past injuries, including the therapist's behavior. For example, a patient who threw a coffee maker at her husband calmly reported that she had only reacted normally after he forgot their anniversary. Patients' association of any feelings of hatred and aggression with an external persecutory object perceived as thoroughly bad makes the "owning" of such emotions so distasteful that some patients would literally rather die through a self-destructive enactment than acknowledge the part of themselves that seems similar to that object. For example, after beginning to see the hatred in her self-destructive actions, a patient said, "I'd rather be dead than think I had anything in common with my father who abused me." Her therapist replied, "You've stated the problem very well. But it may be that to have some measure of aggression in you does not make you as extremely violent and abusive as he was." Working with such patients requires an attitude of acceptance of anger and hatred on the part of the therapist as the patient gains awareness of these emotions.

Because conscious awareness of hatred is often split off, a typical pattern in the early phase of treatment is as follows: As the patient describes enactments of hatred or enacts hatred in the sessions, the therapist—in the spirit of delineating self and object representations—identifies a hateful part of the patient as a part of the self that must be addressed, understood, and integrated. The therapist may describe the tyrannical or persecutory quality of this part of the self. Patients often show a moment of awareness but then utilize the therapist's comment in the service of the hateful part in responding, "See, you're telling me I'm bad, that I don't deserve to live. That's what I've been trying to tell you—I should kill myself." In other words, the patient uses the therapist's comments in the service of a hateful attack against the self (and an implicit attack against the therapist as harmful rather than helpful).

The therapist pursues the analysis and deepens it, pointing out that the patient's hateful part is active right in the moment—distorting the therapist's comment, turning it into a global condemnation, and leaving out the fact that the patient is simultaneously victim as well as persecutor within a dyad relationship that exists in its totality within the patient's mind and defines a way in which the patient relates to himself or herself as well as others. Patients, as well as therapists, have difficulty keeping in mind that the patient has an identification with *both* poles of the dyad and that to talk about the patient as persecutor should not imply that the patient is not victim at the same time. The analysis deepens when the therapist suggests possible interpretations of the hatred—that it may be in response to intense envy in patients who feel they lack what others have and/or that it is defending against awareness of an underlying yearning for ideal caring that makes the patient feel vulnerable and thus must be hidden under the anger and hatred that stem from frustration.

Discussing the intolerance of hateful behavior is the first step in facilitating its tolerance and in the patient's eventually daring to acknowledge pleasure in the sadistic aspects of the persecutory internal object. Helping the patient become aware of his or her pleasure in aggressive affects, as they may emerge in behaviors toward the therapist, is an important step in the patient's tolerance of it. By the same token, for the traumatized patient, beginning to see how he or she attributes to the therapist the characteristics of the abusing person is an important first step in the patient's recognition that he or she carries the "aggressor" inside himself or herself along with the persecuted victim. Dealing with themes such as sadistic feelings must be based on the assumption that all humans share powerful unconscious aggressive as well as libidinal affects. Patients with BPD generally feel affect more intensely than those without the disorder, and therapists should focus efforts on helping those patients develop increasing cortical control. Discussions of issues such as sadistic feelings should be carried out in the spirit that these emotions exist along a continuum that includes the therapist rather than to imply that the borderline patient is fundamentally different or flawed.

Acknowledgment of the possibility of sadistic pleasure in interactions enables the patient to come to terms with the double identification as victim and victimizer, particularly under the influence of the patient's developing awareness of attacks on the therapist who has been attempting to help the patient. This awareness gradually leads to the shift from predominantly paranoid transferences to the depressive transferences characterized by guilt and concern, reparative tendencies, tolerance of ambivalence, and strengthening of the capacity for gratitude and subliminatory functioning.

LATENT AGGRESSION, SPLIT-OFF IDEAL IMAGES, AND THE GOAL OF HEALTHY LOVE

The focus on aggression and hatred in this chapter may lead the reader to believe that hatred is always obvious and up front in this phase of the treatment, but this is not always the case. We emphasize the vicissitudes of aggression in this chapter because of their central role in the dynamics of borderline pathology. However, two things must be remembered. First, patients do not always communicate the most primitive level of their internal world in sessions. Trivialization—reporting relatively unimportant, affectively flat material—is common. Once they are working in the treatment frame, some patients split off their primitive affects for periods of time and engage the therapist on a level at which they address problems in their lives with a degree of observing ego. Patients may do so in a therapeutic way that represents the beginning of functioning at a higher level or in a defensive way that dissociates these problems from the underlying primitive organization of their psyche and establishes a more or less comfortable homeostasis that defends against the more primitive issues. The therapist must always determine whether the patient is addressing issues in a reflective way or trivializing in a defensive fashion. (Trivialization is discussed in more detail in Chapter 7, "Tactics of Treatment and Clinical Challenges.")

Second, aggression represents one side of a fundamental intrapsychic split, and on the other side of the split are libidinal longings that can present in the form of an intensely positive transference based on the image of an idealized object relation. This imagined relation—which, like the aggression-laden one, is primitive and not adapted to external reality—is usually defended against in the early phase of treatment. The paranoid transference found in most patients at the beginning of treatment involves a mistrust and suspicion that would make direct expression of libidinal longings a risky proposition. Even so, these longings, rooted in the idealized object relation, are generally manifested to some degree indirectly, if only through the patient's coming to therapy. The extreme nature of this idealized positive transference[1] is as much a part of the patient's pathology as extreme negative transference insofar as it involves a "pure" representation that does not correspond to the

---

[1]The reader is reminded that this distinction between positive transference and negative transference does not equate to a distinction between "good" transference and "bad" transference. The positive transference is so called because it represents libidinal, or loving, strivings. However, in its extreme form in the split psyche, it is as pathological as the extreme negative transference because it represents an ideal, all-good object that does not exist in the real world.

more complex reality of the world. The two must be integrated into a more complex whole to achieve psychological health and the capacity to love maturely. Like the rest of us, patients have the need to love and be loved. We should note that individuals without personality pathology can temporarily regress to a state of idealization in the phase of falling in love experienced as infatuation. The key to a healthy love relation is to then accept and integrate the imperfections of the object of love. TFP works toward this end. As treatment progresses, the positive affects in the transference generally increase, and the work toward integrating the extreme positive and negative poles of the patient's internal world frees him or her to experience love in a mature way that is not disrupted by abrupt swings between idealization and devaluing.

The aggressively invested object relation that is often the dyad seen first in the therapy generally defends against an underlying libidinally invested dyad. The reverse can also be true: a libidinal "ideal" dyad may defend against the persecutory aggressive one. One of the challenges in treating patients with a split internal structure is that either extreme side of the split defends against the other: there is no solid base but rather the constant potential for a rapid reversal from one side of the split to the other. In clinical practice, the paranoid transference and anxiety about attachment generally predominate early in therapy. Even so, some cases begin with an idealized transference that defends against paranoid fears and aggression. In the case of the more typical paranoid transference, libidinal wishes generally begin to surface after this transference has been worked through to some degree, although there may be evidence of these wishes in nonverbal communication or in the countertransference earlier on (an example of this can be seen in Video 2, "Prevacation Session"). The therapist should note any evidence of the positive elements that emerge and keep in mind that in spite of the patient's suspicion and mistrust, the patient is still there ("There's a side of you that wants to keep this relationship alive"). Also, in discussing aggressive affects, the therapist should not so much emphasize the patient's hostility toward him or her ("You're attacking me") as emphasize the dyad that involves a persecutor and a victim ("This relation seems to be characterized right now by someone who is attacking and someone who's the victim of that"). The part of the patient that seems to hate others also hates himself or herself and undermines the patient's capacity for a good, accepting relationship with himself or herself. In general terms, both positive and negative transferences need to be interpreted to avoid the patient dismissing himself or herself as all bad.

▶ **Video 2–1: Prevacation Session Part 1 (9:24)**

▶ **Video 2–2: Prevacation Session Part 2 (6:12)**

RANGE OF SEXUAL RELATIONSHIPS IN PATIENTS WITH BPO

Love and sexuality do not completely overlap. Sexuality combines libidinal elements and aggressive elements and is, to some degree, a crossroads between the two. The development of a mature and intimate sexual life is a goal of TFP, especially in cases where the patient's sexual life has been stunted or overwhelmingly infiltrated with aggression. We examine issues relating to the sexual history and adjustment of the patient and aspects of sexuality as they arise in treatment.

Human sexuality includes core gender identity, gender role identity, object choice, and intensity of sexual desire (Kernberg 1995). The latter two constructs, object choice and intensity of sexual desire, are most relevant in discussing patients with BPO. The object choice of the patient with BPO may, as a consequence of identity diffusion, involve confusion in object choice and chaotic bisexuality on the behavioral level. Intensity of desire may vary widely, with some patients with severe BPO having little desire.

Patients with BPO generally begin treatment within a defined range of pathology in their sexual adjustments, but within that range there is substantial variation (Table 9–2). The patient's level of sexual capacity and adjustment at the beginning of treatment will define areas of potential improvement. Patients with more severe BPO may present with an absence of the capacity for the central pleasures of normal sexuality. These patients may find no pleasure in any sexual outlet, including masturbation, and no sexual desire linked to any individual. A history of severe traumatic experiences and physical or sexual abuse and the absence of any attachment to a loving parental object often dominate their history. With these patients, the goals of treatment in the sexual realm may be limited. Treatment may first help patients to access a capacity for idealization of another and to express their longing for an idealized relationship. With further treatment and integration of the idealized and persecutory images, the patient may be able to establish a committed attachment that involves affection, but this type of patient may show no capacity for passionate love.

Patients with borderline personality organization with a narcissistic personality structure tend to have a capacity for sexual excitement without the capacity for a deep investment in an intimate partner. Many of these in-

TABLE 9–2.   Range of sexual adjustment in patients with borderline personality organization (BPO)

	Adjustment
High-level BPO	Capacity for sexual excitement and desire; fragile idealizing relationships with part-objects
BPO with narcissistic personality	Capacity for sexual excitement and orgasm; broad spectrum of infantile trends; no capacity for deep investment in love object
BPO with aggression	Dangerous sexual behavior; polymorphous perverse sexuality
Low-level BPO	Absence of sensual pleasure; no pleasure in masturbation; no sexual desire linked to any object; no capacity for sexual excitement

dividuals have never been in love. The notable sexual promiscuity of these individuals is often linked with sexual desire and excitement for a person who is considered by others to be attractive or valuable. With this type of attachment, sexual fulfillment may gratify the need for conquest but may also trigger the unconscious process of needing to feel superior and to devalue the other, resulting in a disappearance of both sexual excitement and interest in the other person.

Patients at the higher end of BPO may begin treatment with the capacity for sexual excitement and erotic desires. These patients may have the full capacity for genital excitement and orgasm linked with a passionate commitment to another. They are able to integrate aggression with love and sexuality, and they have a capacity for a primitive kind of falling in love that is characterized by an idealization of the love object. In fact, intense sexual experiences and intense love affairs with an idealized other may obscure the underlying incapacity to tolerate ambivalence. However, with the splitting mechanisms of BPO, their interpersonal and intimate relationships are fragile and always at risk of being contaminated by split-off, all-bad aspects that may change the idealized relationship into a persecutory one. In the midphase of therapy the question of sex may intertwine with manifestations of the idealized transference and, at times, with the persecutory one.

AGGRESSIVE INFILTRATION OF SEXUAL BEHAVIOR

The sexual behavior of a subgroup of patients with BPO may be self-destructive or destructive to others. These issues must be worked through in the midphase of therapy. Next, we discuss the case of a patient with dissociated sexual feelings whose sexual feelings were hijacked by aggressive motivations (the eroticized transference) (Blum 1973). We then present an example of a patient whose sexual feelings emerged in the context of an idealized transference.

Self-Injury, Dissociation, and Sexuality

The case that follows demonstrates a particularly clear relationship between the patient's primitive defense mechanisms, especially splitting; the patient's behaviors, specifically cutting; and sexual inhibition and its subsequent resolution. Manifestations of splitting are not always as dramatic as in this case, which is more typical of patients with a histrionic quality.

CASE EXAMPLE

Susan, age 26 when she began TFP, had been hospitalized a number of times for cutting herself repeatedly. She was diagnosed with BPD, although her hospital therapist wondered if she had an underlying psychotic illness because her discussion of self-cutting took on a bizarre quality that seemed irrational to him. Susan discussed a fantasy of systematically inflicting so many cuts on herself that she would become totally bathed in blood. Her affect in discussing this fantasy was one of enthusiasm and excitement bordering on ecstasy. Her actual cutting behavior, which was not deep enough to require sutures, included generalized cutting of her arms and legs, along with a particular interest in making cuts on her breasts and vagina.

After discharge from the hospital, Susan started TFP with Dr. Wy. Susan was a virgin at the time of entering treatment. She had dated two boys in high school but had been uncomfortable with them. Her physical contact had been limited to kissing, which she did not enjoy. She did not date after that. Susan graduated from college but did not immediately go on to work because of repeated hospitalizations that interfered with any goal-oriented projects.

After her most recent hospital discharge, Susan began working and was able to maintain a reasonably appropriate job. In therapy, she was quite resistant to working at a deep psychological level. She continued to have urges to cut herself, stating that she refrained from doing so only because she learned from multiple hospitalizations that her cutting behavior disturbed others so much that she would not be allowed to live in peace if she continued to do it. She expressed the opinion that cutting was a pleasurable activity that did not distress her at all. She dismissed any effort to find meaning in that behavior. She also complained about Dr. Wy's "coldness" and repeatedly expressed the wish to return to her prior therapist, a man she described as more "warm and giving." Dr. Wy pointed out that her idea that he was cold seemed to correspond to the understanding in their treatment contract that he would not get more involved with her if she cut herself. Dr. Wy added that Susan appeared not to know how to relate to him except through discussing her cutting.

An initial step toward understanding her behavior came when she was talking about one of her few interests in life, a particular human rights organization. When Dr. Wy pointed out that the symbol of this organization was a candle surrounded by barbed wire, Susan meekly acknowledged that in her fantasies she wished she were the candle. This symbol represented a relationship dyad: the candle as the source of light and warmth and the wire as the persecutor. The key to increasing Susan's understanding was helping her to see her identification with both parts of the dyad. Further discussion established a connection between pain and pleasure that Susan had thus far denied, even though it had been suggested by her practice of cutting herself on her breasts and her vagina. However, after this connection was made, the therapy appeared to come to a stalemate. Susan continued to function at her job but withdrew from social life, spending all her weekends alone in her room at home. She read, sewed, and for periods of time sat in her closet in a blank state of mind.

In the midst of this general sense of blandness in the therapy, Susan reported in a session that she feared dying in a car accident on the way home. She was concerned because when driving to the session, she perceived the taillights of the cars in front of her to be dripping with blood. She described becoming quasimesmerized by this and feared that her distraction with this vision of blood would cause her to lose control at the wheel. Dr. Wy experienced great discomfort and became aware that whatever else the report of a vision of blood and the prediction of a fatal accident represented, it was part of a sadomasochistic dynamic in which the patient was now torturing him. He pointed this out, adding that sadistic feelings may be a more common human emotion than she imagined, and reminded her of the earlier observation that she appeared not to know how to relate to him if the contact were not infused with aggression as it had been with her earlier therapist by means of the cutting. Dr. Wy wondered what other feelings Susan might have for him that were being defended against by the aggression that was, for the moment, the only alternative to blandness in their relations. He suggested that her feelings might include a wish for intimacy and closeness, as represented in the candle image, but that she did not know what to do with those feelings because they were so intertwined with the aggression she tried to deny in herself.

Shortly after this intervention, Susan, who had been in therapy with Dr. Wy for 2 years by then, came into a session one day and announced, "Susan didn't come here today; Renee came in her place." Dr. Wy was taken by surprise and had to pause to get his bearings. He asked if Renee could tell him about herself. The patient explained that she, Renee, dreamed of going out in sexy outfits, picking up men at bars, and having sex with them in ways that would hurt them. However, Renee claimed that "this other girl," Susan, exerted control over her and kept her from doing those things. Renee resented Susan for her prudishness.

In the next session, Susan presented as her usual self. When the therapist asked about Renee, the patient became mildly confused and could only say that she had a sense of this other woman who had recently been trying to intrude in her life. She was intermittently bothered by her but could go for long periods without thinking about her. Over the next weeks, Renee was more or less present in sessions. She was not present at all in sessions in which other material predominated. In some sessions, Susan complained about being harassed by Renee, whom she spoke of as this "other girl" who was bad and who made her uncomfortable, criticizing her and calling her names. In a few sessions, the patient spoke as Renee, describing her contempt for Susan, the prude who kept her chained in.

Dr. Wy understood the situation in terms of split self representations being presented with a histrionic style. This apparent manifestation of dissociative identity disorder (formerly known as multiple personality disorder) did not call for any change in technique because this patient's dissociative identity disorder can be understood as a manifestation of extreme internal splitting of self representations in the transference in which each fragment of self representation is experienced as a separate individual with a different name. The therapeutic challenge remained to understand the need to keep the representations separate and to help the patient overcome this and achieve an integrated identity. Dr. Wy hypothesized that his intervention about other feelings intermingled with the patient's aggression had facilitated the appearance of Renee, who seemed to represent the emergence of split-off material.

Dr. Wy began to wonder with Susan about the role of Renee in her life; he spoke with intentional ambiguity about whether Renee was "another girl" or a part within Susan. Susan said she had no idea where Renee came from but wished she would go away. Dr. Wy noted that Renee's appearance on the scene seemed to coincide roughly with a reduction in Susan's urges to cut herself and with his mention of the possibility that Susan might have a wish for intimacy and closeness. She could see no connection. He pointed out that Renee seemed very interested in sex. Susan said this bothered her because she had no interest in sex. Dr. Wy questioned this stated lack of interest, pointing out that Susan's cutting behavior had a special focus on her breasts and vagina. This observation made her uncomfortable. She responded that "they were just there" but with some awareness that this did not constitute a very convincing explanation. She complained that she "just didn't like talking about sex or thinking about it." Dr. Wy noted that this was apparent but that her efforts not to talk about it or think about it seemed unsuccessful because the issue kept appearing, earlier in a disguised form in her behavior and now in the form of Renee, the unwanted companion. He offered an interpretation that her cutting behavior had worked as a compromise between sexual urges tinged with aggression and prohibitions against them. This behavior simultaneously satisfied sexual and aggressive urges and the need for punishment. It suggested a fusion of sex and aggression in which Susan played the roles of both victim and, less consciously, of aggressor.

Susan was uncomfortable with this interpretation because her libidinal drives were so isolated from her conscious view of herself. However, after this interpretation, Renee faded from the picture. Susan did not announce that she was gone, but after hearing nothing of her for a number of weeks, Dr. Wy inquired after Renee. The patient responded, "It's strange. I haven't thought about her. She just hasn't been around." In the meantime, Susan reported that she had begun to date a man who, it turned out, was the same age and had the same first name as Dr. Wy. For the first time, after clarifying how her aggressive fantasies defended against libidinal material, Susan began to behave in a manner suggesting that libido could predominate over aggression.

The following is a summary of the transference developments in this case:

1. Susan's initial presentation as a relentless cutter functioned in a number of ways in the transference. It was an appeal to the therapist to take care of her because she appeared to be hopelessly ill; a way of subtly torturing the therapist (and thus connecting with him in a sadomasochistic way) because her cutting made others very uncomfortable; and a form of acting out that brought attention to her breasts and vagina.
2. Her bloody visions and fear that she would have an accident driving home from a session were a second way of relating to the therapist through aggression. After the interpretation of this as a possible enactment of sadistic urges and defense against libidinal feelings toward the therapist, Susan began to demonstrate more awareness of the mix of erotic and aggressive feelings within her.
3. Susan's dating a man with obvious similarities to Dr. Wy called for further exploration and understanding, especially because the patient's newfound boyfriend, despite being a generally stable individual, had a minor substance abuse problem, recalling her father's alcoholism.

In summary, this case revealed a situation of sexual inhibition in which split-off aggressively contaminated libidinal impulses were expressed initially in self-destructive provocative behavior and then in a phase of dissociative identity as this major split-off part of the self entered into the patient's consciousness. At each step, the therapist's interpretations helped move the process of awareness and eventual integration forward.

Understanding and Managing Eroticized Transferences: Sexuality and Aggression in the Transference

The key to resolving a borderline patient's possible infiltration of sexuality with aggression and defending against libido by aggression is to focus on the intermingling of the two in the transference. The term *eroticized transference* is more specific than the broader erotic transference. The latter involves loving feelings, whereas the former involves the *appearance* of loving feelings that conceals other affects. In discussing erotic transferences in his paper "Observations on Transference-Love," Freud (1915/1958) spoke of the inevitability of the patient's experiencing love for the therapist and of the need to accept and work with it. To avoid working with transference love would be, in Freud's terms, "as though, after summoning up a spirit from the underworld by cunning spells, one were to send him down again without having asked him a single question" (p. 164). However, after discussing the inevitability of transference love and the need to work with it, Freud pointed out one exception:

> There is one class of women with whom this attempt to preserve the erotic transference for the purposes of analytic work without satisfying it will not succeed. These are women of elemental passionateness who tolerate no surrogates. They are children of nature who refuse to accept the psychical in place of the material…. With such people one has the choice between returning their love or else bringing down upon oneself the full enmity of a woman scorned. In neither case can one safeguard the interests of the treatment. One has to withdraw, unsuccessful. (p.166)

One could hypothesize that Freud was referring to certain patients with severe personality disorders. As we have understood more about their borderline organization and how to address it, we have become less pessimistic about the prospects of working with this eroticized transference. Blum (1973) situated the eroticized transference at the extreme end of erotic transferences and characterized it as "an intense, vivid, irrational erotic preoccupation with the analyst, characterized by overt, seemingly ego-syntonic demands for love and sexual fulfillment" (p. 63). Unlike the erotic transference that expresses primarily libidinal affects, the eroticized transference is one in which a semblance of libidinal affect is used in the service of aggressive affect.

Rather than elaborate fully on the varied forms of erotic and eroticized transferences, we focus here on those variants that are the most difficult to manage. Kernberg (1995) describes how intense erotic transferences may be part of a patient's "unconscious attempts to prevent or destroy the possibility of a steady positive relationship with the analyst" (p. 118). Interestingly, the opposites—love and hate, libido and aggression—can seem to merge in the eroticized transference, but this is not a true integration; it is rather a situation in which one part of the split internal world is appropriated in the service of the other. In the more developed and integrated psyche, there is a capacity for ambivalence and an integration of libido and aggression. However, borderline individuals sometimes manifest a regressive form of pseudointegration in which the aggressive segment of the psyche latches onto aspects of the libidinal segment and recruits them for destructive ends. Love and sexual excitement can be used in the service of aggression in a syndrome of perversity.

We return now to the case of Gabby, who was introduced in Chapter 3.

CASE EXAMPLE

Toward the end of the first year of TFP, after many cycles of appearing to become engaged in the therapy and then pulling away, Gabby began to accept Dr. Tam's interpretation that she was defending against the longing for a loving relationship. She stated, "I guess you're right. It does seem like every time I get comfortable with you, I pull away."

Having thought that this insight would help the patient begin to integrate her ideal and persecutory representations of him and begin to move beyond the paranoid position, Dr. Tam relaxed a bit in the treatment. However, in the middle of a session in the second year of therapy, Gabby got up from her chair, walked briskly to Dr. Tam, and sat on his lap. He had to hold her at arm's length to keep her from embracing him. Nevertheless, she began to unbutton her blouse. Dr. Tam said emphatically that she must return to her chair because this behavior was incompatible with therapy. Gabby stopped unbuttoning her blouse but remained on his lap, vigorously arguing that he had finally helped her see that she could trust another person. She dramatically said that this emergence of trust was a major achievement and that his refusal of her love would be proof that her prior belief that she could trust no one was correct. In fact, if he rejected her, it would be proof that he was lying when he said there could be a positive feeling between people—it would be proof that she was disgusting and that he did loathe her and would reject her, as she always knew. If he rejected her, it would dash all her hope that the world could be different and would confirm her belief that suicide was the only rational choice.

This vignette illustrates libidinal feelings being hijacked by aggressive ones. However, the patient had no awareness of the aggression in her reaction. She projected it onto the therapist. From her point of view, it was he who was rejecting her; it was he who was deceiving her with false kindness; it was she who had been tricked by him into liking him. He had set her up; he had done this to hurt her; she should have known better than to trust him; she was right all along—in her paranoia. The example represents classic, but extreme, acting out and projection: although the patient's words of love constituted an attack on the therapist and the therapy—the acting out of an unacknowledged aggressive identification—the patient's conviction was that the therapist was attacking her by not responding to her. Although this vignette may superficially appear to be positive transference carried to the extreme, the deeper issue is the destructiveness and the attack on boundaries and on the therapy. On the basis of this incident, Dr. Tam realized that Gabby was situated at a lower level of BPO than he had thought previously. Initially, he understood her negative initial presentation as a defense against libidinal strivings. Although he did not totally abandon this formulation, her behavior in this session made him appreciate more fully the force of her aggressive side.

To help organize one's thoughts about complex interactions with borderline patients, it is helpful to schematize them in terms of the self and object relations involved. The schema shown in Figure 9–1 represents the most typical early-to-mid treatment situation of borderline patients presenting with a primarily paranoid transference: they are convinced they will be hurt. If the therapist does not play out the expected role of exploiter/ abuser, the patient has difficulty comprehending the therapist's interest in him or her. Gabby's case presents the complication that the patient's defense against the danger of closeness, involving an unacknowledged identification with the aggressor, is disguised in the language of love. Gabby's attempts at overt seduction both return the situation to the familiar territory of exploiter and victim and place the patient in the exploiter role, albeit without her conscious awareness of that: a repetition of trauma with roles reversed. This situation is an intense and potentially chaotic one because as the therapist sets limits and attempts to interpret the patient's actions, the patient generally experiences herself in the victim role, protesting that the therapist's refusal of her offer is a rejection of her and proof of her worthlessness. It appears to be a "no-win" situation for the therapist. If he responds to the seduction, he abandons all ethical standards and becomes an abuser. If he does not, the patient experiences him as harshly rejecting her.

The first rule in such a situation is to attend to the frame of treatment, as in the following:

Dr. Tam (*literally holding Gabby at arm's length*): We cannot work under these conditions. You'll have to stop unbuttoning your blouse and sit back in your chair, or this session will end.

Gabby: You don't understand. This will help me. You wanted me to trust; now I do, and that will all be gone if you reject me.

Dr. Tam: I agree with you that rejection is the issue, but we have to look at who's rejecting whom and why. And we can only do that if you sit back down. [Gabby sits down.] Something has happened here, and we have to try to understand it before it destroys what we're trying to do here. We've been working together for a year and a half. We've just begun to understand some things. You approach me like this. You say it's going to help. But you know it would destroy what we're doing here, and we have to figure out why you are doing this right now. I have an idea. I believe that you do have tender feelings for me. However, more than anything, I think that scares you. It makes you feel vulnerable. So the only way you can feel safe again is to take charge. The only thing that would make sense to you is if my interest in you is to exploit you. So, to get back to familiar ground, you seem to be taking over the destructive, exploitative role in encouraging me to act it out.

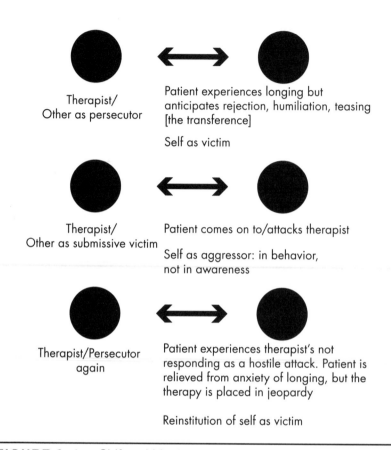

FIGURE 9–1. Shifts within the persecutory dyad in the midphase of treatment of a borderline patient with a predominantly paranoid transference, as seen in the case of Gabby.

Getting back to the overall picture, as the therapy progressed, this situation, which never occurred again so concretely, was dealt with by cycles of limit setting and interpretation. For example, at one point Gabby said she understood that Dr. Tam could not have sex with her if she were his patient. Therefore, she proposed that they end therapy so that they would be free to leave their spouses and start an ideal life together. In this version the dynamics were more contained and included an element of the idealized side of the split internal world. This is a reminder that the idealized segment of the split psyche is as pathological as the persecutory one insofar as it is as unadapted to the complexity of reality. A basic interpretation regarding Gabby's seductive approaches to Dr. Tam was that the fear of misplaced trust and betrayal led her to a reversal of roles in which she tried to gain the upper hand and take control, thus destroying any possibility of a secure and loving mutual relationship. In her world, at this point, the only hope for security in relations is through control. However, her way of forcing control represents an unconscious identification with the figure of whom she is most wary. In such cases, the middle phase of therapy generally represents a conflict between libidinal strivings and aggressive urges. Patients with lower-level BPD may experience a gratification in power and control that they may be reluctant to give up. In Gabby's case, in the later stages of therapy, she was able to acknowledge the aggressive element she brought to relations and was more open to a desire to engage with others positively. She then began the process of integrating this aggression, linking it with libidinal strivings that were more fully explored when the idealized transference became more present. This resulted in, among other forms of sublimation, a very witty and wry sense of humor that simultaneously could be seductive and had a "kick" to it.

Also in the later phase, there was a more advanced manifestation of the erotic transference. The patient began to express a more genuine libidinal longing for the therapist, combining sexual desire with loving feelings, with regret about the impossibility of the satisfaction of this longing. This is a common and challenging situation for therapists. To quote Daniel Hill (1994), "Whereas the choice for the layperson is to reject or not, psychoanalysis relies on the analysis of the transference and the acceptance of paradox; in this case that the love is both genuine and disingenuous" (p. 485).

THE CHALLENGE WHEN INTEGRATION HAS BEGUN AND LOVING AND SEXUAL FEELINGS BECOME MORE STABLE

As reviewed earlier in this section, intense erotic transferences can involve categorical demands by the patient to obtain gratification of these erotic wishes from the therapist or a renewed acting out of self-destructive sexual behavior, such as unprotected sexual promiscuity, while blaming the therapist for this behavior because of his or her lack of sexual response to the patient. In these circumstances, it is important that the therapist work through his or her countertransference sufficiently to be able to discuss the patient's sexual feelings, wishes, and fears thoroughly without undue inhibition or any enactment of erotic countertransference feelings. The need to fully tolerate countertransference emotions and fantasies about the patient without communicating them to the patient, but using them for an in-depth analysis of the dominant object relation in the transference, is as important at this stage as the parallel tolerance of intense hatred in the countertransference at other stages of treatment. In fact, the aggressive and sadistic components of open sexual demands will help to clarify, in the countertransference, the complex nature of the patient's erotic feelings.

It is important that the patient be able to fully express his or her erotic feelings in the transference without experiencing them as a sexual seduction or humiliation and that the therapist, in turn, be prepared to analyze the many aspects of the patient's fantasies of being rejected because of the therapist's maintenance of consistent boundaries in their relationship. Full exploration of sexual demands and fantasies in the transference is an important precondition for the liberation of the patient's sexual life from its contamination by aggressive impulses and for facilitating the patient's integration of his or her sexual life into a mature love relation in external reality.

With regard to countertransference in Gabby's case, the therapist experienced the patient's seduction without any internal sexual response. This is an indication of aggression as the major issue. As the case evolved and Gabby's aggression became more integrated, allowing for the experience of erotic feelings that were not controlled by aggression, the challenge for the therapist was to feel comfortable experiencing attraction in his countertransference without becoming anxious that allowing himself such feelings was itself a breaking of boundaries. These moments can be some of the most challenging in therapy. The patient's expression of interest in the therapist may be direct ("I don't know how to say this, but I've got a crush on you"), joking and ironic ("I'd love to go out with you but I know you'd never be seen in public with someone like me"), or indirect and nonverbal. The most important aspect of technique is to not avoid the material. Therapists have trouble discussing issues of attraction when their feelings are not of the same intensity as a patient's; however, the most rejecting behavior is to give the message that these feelings are taboo. The therapist should proceed with clarification: Can the patient say more about his or her attraction? What are his or her fantasies? If the patient says he or she cannot proceed, that it is too humiliating, the therapist should inquire about the patient's assumptions: What is it about continuing the therapy that is humiliating? Why is the patient convinced that the therapist does not like him or her? What keeps the patient from imagining that if the patient and therapist met in different circumstances, they might not enjoy each other's company or even strike up a relationship? Exploration of these issues sheds important light both on the patient's search for the ideal other and on his or her devaluing of self, both of which frustrate the patient's ability to find an appropriate partner in life. In summary, an erotic transference may be considered both a threat to treatment and an important part of treatment to be worked through.

DEEPENING THE UNDERSTANDING OF SPLITTING AND STRIVING TOWARD INTEGRATION

Evidence of splitting in the patient's internal world may be immediately apparent or may take time to emerge. Movement toward integration is also variable but usually does not begin to occur until a few months into the therapy, at the earliest. When it does occur, the therapist should be prepared for the frustration of experiencing an alternation between partial integration and temporary regressions to the earlier split state. However, the beginning of the integration process signals the patient's capacity to reflect on and change his or her internal world. Appropriate cycles of working through—reflecting the anxiety produced by the shift in defensive psychological organization—can then lead to fuller and more stable integration.

EVIDENCE OF SPLITTING

As discussed in Chapter 7, the therapist should work against the tendency of some patients to remain stuck in an ongoing positive transference or negative transference. This is not an issue with patients who demonstrate their split internal world in early reactions to the therapist. For example, a patient's initial reaction to his therapist's office was, "Wow! This is a big, impressive office. You must be a good therapist. That's what everybody says, and I can tell you're really smart and know how to relate to patients." Two sessions later, the patient said, "This office is so cold and impersonal. It's like you're putting up a wall, hiding behind your degrees and your reputation. If you don't like relating to people, you shouldn't have become a therapist." This patient's reactions demonstrate opposite object representations corresponding to different internal dyads. The therapist in this case should confront the patient about these contradictory responses and ask the patient to reflect on what might motivate the alternating between these different views. (The alternating in this case may likely stem from a narcissistic dynamic in which the patient needs to have "the best" therapist but then cannot tolerate this view of the therapist because it arouses narcissistic envy that makes the patient need to devalue him.)

Some patients, however, begin therapy in a negative or positive transference that remains more consistent. This corresponds to a psychological structure in which one dyad more consistently defends against another. The rhythm of change of transferences varies from case to case; patients with borderline plus infantile-histrionic and schizoid characteristics tend to be rapid cyclers with regard to transference dispositions, whereas those with paranoid, narcissistic, and depressive features cycle more slowly.

The discussion of Gabby's first year in treatment in Chapter 3 provides an example of working with splitting. Gabby maintained a consistently negative transference on the surface for a number of months until an underlying longing burst forth the second time Dr. Tam announced he would be away.

ALTERNATION BETWEEN INTEGRATION AND REGRESSION

CASE EXAMPLE: FIRST EVIDENCE OF SPLIT-OFF POSITIVE AFFECTS

In the sessions leading up to Dr. Tam's departure, Gabby alternated between regressing to a paranoid suspicion and rejection of him (e.g., "It was stupid of me to get upset that you're leaving... I don't know what I was thinking. You're never there for me anyway") and experiencing the distress associated with her underlying attachment to him (e.g., "If you go away, I'll kill myself and it will be your fault!"). In response to this suicide threat, Dr. Tam responded by first addressing the frame. He reminded Gabby that the therapy could not provide a guarantee against her killing herself and that she had a responsibility to seek emergency help if she needed it. He also challenged and explored her attempt to put the aggressive part of herself into him ("and it will be your fault"). Finally, he tried to help Gabby understand her distress. In doing so, he elaborated the dyad of the needy childlike self who longed for a good provider but experienced only disappointment. He also tried to help the patient see her identification with the abandoning object in her way of trying to eliminate her internal image of and connection with him ("killing him off in her mind"), with the consequence of experiencing emptiness and aloneness.

After returning from his trip, Dr. Tam found Gabby once again regressed into her paranoid position. When he contrasted her defiant rejection of any interest in him on his return with the times before his departure when she had felt a connection with him, Gabby replied with hostility, "What are you talking about?" He reminded her of her dramatic reaction when he had told her he was going away. She fired back at him, "I never said that!" This was a clear example of regression from a movement toward integration and a return to a split, dissociated state. Dr. Tam understood that it would still be some time before this patient achieved integration. Five months later, after many repeated cycles of the dynamic described above, Gabby began a session by saying, "I've been thinking about what you were saying...that I fight feeling close to you because I'm afraid that maybe I'll be hurt by you. I think maybe that's true." This was evidence of progress toward integration. Even so, Gabby's regressions to a paranoid position, although less frequent, continued for a long time in response to perceived threats or stressors. By the end of Gabby's therapy, in the fifth year, in reflecting on some of the changes she had experienced, she stated, "You've given me a lot, but you've also taken something away from me.... I used to believe in the perfect love, and I held out for it, no matter how bad my life really was. Now I'm much closer to my husband, but it's not passionate and I know there's no perfect love...and I really miss that idea." Dr. Tam appreciated this layman's description of advancing to the depressive position. As further evidence of her change to that position, Gabby said, "I can't believe the terrible things I used to do to my husband, and sometimes to you, and think they were totally justified. I feel very bad about that now."

FOLLOWING SHIFTING PROJECTIONS: INTEGRATION AND IMPROVEMENTS IN REALITY TESTING

As the patient's internal world becomes more integrated, the distortions of perception based on experiencing the world through rigid internal dyads decrease. Individuals and situations that had previously been threatening become more benign. In a complex process, aggressive feelings and libidinal feelings become both more integrated and more distinguishable as the patient is better able to have a symbolic, linguistic grasp of them and to distinguish inner fantasy from reality. Practically speaking, the patient is able to tolerate negative feelings in the context of a loving relationship, thus allowing for the deepening of relations that would otherwise have been aborted by the sense that any negative emotion poisoned the whole. In addition, the unconscious aggressive feelings that previously infiltrated idealized "loving" relationships without awareness and would lead to sadomasochistic entanglements become accepted as part of the patient's internal world and are both sublimated and more consciously reserved for appropriate settings.

As integration takes place, patients often demonstrate a better capacity to accurately perceive interactions with others. However, in stressful or ambiguous situations, patients may experience a temporary return of splitting defenses. The levels of personality organization are defined in part by the *predominant* use of primitive defense mechanisms. Every individual's use of defense mechanisms shifts to some degree according to the circumstances. Therefore, even as a borderline patient shifts toward a higher level of personality organization with more habitual use of mature defenses, the patient may revert to more primitive defenses, usually under conditions of heightened stress. However, in patients in whom the newfound integration remains fragile, the regression may result merely from ambiguity or lack of clarity. In the following example, we return to the case of Amy, who was introduced in Chapter 8, "Early Treatment Phase."

CLINICAL ILLUSTRATION

Amy's severe self-destructive behaviors showed much improvement when she became aware of and accepted her previously split-off aggressive and sadistic part, thereby taking back her projection. Prior to this awareness, this part of her internal world was expressed either through self-destructive acting out or through experiencing others, by projection, as threatening and harmful. With increased awareness of her own aggressive feelings, Amy allowed herself to experience appropriate anger, stopped hurting herself, and began to function better in the world. Before therapy, she had existed in a limited sphere defined by her illness: her world was that of a patient who lived with her husband and had little contact with the outside world except for the people involved in her treatments.

Amy's situation changed with TFP. First, the treatment contract called for a higher level of activity in her life. Second, as her internal world began to be integrated, she became more comfortable relating to others. The improvement that began by understanding her paranoid transference—her projection of aggression onto the therapist and her aggressive actions toward him—translated gradually to situations outside of therapy (strategy 4, as described in Chapter 3). This change first occurred in the college course she had started as part of her commitment to become more active. Her initial response was to assume that her fellow students disliked her. Over time, she understood that part of this conviction came from the harshness of *her* assessments both of others ("You won't believe what this guy said in class!") and of herself. Before gaining awareness, she had generally denied any harshness toward others, although those opinions sometimes emerged in sarcastic comments, and she experienced harshness toward herself as coming from others, even though she would engage in self-injurious behavior without attributing any meaning to it. This understanding paralleled her experience of her therapist, Dr. Jones.

One result of Amy's improvement, after just over a year of treatment, was her decision to have a child. She was emotionally stable throughout her pregnancy and was a loving and nurturing mother. In general, she was functioning at a higher level. She was not without anxieties, but they resembled those of many young mothers. However, her psychological integration still showed a fragility that could benefit from further therapy and consolidation.

CYCLES OF INCREASING INTEGRATION WITH MORE CONTAINED AND LIMITED PROJECTION

As the patient makes progress, it is important for the therapist to have a sense of the stability versus fragility of the patient's integrated psychological state. This judgment has a bearing on the decision of when to plan the termination of therapy. For reasons that are yet to be understood, the integration is more fragile and subject to regressions to projection in some patients as compared with others. This was the case with Amy.

CLINICAL ILLUSTRATION

Although Amy was generally functioning well, the fragility of her internal integration was apparent in the following areas: 1) her reactions to her own work and 2) her concerns about the safety of her child in certain circumstances. What is important to note is that her concerns began to overlap more with realistic concerns but still could contain an element of exaggeration and distortion based on internal representations that were not yet fully integrated.

An early manifestation of Amy's improvement was her return to a long-standing interest in writing music. As described in Chapter 8, her early treatment focused on the split-off aggressive part of her internal world that underlay her self-destructive acting out. A manifestation of this aggressive part was the harsh, critical voice that attacked her efforts at doing anything (and could attack others as well). This unintegrated part of her internal world paralyzed her every time she began to write a song, and this dynamic (as it related to all of her efforts in life, leading to paralysis) was one of the factors underlying her depressive states. Her treatment involved first acknowledging this aggressive internal part (the "critical judge") and then being able to temper it as she gained control through awareness. The acceptance of and movement toward integrating this part of herself helped Amy advance from identity diffusion to some identity consolidation. The modulation of her internal "critical judge" allowed her to pursue interests that she previously aborted because of her rejection and dismissal of her interests or of her performance at them as worthless. She was able to engage in the creative process more than before. However, she did this in secret, without telling Dr. Jones about it. Then a pattern emerged in which Amy would break her silence about this activity and tell him about a song she had written. Inevitably, she would report in the next session that the discussion about the song made her realize that her songwriting was very bad and that she should give up her efforts.

Exploration of this pattern revealed that Amy managed to fend off the harsh, critical part until she revealed her creative activity to another person. At that point, she was uncertain about whether the harsh judgments she experienced about her work were indeed based on an excessively critical internal part or whether they originated in external reality—that is, in negative opinions from others. Sorting out these distinctions between the internal versus the external source of a thought can be tricky because, of course, a person can encounter harsh judgments from others in reality. Exploring such issues in the transference can help clarify the question. In Amy's case, Dr. Jones focused attention on the pattern of Amy's rejecting her work after she discussed it with him. She stated that discussing it with him brought her out of the illusion that she could compose well and returned her to the "reality" of her lack of talent. In further exploration, Amy acknowledged that Dr. Jones said or did nothing to indicate a negative opinion regarding her work, but she just "knew" that he did not like it. Eventually, she came to understand that assuming that Dr. Jones did not like her work seemed to be the safest position to her. She was at a point where she was able to master her own aggressive response to herself when no other person was involved. However, the involvement with another raised the possibility of the aggression originating *in* the other and, by projection, she assumed this was the case. She required further exploration of the possibility that the response of another to her could be benign, or even positive, before she could control this projective process and further advance her integration of the aggressive part and improve her functioning.

This example demonstrates the importance of technical neutrality. Although Dr. Jones expressed interest in Amy's opinions about her songwriting, he did not provide immediate reassurance in response to her concerns that her efforts were bad. She would probably have experienced such reassurance as a patronizing response offered out of pity, or if the reassurance relieved her at the moment, it would doubtless soon evaporate. It was only by exploring her assumptions about her therapist's response that Amy could come to understand that her doubts were based on the projection of a part of her own internal world and that Dr. Jones might have a genuinely positive response to her work.

The clinical management in this case example is based on Amy's having talent as a songwriter. A therapist might encounter a situation that appears similar but in which the patient is engaging in an activity with little chance of success. In such a case, the therapist's approach would be to explore the patient's capacity to accurately judge his or her abilities and to try to determine whether the gap between the patient's actual talent and level of ambitions represents a narcissistic grandiosity or is the acting out of a self-defeating dynamic. It is because of situations like this, in which similar behavior might be determined by different underlying dynamics, that it is difficult to write a manual that tells the therapist exactly what to do at each moment.

EXPANDING THE FOCUS OF THERAPY IN THE MIDPHASE

In the midphase of therapy, the therapist may need to expand the focus on the transference to increasingly include discussion of the patient's 1) current external reality; 2) pattern of interpersonal interactions over time; 3) past history and the evolving narrative of it as therapy progresses; and 4) fantasies, which become more distinct from the patient's experience of reality. In the first phase of therapy, the emphasis is on identifying the main dyads in the patient's internal world. This is done principally through attention to the transference, although the therapist may also investigate other areas if the patient brings them into the session with intense affect. As therapy shifts to the midphase, the therapist helps the patient explore what, in the patient's internal dynamics, explains the prominence of these dyads and what has kept them from being integrated into a more complex internal world. As these issues become clarified, the work of therapy increasingly addresses the translation of the understanding achieved within the sessions to the patient's outside life, enters into a more refined understanding of the patient, and advances in helping the patient achieve normal satisfaction in work, love, social life, and creative activities. A patient's uneven progress toward integration can be seen in social relations as well as in his or her relation to work. Patients often begin treatment with few social relations, based on their turbulent interpersonal style and/or paranoid assumptions about others. In the course of therapy, both the increased level of life activity and the integration of the internal world that allows more modulated responses to others lead to increased interpersonal interactions. The tentativeness of integration is often seen in this interpersonal sphere as the patient experiences anxiety as he or she moves away from the trusted paranoid position.

A general principle is that as therapy progresses, the therapist gains further in-depth knowledge of the patient's work, leisure, and love life. The therapist then more deeply explores subtle aspects of these areas of the patient's life while continuing to explore the transference. The patient develops a fuller sense of self and others, and the therapist develops a more complete sense of the patient. In doing so, the therapist understands how subtle projections of internal representations that are not fully integrated may persist after the patient's overt acting out has ended. It is essential for the therapist to attend to these projections to help the patient move from a life without borderline symptoms but with significant inhibition to a life of fully satisfying relations. In this sense, TFP goes beyond treatments that focus exclusively on resolving the symptoms of BPD.

CLINICAL ILLUSTRATION

When Amy's son began to attend nursery school, she became highly anxious. This experience exposed her to a new setting, where she encountered many other young mothers. Her immediate reaction was that the other mothers considered her ignorant and inferior. Exploration of this experience uncovered vestiges of her critical persecutory self and revealed not only that there was no evidence that the other mothers saw her in this way but also that Amy harbored hidden devaluing opinions of the other mothers, whom she saw as less devoted and caring than she was to her son. This paralleled Amy's experience earlier in therapy when she returned to college courses. On the dynamic level, this discussion of her reactions to the other mothers helped Amy's efforts to integrate harsh internal representations that served the purpose of supporting an underlying grandiosity. On a more practical level, the discussion allowed Amy to move beyond the negative affects that kept her from establishing gratifying relations with the other mothers. As therapy advances along these lines—with an end of overt symptoms and increasing attention to developments in the patient's external life—the need to carefully attend to the treatment frame decreases.

BALANCING ATTENTION TO THE TRANSFERENCE AND TO THE PATIENT'S OUTSIDE LIFE

The central transference themes often take time to develop. As this is happening, the therapist listens to the material the patient brings to sessions. Some patients discuss their reactions to and feelings about the therapist directly and spontaneously from the beginning of therapy. Others say little about the therapist and talk almost exclusively about other subjects. In this latter situation, the therapist may need to inquire about the patient's experience of the relationship between them or comment on a feeling that is expressed through the patient's nonverbal behavior.

Along with this focus on the transference, however, one of the therapist's roles is to regularly check on the status of the patient's life outside the sessions. This active inquiry into outside life is one of the aspects of TFP (Kernberg, in press) that distinguishes it from more traditional psychoanalytic psychotherapy, particularly from Kleinian psychoanalysis (Joseph 1985). This inquiry may uncover important information regarding how the patient may be enacting important dynamics in his or her life while appearing to be fully cooperative in sessions. For example, a patient may associate freely in sessions but may not have followed up on commitments in the contract, such as getting a volunteer job or attending 12-step meetings. Dealing with such a development was discussed in Chapter 7, in terms of addressing challenges to the treatment. A therapist who does not inquire about a patient's life outside the sessions will not be aware of the acting out. Patients who follow through on commitments regarding outside involvements can bring in important information about the repetition of pathological interactions in new settings. In general, the most effective way to achieve insight into these interactions is through relating the conflict back to the transference, where the data to explore are immediately present. In the following example, we return to the case of Betty, a patient with higher-level BPO who was introduced in Chapter 4, "Assessment Phase."

CLINICAL ILLUSTRATION

Betty took on a volunteer job and, as was her pattern, began to believe that everyone at her workplace was reacting to her with contempt, hatred, and rejection. As in the past, she responded by treating her coworkers with a hostility that she attributed to them. This was crucial to explore because continued hostility on her part (which she understood as defending herself against others' hostility) would likely lead to failure at the job, followed by a renewed cycle of doubt, self-hatred, depression, and suicidality. As is usually the case, questioning Betty's perceptions of her coworkers was not likely to lead to significant insight or change ("You're not there! How can you tell me I'm misinterpreting things? I *know* that when the secretary didn't say 'Hi' to me it meant she hates me!") Although it may help for the therapist to point to a recurrent pattern of such perceptions ("It seems as though this is the same experience you described having at your previous job"), the most productive area of exploration is in the transference. The therapist listening to this material should review his or her experiences with the patient for examples of the same dyad (the "persecuted victim" fearing and resenting the "sadistic tormenters"). It is usually possible for the therapist to then direct the discussion to the interaction between patient and therapist:

Dr. Em: I wonder if there is any connection between how you feel at work and how you felt here in that session after we had discussed the contract. You said that the contract was just to protect me from you. You felt that I had taken an immediate dislike to you and that I was creating barriers to any contact between you and me. You felt I was singling you out and that I didn't set up such strict boundaries with other patients. And it all had to do with the idea that I saw you as inferior and unworthy of my attention.

Betty: Well, I don't think that today. I found this book about therapy with borderline patients, and it says that setting up limits is part of the treatment.

Dr. Em: So, without that external evidence, you might still think that I didn't like you?

Betty: I'm not saying that you like me. You only see me because I pay you.

Dr. Em: So that's the only interest I have in you?

Betty: You'd see anyone who walked through the door who paid you. You're kind of like a prostitute, without the sex. Ha! That's funny. With a prostitute, you at least get sex.

Dr. Em: So, it sounds like you feel I'm exploiting you, taking your money and pretending to be interested in you.

Betty: I don't like talking about this. I'd just got used to coming here, and now you're making me doubt it all again.

In addition to changing the focus from the patient's external life to the transference, this example illustrates the tactic of addressing the negative transference as well as the positive transference. The therapy had slipped into a superficial positive transference that omitted the negative part until the therapist questioned the patient's underlying beliefs about him.

Dr. Em: That's why I think it's important to be having this discussion. Your feeling comfortable with me does not seem to go very deep. We've reached a situation where your doubts had gone underground but still seem very real. You think I'm like a prostitute. That suggests that you think I'm very phony with you and that any interest I seem to have in you is not real. Is that really better than the situation you describe where you work?

Betty: Probably if I paid them, they'd be nice to me too. It's all the same. You probably make fun of me as soon as I leave the office.... You might be making fun of me in your mind right now, behind that sincere look. That's probably what you learn in therapy school—to look sincere when you think somebody's a jerk.

Dr. Em (*in an example of maintaining neutrality and leaving the conflict within the patient*): I don't think there's anything I can do right now to convince you that I don't think you're a jerk. I think that feeling goes too deep. But what we can do right now is to look at the terrible dilemma you're in, and I think it's one you find yourself in again and again, including at the job right now. You're not sure whether I think you're a jerk or not, or whether people in general think you're a jerk or not. And the safest thing is to assume that they do think that. That way you won't get hurt by being nice to people and having them make fun of you or reject you later. So you respond in kind. The problem is that you're not totally sure it is "in kind," and if you're wrong, your going on the attack may have done a lot of damage to what could have been good relationships. Here, for example, you said I was like a prostitute. In therapy, we can explore the feelings and fantasies that go along with that. But if the same kind of aggression came up with a coworker, you might find that you provoke exactly the kind of reaction you expected in the first place.

Later analysis in Betty's case would consider how the patient is the origin of negative and rejecting thoughts about herself and about others. First, suffering from her own self-appraisal, she projects this judgment of herself onto others and sees it coming from them. Second, she can direct her harsh and judgmental part toward others. This results in harsh judgments of others, although her conscious experience of the situation is that she is simply responding negatively to them because of the attack she perceives as coming from them. In other words, she is playing out in the workplace, and in the transference, the dyad of a mocking critic in relation to a despised other that exists in its entirety within her. Also, although she identifies with both parts of the dyad, she consciously experiences herself only as the despised other.

RELATING INTERNAL REPRESENTATIONS, DEVELOPMENTAL IDENTIFICATIONS, AND PROJECTIONS

As discussed in Chapter 3, strategy 3 of TFP is to observe and interpret linkages between object relations dyads that defend against each other. In relation to this, part of the work in the midphase is to track the manifestations of unintegrated or partially integrated representations as they are projected in different settings. This involves discussion of how the perceptions based on these projections were present in the relationship with the therapist, and of how acting on them risks making the feared situation real. In the later midphase, the analysis of representations is linked to considering the *identification(s)* with external objects in the course of the patient's early development that contributed to the internal object representation. In approaching this material, the therapist should keep in mind that each partial identification is with *an aspect* of a person in the patient's life and usually involves some distortion with regard to the actual person. The therapist links the cognitions and affects associated with this identification—which can appear both in the patient's self representation and in object representations—to the projected representation(s) in the transference, the patient's external life, the patient's past, and fantasy material. Later interpretive work might include genetic material, such as the possibility that the patient who projects aggressive affects has difficulty tolerating any identification with past, or present, aggressors. The effort in these interventions is to help the patient appreciate the extent that response to someone new may be based on the triggering of an internal object. These regressions may be considered a retreat into a safe psychological place defined by projection. In the uncertainty and ambiguity of a new situation, a defensive stance seems more comfortable than one that is open to new experience.

As does all psychoanalytically based therapy, TFP has the goal of increasing the patient's awareness and acceptance of prohibited thoughts and feelings. As our examples have shown, discovering these is often through the process of following the projection in all its permutations. In the midphase, as the patient progresses in integrating split-off internal parts, the work of recognizing projections can become more subtle. As the patient's internal world becomes less crude—less all good and all bad—the patient's descriptions of situations that may involve projection become more nuanced with less evidence of distortion. There is a better fit between the internal representations and external reality, but there still may be a gap, especially during times of stress. Therefore, in the advanced midphase, exploration in therapy may go on for stretches of time when it is not clear if the patient is distorting/projecting or describing a situation that is genuinely disturbing. Another way of saying this is that although the patient's reality testing has improved, there may still be evidence of more subtle difficulties in this area. It is in working with these subtle difficulties that TFP helps patients resolve areas of their internal conflicts that may have been initially hidden by overt acting out but that need to be resolved to allow for full appreciation of self and others and optimal functioning in love, leisure, and work.

CLINICAL ILLUSTRATION

When Amy's son was 3½ years old, she began to report concerns about the nanny she had hired. She was uncomfortable with the way the nanny looked at her son at times. She felt that the nanny added a suggestion of sensuality when she let the little boy lick the spoon when they baked together. She also felt that the nanny sat a little too close when she read stories to him. Amy became preoccupied with concerns that the nanny had sexual intentions toward her son and wondered if she should fire her. This situation was more ambiguous than the experiences Amy reported earlier in therapy. Dr. Jones had difficulty distinguishing if Amy was accurately perceiving the situation or if she was being influenced by a projection.

In an effort to see whether Amy's concerns might correspond to an internal issue, Dr. Jones wondered aloud in a way that combined a question with a suggested area of exploration: "It can be confusing and disturbing to think about the kind of things you're concerned about. There certainly are perverse people in the world who abuse children. One thing I wonder about, though, is that as you've become more and more preoccupied with Jennifer's feelings toward Billy, we hear less and less about yours. Of course, I know he's been the joy of your life since he was born, but he's growing fast, as boys do. He's developing more of a mind of his own and more of a character of his own and interests of his own. As he's becoming a person of his own, your feelings about him are no doubt developing and are no doubt complex. That's normal. You may have some regrets, and even anger, about his growing independence from you. You may admire his growing body. These things can be difficult to think about—they may not feel right. But part of our work here is to uncover your feelings, in case they may be relevant here, so that you can know them and manage them better."

Amy was then able to reflect more fully on her emotional responses to her child. The prior work on integrating her libidinal and aggressive affects allowed her to experience some anger about his growing independence and some sexual admiration that could blend in with her predominant love and devotion for him without threatening the bond she felt with him. Part of the patient's reflection on these issues involved her reassuring herself that she could have this range of feelings about her son without engaging in the angry outbursts or the inappropriate touching that were part of her mother's relationship with her.

To summarize, a principle of therapeutic work in the midphase is following projections of the patient's split-off representations as they appear in the transference, in relationships and settings outside the therapy, and in fantasies, and to assume that the patient may present with cycles that repeat the dynamic in a more subtle and contained way.

PATIENT IMPROVEMENT AND THE REACTION

With the structure of treatment, many borderline patients improve their work and/or intimate relations. Progress in these areas can be surprising to patients and even resisted with temptations to dismantle the progress. The progress itself and the patient's response to it can be a theme in the treatment. The therapist observes the progress and is alert to impulses on the part of the patient to undo it. This issue is exemplified in the evolution of the case of Betty.

CLINICAL ILLUSTRATION

In Betty's second year of therapy, she went from her volunteer job to a paid job teaching reading to illiterate adults. After 6 months, she decided she would be more successful if she completed the college degree that she had left unfinished many years before. She enrolled in courses on a part-time basis. She passed the first course with an A. However, in her second course she became paralyzed with regard to writing her term paper, threatening the progress she had made. Exploration of the problem revealed three main themes of which she had not been aware. First, she feared that her initial success aroused the envy of her classmates and that they would begin to gang up on her. This led to further elaboration of the role of envy in her internal world. In a typical way, she could both feel this emotion intensely and, by projection, feel she was the object of it.

Second, Betty became more aware that she associated doing well with losing her therapist. She believed that his interest in her was limited to his role as a helper in relation to a "lowly" impaired patient. Her internal world had no paradigm for an authority figure having an interest in her developing into a healthy equal.

The third theme uncovered in exploration was that Betty's initial success stirred up competitive feelings both with her classmates and with her therapist. Betty, whose internal dyads principally involved an inferior being in relation to a superior one, imagined that competition ultimately involved sadistic subjugation of one party to the other. She had to explore these extreme fantasies before developing the ability to sublimate aggressive affects into more modulated relations with others in academic and other settings.

Although making progress inevitably stirs up concerns about ending the relationship with the therapist, it is easier for a patient to deal with these concerns when the most pathological level of anxiety is explored and the patient can see that it is in his or her interest to grow and move on rather than to remain impaired and dependent. This, of course, involves dealing with issues of mourning related to the depressive position, which are discussed in Chapter 10, "Advanced Phase of Treatment and Termination."

Key Clinical Concepts

- The midphase of treatment is characterized by a decrease in acting out and increased focus on patient-therapist interaction.

- There is generally an evolution of the predominant transference theme from antisocial, narcissistic, or paranoid to depressive.

- Patients achieve greater acceptance and tolerance of their own negative affect but usually with periodic regressions to projection.

- Libidinal longings in the patient generally emerge, along with distortions in the experience and expression of sexuality and romantic love that need to be explored.

- As the therapy evolves, the focus of sessions expands to increasingly include a combination of interest in the patient's 1) internal representations; 2) current external reality; 3) past history and evolving life narrative, especially as it relates to identity; and 4) fantasy material.

- Work in therapy allows for a more nuanced understanding and analysis of problem areas in the patient's love, work, and leisure life.

SELECTED READINGS

Kernberg OF: The psychodynamics and psychotherapeutic management of psychopathic, narcissistic, and paranoid transferences, in Aggressivity, Narcissism, and Self-Destructiveness in the Psychotherapeutic Relationship. Edited by Kernberg OF. New Haven, CT, Yale University Press, 2004, pp 130–153
Ogden TH: Between the paranoid-schizoid and the depressive positions, in Matrix of the Mind: Object Relations and the Psychoanalytic Dialogue. Northvale, NJ, Jason Aronson, 1993, pp 101–129

10

ADVANCED PHASE OF TREATMENT AND TERMINATION

THE ADVANCED PHASE of transference-focused psychotherapy (TFP) corresponds to a sufficient working-through of previously split-off transference developments. At this point in therapy, the patient can tolerate experiencing a fuller range of affect and can better master affects as they arise. The patient's awareness of the interchange of roles with the therapist within a dyad has helped the patient take back parts of the self that he or she traditionally projected. In the advanced phase, interpretive integration of the mutually split-off idealized and persecutory segments of the patient's internal experience proceeds as the central focus in a cycle where decreased internal splitting gives rise to increased cognitive awareness and better affective modulation, which in turn leaves the patient with an improved capacity to reflect and use the interpretive process (as seen in the case of Amy in Chapter 9, "Midphase of Treatment"). The advanced phase is not a clear transition but emerges when the patient begins to accept the awareness that his or her identity includes parts that he or she had unconsciously attempted to reject previously. As described in Chapter 9, even after therapy enters the advanced phase, progression and regression occur as the patient's primitive defense mechanisms diminish or reassert themselves in accordance with the ebb and flow of challenging and stressful experiences in the patient's life.

The time it takes to enter the advanced phase of therapy varies from one patient to another; some patients enter the phase as early as a year into treatment, whereas others may take years to progress that far (Table 10–1). Patients who are less antisocial, paranoid, or narcissistic generally reach the advanced phase more quickly.

CASE EXAMPLE

Greg, whom we described in Chapter 8 ("Early Treatment Phase"), came to understand that his self-criticism and his paranoid fear that his therapist and other people disliked him and were trying to get rid of him was one side of a coin. In the course of therapy, his increasing criticisms of his therapist, Ms. Ot, and other people corresponded to an identification with the harsh critic that he generally experienced as coming from outside. At those times he saw himself as intellectually superior, felt bored with Ms. Ot's "repetitive" statements, and dismissively talked of changing therapists. As he and Ms. Ot explored these two sides of him, Greg came to understand that he could judge, criticize, and "put himself down" in equally harsh terms as he experienced from others. Thus, he became aware of the oscillations of that dyad and recognized that the dyad existed in its entirety in him. In addition, he came to see that the relationship he experienced on the surface between a rejecting, arrogant object and a devalued self, a relationship infiltrated with aggression, was completely split off from a wish to establish a dependent relationship with his therapist, as well as with others, as an approving and benevolent caretaker. This libidinal aspect of his internal world became apparent in fantasies that Ms. Ot would be like a guardian angel watching over him during stressful meetings at his job, keeping him from ever making a mistake. However, moments of harsh criticism toward her returned if he felt she had not listened or understood just right. His lashing out at her at these moments was an example of the damage the idealized internal representation can do when someone does not meet its standards. These reactions undermined the possibility for a dependent relationship with Ms. Ot because real dependency can be experienced only when the patient has advanced from the paranoid-schizoid organization to the depressive (integrated) one. Nonetheless, the emergence of the full range of this material in the sessions was the material they needed to observe and eventually integrate.

In the advanced phase of therapy, Greg was in contact with both the idealized (dependent) and persecutory (arrogant and devaluing) segments of experience without continuing to reenact them in a split-off way. Ms. Ot could then interpret the patient's fear that a more integrated view of her as both benevolent and potentially frustrating, as well as an idea of himself as having serious conflicts around aggression and yet a loving core, would either 1) be intolerable because of the patient's wish for a perfect caretaker or 2) make him feel undeserving of a gratifying or dependent relationship because of his angry and aggressive reactions. In simple terms, Greg was be-

TABLE 10-1.	Changes in the advanced phase of treatment

Ability to experience and reflect on affects that had previously overwhelmed the patient and led to acting out and/or projection

Ability to distinguish raw internal reactions to trigger events from the complexity of the external person and situation

Ability to work with internal fantasies as distinct from external reality

Ability to give up self-defeating patterns outside the treatment and to engage in more consistent and productive investments in personal relations and work

Ability to talk more openly and freely with the therapist about their relationship

Evidence of a changing conception of the therapist and self (patient) in relationship

Ability to accept interpretations from the therapist and amplify them in reference to self and other

Evidence that anxiety and depressed affects can often be resolved in the session by interpretive interventions of the therapist

Evidence of an initially fragile but increasingly dependent transference in lieu of paranoid transference as awareness of projection of aggressive aspects of self increases

Emergence of a clearer self concept and reflectiveness in the relationship with the therapist and others

In BPO patients with narcissistic personality disorder, evidence of dismantling of the pathological grandiose self structure, allowing access to an underlying fragmented identity for more meaningful exploration

ginning to tolerate an ambivalent relationship toward his therapist as both a benevolent but limited caretaker and an authority figure capable of judgment and criticism and a view of himself as having both loving feelings and feelings of frustration and aggression toward Ms. Ot. Previously, these elements had been difficult to merge because of his initial conviction that the harsh, critical element existed solely in her rather than in himself. This had led to both resentment of Ms. Ot's assumed dismissing superiority and to repeated enactments of his rejection of her as a helpful, although limited, figure in favor of the longed-for perfect fantasy version. The integration of love with aggression and hate under the dominance of love marked, fleetingly at first and then more consistently, the beginning of the advanced phase of treatment in Greg's case.

The process of integration does not occur in a linear fashion. Regression to what can seem to be a repetition of the earliest sessions of the treatment—with splitting, projective mechanisms, omnipotent control, and denial of experiences other than those that momentarily dominate the transference—may still occur. However, these regressive episodes no longer last for days or weeks before they can be worked through again or before they come into contact with the split-off opposite segment. They now may be worked through in a series of several sessions and, eventually, in the course of a single session, during which the patient shifts from states of the activation of primitive, split-off, part-object relations in the transference, or in relation to an external situation, to a more complex integrated object relation with more modulated affect. Eventually, the therapist may condense into a few sessions or a single session the progression from 1) recognition of the dominant object relation to 2) awareness of the mutual interchange of self and object representations to 3) integration of mutually split-off affectively opposite dyads with the corresponding emergence of self representations and of object representations with complex qualities. This process continues repetitively throughout the advanced stages of the treatment, with a gradual decrease of the regressive tendencies. If the therapy progresses successfully, a shift occurs from the dominance of primitive, particularly paranoid transferences into advanced or depressive transferences that come to resemble the transference developments in patients with neurotic personality organization and signal the resolution of identity diffusion.

CLINICAL CHARACTERISTICS OF THE ADVANCED PHASE

ANTISOCIAL/PSYCHOPATHIC AND PARANOID TRANSFERENCES RESOLVE

Throughout successful treatment a shift evolves from predominantly paranoid, and the less frequent but more severe psychopathic transference, into depressive transference patterns (see Chapter 9). The psychopathic transference, involving the patient's consciously deceptive behavior in relation to the therapist and the corresponding expectation that the therapist's only objective is to exploit him or her, should be sufficiently resolved for honest communication with the therapist to be possible.

Honest communication does not mean that the patient may not have anxiety about speaking freely, occasional secrets that the patient feels he or she has to keep from the therapist, or temporary suppression of important material out of shame or guilt. It implies, however, that in general, the therapist can rely on the patient's honest communication to resolve such transitory breakdowns of communication in the course of the psychotherapeutic work. One cannot speak of an advanced stage of the treatment before full resolution of psychopathic transferences; we remind the reader that these transferences are the greatest challenge to treatment and are often refractory to treatment especially because antisocial patients are rarely motivated for treatment and usually present because of external pressure. These transferences resolve when the patient is able to question his or her assumption that the therapist is totally exploitative and incapable of empathy and that all relationships are based exclusively on who can exploit the other.

Paranoid transferences still may be present during the advanced treatment stage but now can be resolved within the session or in days rather than in weeks of psychotherapeutic work, and work on these transferences can benefit from a sufficiently strong therapeutic alliance (i.e., a sufficiently strong relationship between the therapist in role and the observing part of the patient's ego) to tolerate paranoid regressions without a threat to the continuity of the treatment. It is in the context of those paranoid transferences that are still present, but no longer overwhelming, that the therapist can see evidence of the patient's tolerance of guilt over his or her aggression and the acknowledgment of ambivalence and reparatory strivings in the transference, signaling movement toward integration.

ACTING OUT OUTSIDE SESSIONS IMPROVES

When the treatment progresses effectively, severe acting out outside the treatment sessions should be better controlled even during the early stages of treatment (3–6 months into treatment), and by the advanced phase the patient's life outside the sessions may have already normalized to a significant extent. In contrast, increasingly intense transference developments are reflected in emotional intensity and possibly affect storms in the sessions. In the advanced stages of the treatment, the patient has become aware of the difference between the therapist's tolerance of his or her regressive behavior in sessions, with the goal of understanding it, and the need to control his or her behavior outside and bring strong reactions to external events into the therapy for exploration rather than act out outside the treatment sessions. Therefore, the threats that were the highest priorities of intervention in the earlier stages—namely, 1) threat to the patient's or others' well-being, 2) threat to the continuity of the treatment, and 3) threat of severe destructive or self-destructive acting out outside the sessions—should have decreased enough to permit the therapist to focus increasingly on transference itself. Many patients tend to split their external reality from the sessions in the early part of treatment, but in the advanced phase the therapist should be able to rely on the patient's communication of his or her experiences outside the session without having to continue to actively inquire about the patient's outside life. In the following example, we return to Betty, the patient with higher-level borderline personality disorder.

CLINICAL ILLUSTRATION

Betty, who had begun therapy talking about the woman who glared at her on the bus, began to develop some friendly acquaintances in the second year of treatment. She described going to a park with two new friends. In the course of the afternoon, she became angry that the friends "were not paying enough attention to her"; at a moment when they were distracted, she left the park without saying good-bye. Although this was a less intense acting out than her initial behavior of yelling at people she thought were dismissing her, Dr. Em discussed it with her as an expression of her acting out aggression that she did not yet recognize (leaving her friends very worried about what had happened to her).

By the next year, Betty was able to recognize, contain, and question this kind of reaction within her: "I'd arranged to have some friends come to celebrate my birthday at a local restaurant. I got there on time, but no one else was there. In the old days, I would have left right away, gone home, and probably cut myself. But I started thinking, 'It *is* raining…maybe it's hard for them to get here. And if I leave and they come, I guess I'd be standing them up.' Part of me wanted to do that to punish them for being late. But then I started thinking that I wasn't suffering only because they were late but because I assumed that meant that they don't give a damn about me. It wasn't easy. I kept wondering if maybe that *was* what was going on. Anyway, they came and we had a good time. It's a good thing I didn't leave because that would have started one of those old cycles of bad feeling."

Sometimes turmoil in the sessions may make it difficult for the therapist to be aware of the patient's improvement outside the sessions. A development in a successful therapy is that the patient comes to trust the therapist enough to remain open about negative reactions that he or she realizes are best hidden from people outside sessions. This is particularly true when the paranoid transference is not fully resolved and the patient is uncertain whether to stay with his or her old instinct of mistrust or anxiously be open to the possibility that his or her wish for a relationship may be reciprocated.

Although Betty was able to wait for her friends at the restaurant, she still responded to Dr. Em's telling her that he would be away for 2 weeks by saying to him, "Just when I was beginning to trust you, you're doing the same old thing! You know my exams are coming up, and if I don't pass them I'll have to repeat the semester, which I won't do! I'll just go back to my crappy temp job until I decide there is no point in living." Even though Betty was able to keep these reactions to herself in other relations, she could continue to explore them in therapy. She needed to further explore her wish for an ideal other who would be there whenever she wanted before she could fully move beyond her reaction that a disappointment was the same as total rejection by the other.

In some cases, when the transference is negative, the improvement outside the sessions may be so dissociated from the material in the sessions that the therapist may not be aware of and thus may not be able to take into account the patient's changes in significant areas of his or her relationships. An example occurred in the fourth year of Betty's therapy. Although she had made progress, she could still regress to moments of negative transference. This example involves progress in the work and relational life of this woman who had entered treatment after a long period of unemployment because of conflictual relations with others.

> Betty began a session by stating with a demoralized tone, "I had another fight with my boyfriend. I may as well kill myself." Dr. Em was concerned because this was Betty's first mention of suicide in many months, and his facial expression probably reflected his concern. Betty, likely having noticed Dr. Em's anxiety and concern, went on by saying, "But then again, I've been getting along really well with my colleagues for the first time ever so maybe I should hold off on killing myself." Dr. Em had been unaware of this positive development that apparently dated back for some time. This is an example of how the interchanges in the advanced phase can be complex. Betty began the session disappointed with herself ("another fight with my boyfriend") but attempted to free herself of self-directed anger by attacking the therapist ("I may as well kill myself" = "you haven't done your job and helped me"). However, when she noted Dr. Em's anxiety, her level of integration allowed her to feel concern for a now-valued relationship and to worry about her attack on him rather than to push him further away out of disappointment, anger, and envy. Her comment that relations with colleagues were good for the first time showed that she could limit her aggression when it threatened a relationship that was now still valuable in spite of a moment of disappointment—it was an attempt to repair the damage done by her attack that allowed Dr. Em insight into a burgeoning positive area of her life that she had heretofore kept from him. Dr. Em and Betty could now move on to explore both this positive development in her life and the meaning of her having kept it to herself until then.

RELATIONSHIP WITH THE THERAPIST DEEPENS AS PROJECTION DECREASES

Evidence of the patient's capacity to internalize the therapist will be demonstrated in the form of improved reflecting on his or her own affects, perceptions, motivations, and actions. In addition, other relationships in the patient's life will acquire a sharper, more realistic, more alive quality as they are described in the sessions. More subtle contradictions in the patient's behavior may emerge that were previously ignored by patient and therapist. New information may be forthcoming, such as secrets previously kept from the therapist. The relationship with the therapist now deepens; the patient appreciates more appropriately the therapist's contribution to the therapy and develops a more empathic, realistic observation of the therapist as a person with limitations but goodwill. The patient's capacity to recall the shared history of the relationship with the therapist increases. Mutually contradictory transference dispositions tend to get mixed up, only to be resolved in the same session and to acquire a new emotional depth and complexity. Patients are able to work more autonomously in the sessions. The therapist's role evolves from one of primarily clarifying, confronting, and interpreting to one of being witness to the patient's improved capacity to reflect on his or her own issues, making only occasional reminders of pathological patterns at times of regression under stress.

> As Betty got more involved with work, she started a session saying, "I'm really busy, maybe stretched too thin. Sometimes I don't have time to call people, but I still worry about people not getting back to me on time." Dr. Em responded, "It's a familiar theme but it seems less intense now." Betty replied, "Right, it's still hard to trust people, but if somebody doesn't respond right away, I try to be patient now and think about it."

Regarding shifts in the interpretive approach and other techniques in advanced stages of the treatment, the therapist may be able to increase the linkage of present transference developments to unconscious, past pathogenic object relations. In other words, the therapist can increasingly include genetic interpretations involving the patient's history along with the here-and-now interpretations that predominate in the early and middle phases of treatment. This is most effective when the patient makes the link himself or herself. There may be an increase in the patient's capacity to use free association and dream interpretation, and the therapist is now able to rely more on the observing part of the patient's ego in formulations of transference and other interpretations. The relationship between the sessions and the patient's external life may become more fluid and natural, in contrast to earlier dissociation between these two areas of the patient's experience.

For example, Gabby said to Dr. Tam, "It's hard for me to believe the violent things I used to do to my husband, and sometimes to you [e.g., she had once thrown Dr. Tam's briefcase across the office], thinking they were totally justified. Now I see how much I can hurt others. I used to think I was the only one who ever got hurt." This linking of Gabby's reactions to her husband and to Dr. Tam shows how her movement from paranoid-schizoid organization to the depressive organization, characterized by the remorse that accompanies the acknowledgment of aggression, affected her experience across relationships. At this point, Dr. Tam could better help

Gabby integrate her aggressive affects and gain mastery over them in terms of how to express and direct them.

In most cases, as the patient enters the depressive organization, mourning of the ideal object precedes remorse over the patient's own aggression. In terms of the analysis of the content of the patient's conflicts, as termination approaches, the focus may be on these more advanced mourning reactions characteristic of the depressive position—with its themes of awareness of the patient's needs, desires, and aggressive affects. Changes in the patient's relations to parents, siblings, and other family members may occur in the context of a mental reorganization of the patient's past, and patients may come to terms with traumatic circumstances of the past.

As the patient moves into the advanced phase of treatment, the atmosphere of the individual sessions gradually shifts to a reduction of the dominant primitive defense mechanisms responsible for earlier distortions in the transference. The patient's relationship with the therapist becomes closer to that of a psychotherapeutic session with a more integrated patient dealing with neurotic conflicts. The patient more easily talks freely at the beginning of the sessions, without consistent challenges to the boundaries of the psychotherapeutic relationship or paranoid fear of humiliation, rejection, and abandonment. The patient's greater access to fantasy and sharper awareness of his or her psychosocial reality facilitate longer stretches of a narrative in which significant subjective experiences are verbally communicated in contrast to the previous dominance of nonverbal communication and intense countertransference reactions provoked by dissociated elements in the patient. The patient's observations of his or her own behavior and that of important people surrounding him or her have a more balanced, less chaotic, less distorted, and less rigidly restrictive quality.

In the relationship with the therapist, the patient may anticipate the therapist's comments, thus signaling the patient's internalization of aspects of the therapist's attitudes toward him or her and an increase in his or her own observing (reflective) capacities. This strengthening of the patient's observing ego is apparent in his or her reaction to moments of regression in the transference or in relation to an external event that provokes a return to an unrealistically idealized or persecutory view of the reality. For example, Betty was able to say, "What you're saying, it's making me upset. It makes me think again that you're disgusted with me and want to get rid of me, though I know that's not true." These comments demonstrate the return of a gut reaction that is now tempered by Betty's reflective work and interpretation. Betty showed evidence of similar affect modulation tempered by cognitive effort when she said, "My boss gave me some suggestions. Before I would've thought it was all criticism. Now I realize they were interesting ideas. I still have a negative reaction, but now I think about it. I used to think all the attacks I saw were right. I wanted to leave therapy because I thought you were taking me away from the truth when you questioned them. Now the truth seems different—but this [positive view] better be real! I guess there's no way to know the absolute truth." This final comment is evidence of deep psychological change in that it shows that Betty has developed her observing ego to the point where she realizes that every experience requires reflection before an accurate appreciation can be achieved.

These changes allow for modifications in technique. The therapist may feel more at ease in being direct with the patient, as in presenting the patient with more direct reflections about his or her difficulties that may be painful for the patient, without the patient experiencing the interpretation, or the simple statement of a difficult reality, as an attack or devaluation. The therapist may also become more direct and open in the sense of being less cautious or tentative in formulating interpretations, with the assurance that the patient has become able to reflect more independently on interpretations in the context of the history of the exploration of problems in the treatment. Finally, the therapist simply has to do less because the patient's increased capacity for reflection allows him or her to do the work of correcting distortions. At these moments, the therapist may have the role of validating or confirming the patient's own observation.

> **Betty:** It was a major thing to talk to my boyfriend—now we live like couples do, without stress *all* the time. I used to think my future depended on him. Now I don't feel so burdened.
> **Dr. Em:** In the past your way out of the burden seemed to be suicidal ideation and actions. I guess you see there are other ways. Also, the burden seems now like it was mostly in your head, doesn't it?
> **Betty:** That's true—at work, the work doesn't stress me, but the demands in my head do. And I'm doing well with friends now—I just say to myself, "hold on, they'll get back to you."
> **Dr. Em:** You used to think you were untouchable.
> **Betty:** Yes (*laughs*), now I realize people can be busy—I can be busy! The only thing that has changed—now I cut people some slack…, and I cut *myself* some slack!

If, over the course of the therapy, the therapist has consistently reflected back to the patient the evidence of his or her conflicts (the technique of confrontation) without giving in to the patient's unconscious efforts to control the therapist to support the patient's primitive defenses, and if the patient has learned that to be encouraged to reflect on previously unacceptable or intolerable aspects of his or her personality does not mean that he or she is being attacked or devalued, the patient will now be much more able to listen, less afraid of his or her own negative transferences, and more able to observe and modulate what was previously split off from awareness and thus not subject to cortical control. In general, the decrease of primitive mechanisms implies a greater awareness of and tolerance for internal contradictions and conflicts on the patient's part and a strengthening of the patient's ego in terms of impulse control, anxiety tolerance, and capacity to reflect on the internal contradictions. Nonspecific manifestations of ego weakness decrease as higher-level defensive operations start to become predominant. Independent work by the patient in some areas of conflict begins to emerge, and the therapist may take more of a listening stance, receptive to the patient's autonomous work in the sessions and able to help the patient strengthen it.

CLINICAL ILLUSTRATION

Betty had been waiting to hear from a job she was excited about but had become cynical and dejected when she did not get any response for a few weeks.

Betty: I heard from the school—I got the job. I decided to take everything that way now, like friends—give them the benefit of the doubt. I realize I have to be active and not just wait to get approached. But I still feel a little lost….

Dr. Em: That's not surprising; you're building an adult identity.

Betty: And trying to change the way I think. I realize that people might react to me in a certain way because of something going on in *their* life.

Dr. Em (*with a smile*): So it's not all about you?

Betty: Right, it's ironic; it's like I had the opposite of narcissism—it was all about me, in negative.

Dr. Em: I could have imagined you having an angrier reaction when you didn't hear from the school.

Betty: Me too.

Dr. Em: That could have destroyed the opportunity you have now, and you could have been left feeling hopeless.

Betty: I think about the trip to the park with my friends. I couldn't think of what to say at the time so I got angry and left. I couldn't say what I wanted or needed. I was afraid of people not liking me. I didn't realize I was doing something that might make them not like me.

Dr. Em: That fear of people not liking you seems to correspond more to an image of yourself that you have inside of you rather than what's in them.

INDICATORS OF STRUCTURAL INTRAPSYCHIC CHANGE

There are a number of indicators of structural change manifested by the patient that can be used as markers in the advanced stage of TFP.

EVIDENCE OF THE PATIENT'S PROGRESS TOWARD SELF-OBSERVATION

Patient statements demonstrate the capacity to observe and reflect on gut reactions that would previously have dominated the patient's thinking to the exclusion of alternative and more realistically nuanced perspectives as demonstrated in the above examples from the case of Betty.

EXPLORATION OF THERAPIST COMMENTS

The patient's statements now demonstrate either an expansion or a further exploration of the therapist's comments. The issue here is not whether the patient agrees with an interpretation or goes along with the suggested subject for exploration but the extent to which the patient gives himself or herself the chance to reflect on what the therapist has said instead of immediately and automatically rejecting, denying, avoiding, or contradicting the therapist's comments. We also emphasize that the issue is not whether the transference is positive or negative but whether there is some degree of cooperation in clarifying what is going on, in contrast to either a categorical rejection of exploration or a thoughtless acceptance of, submission to, or lip service to the therapist's suggestions. This ability to move from blanket reflection to exploration of the therapist's comments is of particular importance in the treatment of patients with severe narcissistic personalities.

CONTAINMENT AND TOLERANCE OF THE AWARENESS OF AGGRESSION AND LOVE

Insofar as borderline personality organization is linked with difficulties with primitive aggression and its impact on the integration of positive and negative affects (regardless of whether the intensity of aggressive affects derives from genetic, constitutional, and temperamental factors or is secondary to neglect, trauma, or witnessing of abuse), the dominant unconscious affect associated with such severe aggression is hatred. The patient's psyche is marked by a characterologically structured hateful relationship between a traumatized self and a sadistically perceived object, with a fundamental motivation of destroying the object that is seen as inflicting pain, making it suffer, or controlling it. In addition, projection leads to corresponding fears of the object's hatred toward the self. Interference with the experience of libidinal, affiliative, loving affects is clear. The process of overcoming the internal split and bringing affects of aggression and hatred into an integrated self includes the patient's becoming aware that these affects are part of the human experience and that, if integrated and mastered, they do not destroy any possibility of experiencing oneself as a decent human being and experiencing gratifying relationships. Containment and tolerance of the awareness of aggressive and negative affects, in contrast to their expression by acting out, somatization, or destruction of the communication with the therapist, is a sign of an advanced stage of treatment.

The decrease of manifestations of aggression is seen in changes in its direct expression in sessions, in a decline in aggressive dismissals of whatever the therapist offers, and in the reduction in sadomasochistic transferences. In addition, negative therapeutic reactions as the expression of unconscious envy of the therapist (i.e., the need to defeat the therapist's efforts) resolve, as do characterologically anchored self-directed manifestations of hatred, such as suicidal, parasuicidal, and self-injurious behaviors; substance abuse; eating disorders; severe self-destructive sexual behaviors; and/or relentless self-loathing.

At this stage of the treatment, the most destructive aspects of the patient's sexual behavior should be under control or, in those cases characterized by an inhibition of sexuality, sexual feelings can now be experienced. In the early stages of the treatment, the dominance within some patients' sexual behavior of severe aggressive and self-aggressive trends interferes with all intimate love relationships. This could consist of promiscuous, unsafe sex; sadomasochistic sex; or, more subtly, serial affairs that are based on the quest for the ideal object and that destroy the possibility of any in-depth relationship. Alternatively, in some cases these patients present an absence of all sexual engagements. A general increase demonstrated in sessions of the patient's concern for his or her love life and sexual interactions indicates an improvement in the patient's functioning in the sense that sexuality is no longer dominated by aggression and libidinal desires are no longer overshadowed by paranoid fears.

A potential problem in the advanced stages of treatment, however, is that in cases of severe primary inhibition of the sexual response, such inhibition may increase as the patient's general functioning improves and repressive mechanisms replace more primitive dissociative or splitting mechanisms. This is a complication that may require modification of the psychotherapeutic approach, such as combination with sex therapy once the patient's severe inhibition of sexual desire has been sufficiently reduced to make the unconscious dynamics of this primary sexual inhibition clarified enough to permit an integration of psychodynamic psychotherapy and sex therapy.

TOLERANCE OF FANTASY

The tolerance of fantasy and an increase in the symbolic awareness and containment of previously dissociated or acted-out affect states allow the patient to experience and play with emotions that he or she previously experienced as too threatening to allow into awareness and/or that he or she felt had to be hidden from the therapist. This can be particularly relevant in the treatment of a borderline patient with narcissistic personality for whom an issue is the extent to which the patient may openly reveal free associations that are not under his or her control, with the implicit perceived danger that the therapist may gain understanding about what is going on in the patient's mind before the patient is fully aware of it. The need for omnipotent control tends to inhibit free association and reduce the availability of fantasy material.

CAPACITY TO USE INTERPRETATION OF DEFENSE MECHANISMS

During the early stages of the treatment, interpretations are often effective in initiating a questioning of entrenched positions in spite of apparent dismissal of them or a premature acceptance on the patient's part. In the advanced phase of the treatment, the effect of interpretations includes an increase in the patient's capacity for self-awareness and self-exploration as a consequence of interpretation. The increased capacity to take back what has been projected is precisely what may be expected in the advanced phase of TFP.

CASE EXAMPLE

In one session with a patient who sometimes viewed her therapist as someone who was friendly and at other times viewed the therapist through a projection of an internal image of a sadistic stepmother, the therapist commented, "This raises the question whether I am indeed two different persons or whether you see in me something you are struggling with inside of you. Part of this person is friendly and nice, trustworthy. The other part is a hostile, sadistic person who enjoys provoking while acting innocent and yet is totally blind to this aspect of her personality." The patient commented, ironically, "Does that sound like somebody we know?" When asked whom she had in mind, the patient wondered whether it was herself or her stepmother, and the therapist responded that the patient seemed to be aware of having some aspects that her stepmother represented of which she had not been aware before and that her awareness could help her manage these aspects of herself that had tended to emerge in uncontrolled and damaging ways. The patient returned to this interpretation later on, using it to help gain mastery over aggressive and controlling tendencies of which she was now more aware.

The following is an example from the case of Amy:

CLINICAL ILLUSTRATION

After Amy's overt acting out of aggressive affects ended (as described in Chapter 8), a regular characteristic of her interactions with Dr. Jones was a dismissive and devaluing attitude, often accompanied by a piercing look and a wrinkling of her nose as though in the presence of a very unpleasant smell. After observing this behavior over a period of time, Dr. Jones commented on it.

> **Dr. Jones:** It hasn't been a part of our discussion, but it might be relevant to think about the feelings you are communicating through your look and gestures. There's something in your way of looking at me, the way of wrinkling your nose, and a tone of voice that suggests a rejecting and condescending way of feeling about me.
>
> **Amy:** You're kidding! You *always* have an arrogant and condescending look in relation to me. Because it's always so present, I don't even bother to mention it; I just figure it's part of who you are.
>
> **Dr. Jones** (*who decided to proceed with the therapist-centered approach to interpretation*): I wasn't aware of that. Could you tell me more about it?

The two continued to discuss the theme of Dr. Jones's "condescension" periodically over the next sessions. Then one day, Amy said, "We may have some things in common; I think we're both highly critical." Dr. Jones understood this as Amy's having needed to spend some time getting comfortable with reflecting on a highly critical part of a person. Dr. Jones's ability to think about this, without accepting it or denying it in himself, may have signaled to Amy that one can reflect on a characteristic of the self without being totally overwhelmed by it. She eventually could consider this part of herself.

SHIFT IN PREDOMINANT TRANSFERENCE PARADIGMS

The movement from one predominant transference pattern to another is not linear but is characterized by an alternation of progression and temporary regression to the earlier predisposition because each newer and more positive perspective is relatively unfamiliar to the patient and provokes a measure of doubt and anxiety. This indicator of structural change may be considered the most fundamental marker of the patient's evolution through treatment. As we emphasize in Chapter 9, antisocial or psychopathic transferences, should they be present, evolve, in successful therapy, into paranoid transferences. The paranoid transference, while recognizing the possibility of motivations in the therapist other than the exploitation assumed in the antisocial transference, is still fundamentally negative because it is based on the projection of negative affects and motivations. In successful cases, the exploration of the paranoid transference allows more access to the idealized segment of the split internal world, in addition to the recognition of the intrapsychic origin of aggressive impulses previously projected. As this material emerges, questions about the radical separation of these aspects of the patient's mind can be more fruitfully addressed.

A depressive transference—characterized by mourning the loss of the ideal object and experiencing remorse as awareness of aggressive affects increases—emerges in connection with the overcoming of splitting operations and the development of a more integrated and normal ego identity. In practice, this shift is illustrated by the appearance of new, more complex and differentiated aspects of self and objects, as well as the emergence of new relationships that transcend the rigid patterns of the repetitive early ones. Although the development of the depressive transference is a major advance, it involves conflicts around aggression, guilt, and loss that benefit from further work in therapy.

CLINICAL ILLUSTRATION

Amy, who initially experienced Dr. Jones as an indifferent robot, entered a phase in which she oscillated between experiencing him as a powerful sadistic figure and as a benevolent fatherly figure who offered the promise of peace and harmony. Over time, she began to experience him as a friendly yet strong and sexually seductive fatherly figure, a new constellation that emerged as the split-off primitive transferences began to integrate into a more complex whole. In this context, new aspects of her evolving internalized relationship with father figures emerged that had a markedly oedipal quality, in contrast to the pre-oedipal denial of all sexuality in the image of the idealized warm and giving yet "sanitized" father.

The following case also illustrates a patient's clear shift into a depressive type of transference:

CASE EXAMPLE

A patient who had severe antisocial features and who had perceived her therapist for a long period as a persecutory, sadistic moralizer against whom she had to protect herself through a combination of secrets and manipulation, gradually began to acknowledge and feel guilty about her dishonesty and also felt guilty about mistreating her therapist, whom she now perceived as reassuringly maintaining their relationship in spite of her indirect attacks on him. She began to perceive him as a strict but concerned father figure, very different from what she now, probably realistically, became aware of as the manipulative and dishonest father in her past. She became depressed, with a profound conviction that she did not deserve to be loved by the therapist and taken care of by him and a quiet despair that coincided with an effort to repair relationships with former friends whom she had treated badly and whose friendship she was now trying to recover. In this patient, the development of an integrated yet severe superego and the related expression of guilt feelings toward the therapist coincided with a sense of incapacity to repair such guilt that constituted an entirely new transference constellation, requiring exploration as to the source of the sense that forgiveness was impossible.

Perhaps the most dramatic shift in transference dispositions in the advanced phase of treatment is the case of the breakup and working through of the pathological grandiose self in the transference of patients with narcissistic personality disorder and, particularly, in patients with the syndrome of malignant narcissism (Diamond et al. 2011; Stern et al. 2013). In these cases, the defense against the blend of aggression and emptiness that the pathological grandiose self provides gives way to a capacity to experience and explore the internal fragmentation that has been defended against. This development can lead to the patient's appearing more classically borderline while moving from an aloof and dismissive transference to a more engaged, anxious, and preoccupied one. A narcissistic patient whose initial stance in the therapy was to treat her therapist as hired help ("This is not a relationship—I just hire you") shifted to fragmented experiences of intense affect in relation to him. These states ranged from neediness and rejection ("I can't believe you can't give me an extra session tomorrow") to comfort and gratitude ("Somehow there is a strange kind of love in this relationship"), making it possible to work with the fragmentation of the patient's internal world that had been covered over by the dismissive grandiose self.

However, the dramatic, positive development seen in the dismantling of the pathological grandiose self does not occur with all narcissistic patients. Some, particularly those with the syndrome of malignant narcissism, improve to the extent that ego strength develops in the context of all the various indicators mentioned, but with a simultaneous consolidation of the pathological grandiose self at a higher, more adaptive level, and the utilization of this better functioning pathological grandiose self as a defense against further change in the treatment. In these latter cases, significant symptomatic changes evolve outside the sessions, and a decrease of severe turmoil occurs inside the sessions as well. However, there is also a subtle yet stubborn resistance to further change that, when matched with an often impressive improvement in the patient's total functioning, may lead to the therapist's conclusion that this is as far as the patient can get in treatment. In such cases, the therapist may move toward termination, with the potential recommendation to the patient for further treatment, possibly even psychoanalysis, later on if the remaining narcissistic personality structure predisposes the patient to severe difficulties in sustaining intimate relationships.

IMPEDIMENTS TO AND COMPLICATIONS IN ENTERING ADVANCED STAGES OF TREATMENT

A complication in the advanced stages of treatment may be linked to the improvement itself, the move from a paranoid into a depressive transference, with the development of unconscious guilt over being helped, especially when experiencing remorse for aggression ("I'm too bad to be worthy of this") and an unconscious tendency to avoid further improvement as the price being paid for the improvement obtained thus far.

CASE EXAMPLE

A patient, after years of treatment in which she was chronically confined to her home or in a psychiatric hospital, with severe self-mutilating tendencies, total incapacity to study or to work, and extreme sexual inhibition, was able to resume her studies, successfully pursue a professional career, marry, and have children. Nevertheless, she continued to have a severe sexual inhibition that she now had no desire to explore further, reflecting an unconscious guilt-based way of punishing herself for triumphing over her siblings, as she was doing so much better than they were.

This type of negative therapeutic reaction out of unconscious guilt needs to be differentiated from the negative therapeutic reaction out of unconscious envy of the therapist, which is typical of patients with narcissistic pathology. The latter usually appears in the early stages of psychotherapeutic treatment and can be resolved through interpretation of the patient's perception of the therapist's ability to help him or her as a demonstration of the therapist's superiority. In such cases, the patient's worsening condition may be a response geared to avoid the humiliation of acknowledging or submitting to the therapist's supposed superiority.

Another complication is intense erotic transference, as discussed in Chapter 9.

TECHNICAL APPROACHES DURING THE ADVANCED PHASE OF TREATMENT

The need to analyze the dominant transference developments systematically—in the sense of the gradual steps of interpretive integration of split-off transferences into their integrated counterparts—continues to be a major technical strategy during the advanced phase. The attention to every opportunity in which mutually split-off idealized and paranoid transferences can be integrated is the major concern at this stage of treatment. The effectiveness of this approach will be signaled by the strengthening of the patient's depressive transferences, with related deepening of the affective relationship of the patient with the therapist, the integration and maturation of affective responses, and the development of continuity in the relationship. Deepening or new areas of interest and commitment that were previously impossible because of the syndrome of identity diffusion may now be explored fully. The following may begin to absorb the attention in sessions: the patient's relationship to his or her broader social and cultural background; the patient's linkage with vocational, cultural, religious, artistic, and intellectual interests and pursuits; and, in particular, the more complex relationships with the patient's intimate partners. However, these developments may continue to be affected by the still-evolving integration of the projected negative elements of the patient's internal world.

CLINICAL ILLUSTRATION

Betty developed an interest in becoming an art therapist in the course of her treatment, carried out the corresponding studies, and started to work in a psychiatric treatment center. However, this interest, based in part on an identification with positive qualities she perceived in Dr. Em, was happening before the patient had fully integrated idealized and persecutory internal representations. Unconsciously, this interest also acquired a negative meaning of imitating what she considered the "phony" interest she believed mental health professionals had in their patients, based on residual paranoid transference and an element of an underlying idealized transference that would see "saint-like" devotion as the only authentic commitment. A lack of full commitment to her work led to her losing her position because of carelessness in interactions with patients. In therapy, exploration of both the residual paranoid and idealized transferences was possible. In discussing instances of carelessness toward patients, Betty said, "I got the feeling I couldn't give them enough. Some of them wanted me to take their projects home with me to evaluate and critique. I wondered how you do this work and figured that you must just pretend interest, or how could you survive?"

Abandoning her attempt to function as the ideal caretaker, Betty retreated into a position of questioning the genuineness of her own as well as her therapist's goodness. Dr. Em helped her see that what was unrealistic in the picture was not her sincere wish to help others but rather her patients' expectation that she was limitless (inexhaustible). With a bit of humor, Betty said, "So I'm not the only one who can live in that unrealistic place?" She realized that rather than "throw in the towel" in response to her patients' demands, she could now rely on her increasing sense of what can realistically be expected in a relationship because she had come to accept that Dr. Em had a sincere commitment to her while having other commitments in his life. Betty's interest in art therapy evolved into a commitment to an area of genuine interest. Moving from reacting in terms of idealized expectations and paranoid projections to the development of a general new area of concern and expertise represented a broadening of her identity, and her adjustment to this new field of activities occupied an important part of the sessions during the advanced phase of her treatment.

RISK OF A CHRONIC COUNTERTRANSFERENCE ACCEPTANCE OF A LIMITED VIEW OF THE PATIENT

It is important that the therapist reexamine in his or her mind on a continuous basis whether the routine ongoing contact with any particular patient may have led to a narrowing of his or her perspective regarding this patient's overall conflicts, life situation, and potential. In other words, it is important for the therapist to resist being lulled into accepting the patient as he or she is, with a consequent subtle restriction of the treatment goals and the potential to experience life fully. Instead, the therapist should continue to reexplore the patient's present and potential future functioning. In relation to this, the connection between learning in the sessions and the patient's utilization of this learning outside the sessions becomes very important. A general attitude of impatience (vs. complacency) in each session combined with great patience in terms of the long-term working-through of dominant problems becomes important. Impatience in each session leads to maintaining the momentum of work in opposition to the patient's subtly learning how to maintain the equilibrium in the sessions and serves as a protection against a natural tendency of the therapist to relax because things seem to be going well.

EVOLUTION OF TECHNIQUES

As therapy evolves, there is the possibility of more direct and less cautious interpretive statements. At a certain point, more complex, advanced neurotic transferences may emerge, such as typical oedipal fears and fantasies, including rivalries regarding other patients, colleagues, or people whom the patient imagines in the therapist's life, that reflect the more organized psychological structure. The therapist needs to be alert to the fact that attention to such advanced neurotic transferences may need to be temporarily put aside in order to pay attention to regressions to primitive transferences that take priority over the more elaborate transferences that now evolve. The general principle that paranoid transferences need to be addressed before depressive ones holds particularly true at this advanced stage of the treatment.

In addition, new aspects of the patient's material may acquire relatively more importance. Genetic interpretations may link the unconscious present with the unconscious past and contribute to integrating the patient's life history in the context of an increased capacity for self-reflectiveness about present and past experiences. It remains true that one overarching view of therapy is that it helps the patient establish a coherent life narrative. The patient's way of discussing the past loses a defensive quality in favor of a more genuine curiosity and access to authentic painful affects that were previously defended against. The patient's increased capacity for reflectiveness should become evident in his or her increasing in-depth evaluation of others, particularly in the context of relations with sexual partners, close friends, and family members.

CLINICAL ILLUSTRATION

In the initial phase of therapy, Betty had repeatedly described her demanding and often disapproving father as "worse than Stalin." In the termination phase she could elaborate a more balanced view: "I guess he did his best for us, but he was very limited. He couldn't deal with his own emotions, so he focused on his work—and on ours [referring to herself and her brothers]." Interestingly, Betty also somewhat sheepishly reported in the termination phase that she had been reading about Stalin and that "I guess I had a little bit in common with Stalin—the way I used to 'eliminate' people if they looked at me the wrong way." Although the statement is dramatic, it communicates Betty's ability to acknowledge and integrate an aggression that she had previously split off and both projected and acted out.

In the termination phase, dream analysis may take the more classical form of inviting the patient to free-associate regarding the components of the manifest content of the dream and connecting these associations with the patient's style in communicating the dream, as well as with the dominant transference at that point. This fully developed dream analysis is in contrast to the earlier selection of partial aspects of the manifest dream as elements to be integrated with transference interpretations (i.e., focusing on "why the patient is telling me this material at this point") (Koenigsberg et al. 2000c).

The patient's reactions to separations from the therapist—on weekends, over vacations, and in the case of illness or unexpected disruptions of the treatment—need to be explored very carefully because they will also illustrate progress toward the predominance of depressive transference reactions. Reactions to separations in the earlier stages of the treatment may take the form of severe separation anxiety, panic, anger, and regressive behavior with a paranoid coloring, or, in the case of narcissistic pathology, a complete denial of the dependency on the therapist with a tendency to express indifference. In patients who have shown movement toward internal integration, there tend to be more depressively tinged separation reactions, with mourning processes and feelings of sadness and loss rather than panic over being abandoned and mistreated. The systematic analysis of these sep-aration reactions in terms of the images of self and other that are involved, in turn, further help to explore the patient's evolving internal representa-tions and move from simplistic negatively tinged ones to more complex and integrated ones.

CLINICAL ILLUSTRATION

Early in therapy, Amy reported, "It's horrible for me every time you go away; I picture your plane blowing up as soon as it takes off." Dr. Jones helped Amy understand the aggression that was involved in her experience of loss and how it was linked to her inability to maintain a sense of internal connection. He suggested that the level of her anger at him for not being permanently available attacked and destroyed the image she had of him in her mind. In the termination phase, her reaction to separations was more benign but mixed with depressive anxieties that were explored: "I know you need a break—everyone does sometimes. But you probably especially need a break from me."

TERMINATION

The issue of termination of TFP is connected to the patient's entire psy-chotherapy because the way in which the patient can accept termination is a fundamental indication of the general level of psychological structure that the patient has achieved. Insofar as termination has to do with the dynamics of separation, we work on the psychology of termination from the very be-ginning of treatment in discussing the patient's reactions to all interrup-tions. The nature of the patient's reactions always gives an indication of where the patient stands in terms of the severity of his or her illness. One can describe normal and pathological levels of reaction to separations in general, which reflect the degree to which the patient's internal world is split or integrated.

THEORETICAL CONTEXT: NORMAL AND PATHOLOGICAL SEPARATION

If an individual separates from a meaningful relationship, a normal reaction is to feel the loss, and the more definitive the separation, the more serious the experience of loss. A normal reaction is a mourning reaction; the proto-type is the mourning for somebody who was loved. What happens con-sciously and unconsciously in mourning has been explored in psychoanalytic theory. Freud (1917/1958), in "Mourning and Melancholia," described the differences between normal and pathological mourning, concluding that normal mourning includes a period of sadness and normal depression without guilt in relation to the loss of the object. If someone dies, we are sad, and then we experience a process of introjection of the lost object, a reconstruction of the person inside our own mind—of all the things that we loved that are missing—and in subtle ways we become to some degree, or take over the characteristics of, the lost person. This process goes on simultaneously with a healthy narcissistic gratification of being alive, of being "here" in contrast to the person who has been lost. The combination of introjection of the lost object and narcissistic gratification with one's own aliveness gradually permits the working-through of the process of mourning and generally ends in 6–12 months.

In contrast, in pathological mourning the depression is very severe, lasts longer, and is accompanied by feelings of guilt. This guilt is considered related to unconscious hostility and ambivalence toward the person who was lost. It is related to aggression toward the object that, before its loss, was already experienced (perhaps unconsciously). Now, as part of the process of trying to identify with and internalize that lost object, the aggression previously directed toward the object is directed inside the self. This stymies normal mourning and healthy identification with the person who was lost. The attacks on the internalized object—now part of the self—prevent the normal narcissistic gratification of being alive and bring about an unending suffering: continued depression.

Klein (1948) modified Freud's theory in ways that are relevant to the treatment of borderline patients, to understanding separation anxiety, and to normal and pathological mourning reactions at the termination of treatment. Klein suggested that in normal mourning there is a repetition of a very early stage of development in which the original splitting of idealized and persecutory relations to the object may be surpassed, with an integration of all-good with all-bad representations of the object and of all-good and all-bad representations of the self. This is, of course, the trajectory we hope to see in therapy. Primitive defensive operations of splitting and related mechanisms are overcome in an integration that brings about the awareness that oneself is not all good or all bad but a mixture of good and bad experiences and characteristics. With this recognition of the complex nature of the self comes the awareness that significant objects (e.g., caretakers) are similarly complex. With this awareness, one recognizes that the aggression one has at times expressed because of perceived attacks by the other was directed toward an object that is not all bad but a mixture of good and bad. A sense of guilt ensues as the aggression that had seemed fully justified is now questioned. Projective mechanisms decrease at that point—one does not project all aggression on the outside but acknowledges one's own share.

At that point, the capacity for guilt develops as a normal affect, as a consequence of that integration of good and bad that involves the loss of the idealized and "pure" self and idealized object. When one's relation to one's own aggression changes from projection to acceptance and recognition, there is a shift in one's attitude toward demands and prohibitions. What was previously experienced as solely belonging to the object and as attacks from the outside are now experienced as internalized demands in the self that have to be fulfilled. In this way, the first primitive layer of the superego—the internalized demands and prohibitions—is established, and the internalization of the *demanding* aspects of the objects in the form of a primitive superego is the source of these feelings of guilt (Jacobson 1964). According to Klein, guilt feelings are not directed against the internalized object, as Freud said, but against the self because the self is recognized as having been aggressive to the object that, at times, was perceived as all bad when in fact it was a mix, and possibly a more benevolent than persecutory mix.

There is a simultaneous consolidation of an internal object that is neither all good nor all bad but integrated and ambivalently but realistically loved. This corresponds to a stable internalization of the good-enough, more realistic other, with ambivalent feelings in which love is generally stronger than anger or aggression. This object therefore can be accepted internally and incorporated without fear, rejection, or attack. This acceptance of the external object as a stable internal object establishes an internal world of object representations that provide security and an internal sense of safety and stability to the self. At the same time, in this depressive position of relinquishing the imagined ideal object and accepting ambivalent and aggressive affects, the other is still there, alive outside, not lost but perceived in different ways.

The feelings of guilt that accompany the ambivalence lead to wishes to repair the relationship with the other and wishes to do good things—what Klein (1948) called *reparation*, which she saw as the origin of subliminatory tendencies in general. Feelings of gratitude become prevalent at this point. The patient longs to establish a good relationship with the external object.

Pathological mourning, according to Klein (1948), not only was characteristic of a pathological reaction to a real loss but also constituted the dynamics of a form of depressive illness. The aggression toward a lost object would be so intense that the internalization of the lost object as a representation in the superego would have sadistic qualities, leading to a sadistic attack on the self. In other words, pathological guilt feelings would acquire fantastic, extraordinary characteristics. The individual who suffers from a pathological mourning process feels that he or she is the worst sinner in the world, possibly reaching delusional extremes. There is a cruelty of the superego, demands for perfection, and hatred of one's natural impulses. That attack is accompanied by a sense of having destroyed the good nurturing object, so what is destroyed is not only a good feeling of self but also a sense of a good internal object. It is as if one has lost everything. The good object has been lost externally and internally—a victim of the self's aggressive response. When Amy commented to her therapist, "It's horrible for me every time you go away; I picture your plane blowing up as soon as it takes off," she felt a sense of emptiness—a fantasied destruction of the internal object as well as of the external one. This involves intense separation anxiety in that the separation is associated with emptiness rather than internalization.

In pathological mourning, the feelings of internal emptiness and loss intensify the sense of guilt, and there is a vicious cycle of guilt because of the destruction of the internal object in addition to the loss of the external object, and even more attacks on the self occur as a consequence. As a secondary defense against that sense of despair, guilt, emptiness, and void, the individual may regress to the paranoid-schizoid position in which the primitive defenses of splitting, projective identification, omnipotent control, and a general disorganization of the self take over. Under these conditions, hypomanic defenses against guilt may evolve, with exaggerated qualities of feelings of triumph, contempt, defensive identification with an idealized lost object, a sense of omnipotence, and denial of any mourning or any need. A kind of compulsive engagement in multiple relations evolves—a hypomanic relation to reality without true engagement with others. Thus, for Klein (1948), depression and hypomania were the extreme manifestations of pathological mourning.

TREATMENT TERMINATION: NORMAL, NEUROTIC, AND BORDERLINE PERSONALITY ORGANIZATION

When long-term treatment ends satisfactorily, a normal person experiences a sense of sadness, loss, and mourning but, at the same time a sense of freedom and well-being. The behavior is very much like what Freud (1917/ 1958) described for normal mourning. The individual feels a sadness that is not excessive and has an appreciation for what he or she has received from the therapist, as well as the sense that now he or she can go on without the therapist.

In the case of a person with neurotic personality organization, who has excessive superego pressures and excessive guilt, the mourning is more intense. This individual experiences an intense sadness and idealization of the therapist, a sense of having been unworthy of all the love and everything that has been received, and a tendency to cling to the relationship without being able to let go. This person demonstrates a mild form of the pathological mourning reaction described by Klein (1948).

For patients with borderline personality organization, even minor separations—including the therapist's absences because of illness, vacations, or holidays—generally provoke severe separation anxiety. Instead of sadness, intense anxiety and fear of abandonment are experienced. These patients regress into the paranoid-schizoid position. Because of their intolerance of normal ambivalence, they experience problems with maintaining a benign internal image. Sadness is not prominent because these patients have not achieved the integration into the depressive position that makes it possible to hold on to a positive image of the disappointing object. The separation anxiety is immediately interpreted by the patient as a consequence of the frustration from the therapist that represents an attack from the object who is gone and who, by going, becomes the persecutory object. The attacker-victim dyad can shift, in cases where the patient relentlessly attacks the therapist for leaving, but the conscious or unconscious experience is of being attacked by the therapist—an attack that creates a reactive rage toward the bad object. This rage is directed not only at the external object but also at its internal representation. The therapist's good image is revengefully destroyed, leaving the patient with nothing to hold on to, which explains the desperate sense of loss and emptiness that accompanies separations in the early phase of therapy. The patient feels attacked, enraged, and also emptied out internally, as if he or she has lost the therapist completely. The sense of emptiness is accompanied by fear of revenge from the therapist because of the patient's rage toward him or her. This fear also increases the sense of loss. The patient has fantasies of being mistreated and fear of the rage against being mistreated; under more extreme conditions, a fragmentation of emotional experiences may evolve, leading to a kind of schizoid emptiness and indifference.

Even more severe is the reaction of patients with narcissistic personalities to the therapist's absence. In these patients, the pathological grandiose self and the defenses against dependency are manifest in an immediate protective devaluation of the therapist. This is like a characterological derivative of the hypomanic reaction to loss mentioned before. An immediate devaluation of the therapist may be reflected in the patient's feeling perfectly all right, not feeling anything, or feeling that he or she never needed the therapist anyway. In such cases, the patient seems to have locked the therapist away in the closet for the period of absence. When the treatment starts again, the patient opens the closet and lets the therapist out. One patient, who had no reaction to the therapist's being away for a month, said on the first day of resuming therapy, "To continue what I was talking about in the last session...." Another narcissistic patient said, "I hear from my friends that they missed their therapist. I don't miss you at all. I like you; you are a nice person, but if you died tomorrow, I would be angry that I had lost all this time and that I would have to look for a new therapist, but I wouldn't feel anything in particular."

TECHNICAL IMPLICATIONS

Analysis of Separations During Treatment

When a patient demonstrates pathological reactions to separations, the therapist needs to explore and analyze them. Doing so throughout the entire treatment helps the patient be prepared for the end of the treatment. The therapist needs primarily to analyze whatever reaction the patient has to separations in terms of the unconscious object relations that underlie the patient's feelings of depression, anxiety, rage, or indifference. In the case of borderline patients, analysis of separation anxiety often reveals that in the patient's fantasies, a separation is really an attack from the therapist and a sign of indifference and irresponsibility on the therapist's part. The projection of rage onto the therapist parallels the patient's feelings that he or she is being abandoned and that the therapist is interested in only his or her own well-being, leaving the helpless patient behind while the therapist goes on to gratify his or her own desires. The patient may feel a secret hatred of the therapist and an unconscious wish to ruin the therapist's time away and may wish to make the therapist feel guilty at every step for leaving the patient alone. Any separation that evolves with unconscious rage because the separation is experienced as an attack and with the unconscious destruction of the image of the good therapist—leading to a deep sense of internal emptiness—needs to be explored and worked through in the course of the treatment. This work involves exploration of the patient's suspicion of the therapist's bad intentions, the resentment and envy of the therapist's good life and wishes to destroy it, and the sense that the good image of the therapist inside has been destroyed by the patient's own reaction of hatred.

In the case of a neurotic depressive reaction to separation (by the end of TFP, the patient ideally will be at this level or higher), the sadness over the therapist's going away needs to be explored in terms of the patient's unconscious feelings of guilt for having contributed to the loss caused by the separation. The therapist is no longer seen as indifferent and rejecting but is seen as concerned and dedicated to help. The patient's guilt may be rooted in the belief that the intensity of his or her needs and demands has overwhelmed the therapist's capacity to help and has exhausted the therapist. The patient may feel that his or her needs make him or her not good enough to receive the therapist's help. In the context of any separation, the therapist has to analyze depressive anxieties that may be very similar to those that are generally found more intensively at the end of the treatment. The fantasy behind the depression is that the patient is too demanding and does not deserve that good therapist. There is a movement at times between these manifestations of the depressive position and partial regression to the paranoid-schizoid position of idealization and devaluation in the form of an idealization of the therapist and devaluation of the self. At the end of the treatment, feelings of guilt may lead the patient to feel that he or she does not deserve autonomy and health; this is linked to the fantasy that the therapist has had to stop the treatment because the patient's demands have exhausted the therapist. The therapist, in the patient's mind, deserves a respite from such a patient who has taken so much. In the extreme form, the patient may feel that to grow up at the end of the treatment—to become independent—implies the death of the therapist insofar as the patient has depleted him or her. These depressive fantasies may be the focus of the interpretive work in the termination phase.

Analysis of Separation at End of Treatment

Many patients have mixed paranoid and depressive anxieties, and the general rule applies that the therapist should interpret the paranoid reactions before the depressive ones. If the depressive anxieties are interpreted first, the paranoid reactions tend to go underground. In contrast, if the therapist first analyzes systematically the paranoid reactions, the depressive ones are strengthened—as the object being lost comes to be seen more realistically and is therefore more valued—and become more evident and can then be explored. Thus, it is very important in all separations for the therapist to analyze the patient's fantasies that the therapist is leaving because of indifference, greed, callousness, or secret depreciation of the patient before addressing, if present, the fantasies that the separation is due to the therapist's having become exhausted or damaged by the patient because of the therapist's inability to tolerate the patient's neediness, badness, or aggression.

THE REALITY OF ENDINGS

In all cases it is important for the therapist to help the patient tolerate his or her ambivalence toward the therapist and to link that tolerance of ambivalence with the analysis of the mutually split object relations typical of borderline patients. It is important to tolerate mourning processes and to permit their development rather than trying to eliminate or avoid them. It is important to realize that they are unavoidable and necessary. Gradually decreasing the frequency of the treatment hours to get the patient accustomed to separation is not a desirable technique. Instead, the ideal technique is to maintain the same intensity of treatment until its termination and to work through separation anxiety and mourning as much as possible before the treatment ends, with the understanding that after the end of the treatment, the patient will have to undergo a period of mourning. The more intensely the therapist analyzes separation anxiety and mourning reactions before the end of the treatment, the better able the patient will be to continue to work through those reactions alone after the treatment ends. It is important to remember that mourning reactions are growth experiences. They repeat the experiences of growing up, leaving home, and going to college, and everybody has a potential for those experiences. Although it is important to acknowledge the reality of the termination, patients often ask about the possibility of returning at some point. When we are asked that question, we respond that we are available for consultation in the future and that if the situation calls for it, it would be possible to take up the therapy process again.

THERAPIST COUNTERTRANSFERENCE

The therapist's countertransference is often a good indicator of the dominant characteristics of the patient's transference during termination. When paranoid reactions to separation or termination dominate, the countertransference may be a paranoid reaction to the patient. The therapist may feel that the end of the treatment means that the patient is escaping from therapy, devaluing it, or denying how sick he or she is and that the patient is attacking the therapist by ending the treatment. When the transference is predominantly depressive, the countertransference may be predominantly depressive as well, and the therapist may feel that he or she failed the patient, that the patient deserved better than what he or she received from the therapist, that the therapist is indeed abandoning the patient, that the therapist should have loved the patient more or understood the patient earlier and better, or that the patient is right to be disappointed. In the case of narcissistic devaluation of the treatment on the part of the patient, the therapist may experience narcissistic defenses in his or her own countertransference, considering the patient to be hopeless or impossible—in short, developing an internal devaluation of the patient that must be factored into the therapist's understanding of the patient's internal world.

TIMING OF TREATMENT TERMINATION

An important consideration is when to terminate treatment. Ideally, termination would not occur until there is both satisfactory symptom resolution and structural psychological change in the form of integrating previously projected parts of the self, as reflected in significant personality change, with treatment and life goals achieved in terms of work, love, and recreational and creative pursuits. Practically, the therapist has to evaluate on an ongoing basis whether optimal treatment goals have been achieved.

In the case of possible stalemates, when the therapist cannot decide whether the patient has reached maximum benefits or whether a stalemate has to be resolved, a careful evaluation of the transference and the countertransference may provide an answer. Extended stalemates are reasons for consultation rather than for making an immediate decision about ending the treatment. In general, in cases where secondary gain has not been analyzed sufficiently or where the treatment tends to replace life, great resistances by patients to end the treatment may evolve. In these cases, the analysis of secondary gain or of treatment replacing life is central to the work of therapy and part of a preparation for an appropriate termination of the treatment.

For practical purposes, it is always important to prepare for the termination of treatment ahead of time, to be predictable, and to inform the patient where he or she stands in his or her treatment. In any extended psychotherapy, the decision to terminate should be made at least 3 months ahead of termination, and ideally the decision is made jointly by patient and therapist. The same amount of time is also required before the transfer of a patient whom a therapist has been seeing for a year or more in a psychotherapeutic relationship (e.g., in the setting of a training program). For treatments that last several years, a 6-month period of termination is desirable. It is important for the therapist to observe the reactions of the patient to the decision making about when the end of the treatment will occur.

Key Clinical Concepts

- Integration is not a linear process but rather is a stepwise process with movement toward integration interrupted by periodic regressions that represent a temporary retreat to the more familiar position of splitting and projection. If therapy is progressing, the regressions can be dealt with more quickly and effectively over time.

- Termination issues are foreshadowed by any experience of separation in the course of the therapy.

- The termination phase may be marked by a mix of paranoid themes or by depressive themes; it is important to address the former before the latter.

- The psychological integration achieved by termination allows the patient to assess internal reactions and put them in a broad context.

SELECTED READINGS

Freud S: Mourning and melancholia (1915/1917), in The Standard Edition of the Complete Psychological Works of Sigmund Freud, Vol 14. Translated and edited by Strachey J. London, Hogarth Press, 1957, pp 237–258
Klein M: Mourning and its relation to manic-depressive states, in Contributions to Psychoanalysis. London, Hogarth Press, 1948, pp 311–338

11

TRAJECTORIES OF CHANGE IN TRANSFERENCE- FOCUSED PSYCHOTHERAPY

POSITIVE CHANGE in personality function is a process that takes place over time. With their substantial difficulties in relationships, individuals with severe personality disorders need time to gradually develop trust in the therapist and to begin the process of examining their patterns of interaction and of using affect regulation and contextualization in their daily lives. Brief therapy is not appropriate for these tasks. Thanks to Linehan (1993) and her groundbreaking research on the treatment of borderline personality disorder (BPD), it is now accepted that long-term treatment is necessary for patients with BPD.

We have identified both clinical and empirical patterns in the progression of this change process across time and in relation to various domains of dysfunction. These patterns of change are important for the therapist using transference-focused psychotherapy (TFP) because they can inform the therapist of the progression or lack thereof in the individual patient. In general, control over self-destructive behaviors must increase in order to provide a context in which the patient can reflect on his or her dominant representations of self and others that guide emotional responses and interpersonal behaviors. The interaction between the TFP therapist and the patient provides the opportunity to examine these powerful affect-driven internalized representations, a curative process that takes time to evolve. In this evolving process, the gradual integration of positive and negative affect states, in the context of the corresponding object relations dyads, underlies these curative effects.

In Chapters 8–10, we have described the typical issues that arise in the early, middle, and advanced phases of TFP. When one combines the goal for personality change across time with the fact that borderline patients begin treatment at different levels in their development, it becomes clear that the domains and rates of change in treatment are quite variable across individual patients.

A major theme in the research and clinical work we do with our colleagues is the diversity of borderline patients (Lenzenweger 2010) and the diversity of psychological and neurobiological processes involved in the adjustment of the individual patient. Throughout this book, we have used the concept of borderline personality organization (BPO), a concept based on object relations theory, as well as the definition of BPD as first presented in DSM-III (American Psychiatric Association 1987) and further elaborated in subsequent editions of DSM. Patients diagnosed with BPO and those diagnosed with BPD are similar in some respects but may be quite different in others. This diversity among the patients ensures that the trajectory of change in each patient will be unique.

A number of factors contribute to the diversity in patient change in TFP: 1) empirically identified subgroups of borderline patients; 2) patients beginning treatment at different points of development and levels of adjustment, as captured in part in our concepts of high- and low-level borderline organization; 3) the progression of transference patterns seen in the course of TFP; 4) patient attachment styles and their progression in relation to self and the therapist; and 5) patterns of change that involve the therapist as he or she relates over time to the individual patient. These five factors each deserve some consideration, but they are not totally independent of one another. In fact, the areas of overlap may be especially important. As described later in the section "Empirically Derived Trajectories of Change," one of the empirically derived predictors of change in treatment is level of identity diffusion, a construct that is central to the identification of high- and low-level BPO.

EMPIRICALLY DERIVED SUBTYPES OF BORDERLINE PATIENTS

Although factor analysis of the diagnostic criteria for BPD can identify salient dimensions across individuals, it is not the most effective statistical approach to identifying clinically relevant subgroups of these patients. With our colleagues (Lenzenweger et al. 2008), we investigated the diversity of patients with BPD using a model-based taxonomy (described in Chapter 2, "Empirical Development of Transference-Focused Psychotherapy") combined with advanced statistical methodology called *finite mixture modeling*. We used the dimensions of aggression, paranoia, and antisocial traits as specified in the object relations model of personality pathology, defining high- and low-level BPO to statistically generate subgroups of patients. Three phenotypically distinct groups of borderline patients were identified within the overall BPD category. Group 1 contained individuals who showed comparatively low levels of paranoid, antisocial, and aggressive features. Group 2 was composed of individuals with higher levels of paranoid features and comparatively lower levels of antisocial and aggressive features. For these individuals, aggression is projected rather than directly expressed as by individuals in group 3. Finally, individuals in group 3 had higher levels of antisocial and aggressive features and relatively low paranoia. It is important to note that these three groups are different not only in terms of severity but also in relation to paranoid, antisocial, and aggressive features. This finding is quite consistent with the object relations model and can be interpreted as reflecting the way aggression is defended against and manifested (e.g., inwardly experienced or outwardly expressed).

We also examined hypothesized associated features of the members in the three groups and found evidence to support the hypotheses. Individuals in group 1 (comparatively low on aggression, antisocial aspects, and paranoia) were characterized by less negative emotion, less childhood physical abuse, and better social and work functioning. Members of group 2, the paranoid group, experienced less social closeness and reported higher rates of childhood sexual abuse. Patients in group 3, the relatively high aggressive and antisocial group, showed a breakdown of behavioral constraint with overt aggression, high impulsivity, and high identity diffusion. These results have been replicated (Hallquist and Pilkonis 2012; Yun et al. 2013), suggesting that these subtypes may be important to guide further efforts to understand underlying endophenotypes and genotypes.

TREATMENT IMPLICATIONS

The immediate implication of these findings of important differences among borderline patients is the need for a careful and detailed assessment of patients prior to intervention, with an eye to possible differences in the process of change and the treatment prognosis. Group 1 may present as more depressed initially. Group 2 may have more anxiety in the context of the attachment that develops in the therapeutic relationship and may be more prone to have aggressive reactions in the therapy or to drop out because of this anxiety; therapists should be attentive to the potential for this type of anxiety and the need to tactfully address and interpret it. Group 3 is the most disturbed group in terms of multiple disruptive behaviors, aggression, and mistrust of others; these are the patients who meet the criteria for low-level BPO. They may require more attention in the contracting phase.

PATIENT ADJUSTMENT AT INITIATION OF TREATMENT

The diversity of patients at a borderline level of organization has been described in the object relations' nosology and in Chapter 4, "Assessment Phase." The initial clinical assessment provides the therapist with information about what particular zone of adjustment the patient is in at the beginning of treatment.

HIGH- AND LOW-LEVEL BORDERLINE ORGANIZATION

We use the concepts of high- and low-level borderline organization to clarify some of the patient diversity. Patients at a high level of BPO begin treatment with some measure of an internal moral guidance system and with conflicts in relationships but without overwhelming aggression and projection of aggression. These patients are more likely to be involved in relations with others, albeit conflictual ones, and to be involved in some work. In Chapters 8–10, we presented the case of Betty as a prototypical high-level borderline patient in her trajectory of change in TFP. At the time of beginning therapy, Betty was highly involved in angry and conflicted relations with members of her extended family. Although she had been unemployed and inactive for months, she started a meaningful half-time volunteer job the week after the issue of work had been discussed in the treatment contract. In the course of therapy, libidinal longings became visible relatively quickly beneath her surface angry and paranoid presentation. Although the sessions were often fraught with intense affect, she never presented as a risk for dropout. Over the years of therapy, she completed graduate education, settled into a steady relationship, and expanded her circle of friends and cultural interests.

In contrast, patients at a low level of borderline organization are deficient in terms of moral functioning and exhibit higher levels of aggression in their relations with others and their perception of aggression coming from others. In Chapters 8–10, we presented the case of Amy to represent a prototypical low-level borderline patient. Amy's initial levels of aggression, manifested in her serious self-destructive actions, were the intense focus of early intervention (Chapter 8, "Early Treatment Phase"). As she came to recognize, own, and more adequately tolerate her aggression, she moved to a higher level of adjustment (i.e., no longer in the borderline level of organization) and became involved in wider areas of life, having a child and furthering her education (Chapter 9, "Midphase of Treatment").

PRETREATMENT EXTENT OF SYMPTOMS AND FUNCTIONAL DEFICITS

As described in Chapter 4, borderline patients have different levels of adjustment and development before treatment begins, and this can vary in nature and extent within the categories of high- and low-level borderline organization. This variation also has a powerful impact on the subsequent focus and process of treatment. The most obvious impact on the subsequent treatment is the relative salience of self-destructive behaviors in which the patient is currently engaged. These behaviors, ranging from lethal suicide attempts to relatively nonlethal cutting, are the first to focus on. Other behaviors include substance abuse and physical attacks on others, often in intimate relations. Patients without current suicide attempts and self-destructive behaviors are often under more behavioral control and are easier to engage in a self-reflective therapy. Nevertheless, patients who begin therapy with a narcissistic personality disorder structured around a pathological grandiose self can have as much difficulty developing reflective capacities as highly acting-out patients.

TREATMENT IMPLICATIONS

There are implications for treatment depending on the state in which the patient begins TFP. Those patients with the most behavioral dyscontrol—suicidal behavior, substance abuse, impulsivity, physical aggression—will require therapeutic management of acting out by an active TFP therapist through an emphasis on contracting and limit setting, followed by interpre-

tation of the acting-out behavior. Only with control of these acting-out behaviors can the treatment proceed to an understanding of the connection
of the behavior to the patient's underlying mental structure as it plays out
in relations between patient and others, including the therapist.

DOMINANT TRANSFERENCE THEMES IN TFP

In Chapter 9 we emphasized that during the midphase of TFP, transference
patterns exhibited by borderline patients are expected to progress from paranoid transference patterns to depressive patterns. In the most severe cases,
an antisocial transference precedes the paranoid transference. In cases of
narcissistic personality disorder, a narcissistic transference based on the internal structure of the pathological grandiose self must be worked with to
advance to the more disorganized but accessible paranoid transference
most typical of BPD. (For further elaboration of therapy with narcissistic
personality disorder, see D. Diamond, F.E. Yeomans, and B.L. Stern, A Clinical Guide for Treating Narcissistic Pathology: A Transference Focused Psychotherapy, in preparation.)

TREATMENT IMPLICATIONS

We have made clear throughout this treatment manual that the TFP therapist is constantly aware of the dominant transference theme activated in the
treatment. Therapeutic techniques will vary to some degree according to
whether the patient enters therapy with a predominantly antisocial, narcissistic, or paranoid transference, with more structure in the first, more thera-
pist-centered interpretations in the second, and standard TFP in the third.

ATTACHMENT

Object relations theory and attachment theory have notable similarities
(Calabrese et al. 2005), which is hardly surprising because Bowlby (1988),
the first attachment theorist, explicitly saw attachment theory as a variant of
object relations theory. Both orientations focus on the ways people symbol-
ize their relatedness to others, and both theories posit that the perceptions
of self, others, and relationships are the most important and influential attitudes that people form. Although there are important differences between
the two orientations that have treatment implications (Kernberg et al.
2008), we focus here on the ways that both have influenced our therapeutic
assessment and conceptualization.

   Major contributions of attachment theory are the reliable measurement
of the nature of attachment and the demonstration that there are different

identifiable patterns of insecure attachment. Our clinical experience with TFP is that the differences in attachment style or state of mind have treatment implications. We noted in Chapter 2 that patients with BPD experience a combination of intense negative and positive affect states, harbor malevolent perceptions of others, lack trust of others, and are vulnerable to painful perceptions of rejection. However, this combination does not lead to just one outcome but rather takes on different phenotypic features depending on factors such as levels of effortful control and each person's individual, unique experience with caregivers during the developmental years.

Patients with BPD have insecure attachment organization (Fonagy et al. 1996; Levy et al. 2006; Patrick et al. 1994) and deficits in reflective functioning or the ability to think about self and others in mental state terms (Levy et al. 2006). These features are relevant to the treatment of these patients because the patients' internal working models of attachment with others affect a number of important aspects of the therapeutic process, including 1) extent of reporting of symptoms, 2) capacity to engage in and utilize the treatment relationship, 3) quality of the therapeutic alliance, and 4) treatment outcome.

In brief, patients with preoccupied states of mind report higher levels of symptomatology than do those with autonomous or dismissing states of mind. This reporting style could conceivably influence the patient's self-report on symptom state across the treatment span. Secure individuals are more involved in treatment than those with unresolved and dismissing status (Korfmacher et al. 1997). Patients with BPD are by nature insecure in their attachment status, creating one of the initial challenges to treatment.

The treatment process may be influenced not only by the patient's attachment state of mind but also by the therapist's own attachment state of mind toward the particular patient. Dozier et al. (1993) found that clinicians with a more secure state of mind were more likely to appropriately challenge patients' strategies for relating.

With our colleagues, we investigated the diversity of borderline patients in terms of their attachment styles both on the Adult Attachment Interview (AAI; Hesse 2010; C. George, N. Kaplan, and M. Main, "The Berkeley Adult Attachment Interview," unpublished manuscript, University of California, Berkeley, 1996), which focuses on the subject's internal representations of relations with parental figures, and with self-report questionnaires that assess the interaction with peers in intimate relations (Levy et al. 2006). Although borderline patients are predictably insecure (as opposed to secure) in their attachment style, there are important differences among those individuals with insecure attachment. Individuals classified as *dismissing* devalue the importance and impact of attachment relationships. They are low in coherence of mind because of the vagueness and inconsistency in their descriptions of relationships. Individuals classified as *preoccupied* are detailed in their descriptions of relationships and related feelings but describe early relationships as overinvolved or guilt inducing. They have a tendency toward incoherence in their descriptions, which are often lengthy and confusing. Those patients classified as *unresolved/disorganized* have lapses in the monitoring of reasoning or discourse when discussing experiences of loss and abuse. Patients are designated *cannot classify* when their discourses combine contradictory or incompatible attachment patterns or when no one single state of mind with respect to attachment is dominant.

The instruments that have been developed to assess attachment states of mind, attachment categories, and the related concept of reflective functioning enable therapists to ask a number of questions in relation to borderline pathology and TFP. In addition to these instruments, with an interest in the attachment that evolves between patient and therapist, we and our colleagues have developed the Patient-Therapist Adult Attachment Interview (PT-AAI; Diamond 1999) to measure these issues. Important questions to consider, as discussed in the subsections below, include the following:

- What are the dominant attachment patterns of borderline patients?
- Does the attachment state of mind of the borderline patient add understanding to the process and outcome of treatment? For example, do preoccupied versus dismissive attachment states of mind make a difference in the process and outcome?
- Does the patient's attachment state of mind toward early caregivers relate to the dominant transference themes in TFP?
- Does the patient's attachment state of mind toward early caregivers relate to the patient's attachment state of mind toward the therapist?
- Do TFP therapists demonstrate various attachment states of mind toward different patients with BPD?

CHANGE IN ATTACHMENT ORGANIZATION AND REFLECTIVE FUNCTIONING IN TFP

In a randomized clinical trial comparing TFP, dialectical behavioral therapy, and a psychodynamic supportive therapy (Clarkin et al. 2007), we and our colleagues (Levy et al. 2006) used changes in attachment organization and reflective functioning as putative mechanisms of change. With AAI data on 56 patients with BPD both before and after 1 year of therapy with one of the three treatments, we were able both to investigate pretreatment attachment status of a large group of patients with BPD and to examine change in attachment status after 1 year of treatment.

In a three-way classification scheme (secure, preoccupied, and dismissing) based on AAI data prior to treatment, we found almost equal numbers of patients in the preoccupied category (50%) and the dismissing category (45%). There were significant changes in both attachment patterns and reflective functioning during the course of 1 year of psychotherapy. The percentage of patients classified as securely attached at the end of TFP significantly increased, whereas no significant change occurred for patients in the other two treatment conditions. In addition, patients in TFP significantly increased in narrative coherence at the end of treatment (controlling for coherence at the beginning of treatment). This effect was not seen in reference to the other two treatment conditions.

Finally, we examined the influence of the three treatments on reflective functioning as rated from the material on the AAI. Reflective functioning is the capacity to interpret and make sense of the behavior of oneself and others in terms of intentional mental states such as thoughts, feelings, and beliefs. Given the focus of TFP on the internal representations of self and others, we hypothesized that TFP would result in a significant increase in reflective functioning as compared with the other two treatments. As hypothesized, patients in TFP significantly increased in reflective functioning during 1 year of treatment, unlike patients in the other two treatment conditions.

INTERACTION OF PATIENT ATTACHMENT TO THERAPIST AND THERAPIST ATTACHMENT TO PATIENT

With the data on the 56 patients with BPD just described as a background (Levy et al. 2006), it is instructive to examine two representative cases in some clinical detail. To further the understanding of patient attachment status and the process in TFP, we and our colleagues (Diamond et al. 2003) examined in detail five borderline patients and their attachment status toward the beginning and at the end of 1 year of TFP. The AAI was used to assess the patients' attachment state of mind. In addition, we used the PT-AAI to examine the patients' attachment state of mind toward the therapist and the therapist's state of mind toward the patient. We hypothesized that the relationship that evolves in the particular patient-therapist dyad would be somewhat unique and important in the process and outcome. With this dual focus on both the patient's attachment state of mind toward early caregivers (AAI) and attachment state of mind that evolved toward the therapist in TFP (PT-AAI), we can monitor the patient's combined internal working models of both early caregivers and the TFP therapist as they arise in the treatment relationship.

To pursue an in-depth description of attachment and the therapeutic process, we contrast here Patient A, a patient with initial levels of unresolved and insecure state of mind (preoccupied) who changed to a secure state of mind after 1 year of treatment, and Patient B, a patient with unresolved and insecure state of mind (dismissing) whose categorization after treatment was changed to *cannot classify* or *mixed states of mind*. Both patients had the same therapist.

CASE EXAMPLE: PATIENT A

Patient A, some of whose characteristics were included in the composite case of Amy in Chapters 8–10, was 23 years old when she was referred to TFP. At the point of entering TFP, she was married, unemployed, and exhibiting serious acting out, with major difficulties in her social and intimate relationships.

At 4 months into treatment, Patient A's AAI revealed a primary attachment classification of unresolved and a secondary classification of preoccupied, with specific subtypes of 1) fearfully preoccupied with traumatic events for which she showed loss of memory and 2) angry/conflicted. She demonstrated a breakdown of discourse strategies in the AAI, and the content revealed memories of violent behavior by her father. In the adjectives she chose to describe early attachment figures, she showed a rapid oscillation between positive and negative evaluations of others, raising hypotheses that these extreme positive and negative evaluations would color the transference in TFP.

At 1 year into TFP, Patient A's AAI revealed a classification of secure autonomous, with a secondary classification of unresolved. She remained on the preoccupied end of the secure category, manifesting some moderate anger and resentment toward attachment figures. However, her discourse at this point was coherent, contained, and at times humorous.

Given Patient A's scores and performance on the AAI that capture her attachment state of mind toward early caregivers, it is interesting to examine her attachment state of mind toward her therapist. She demonstrated a secure state of mind with regard to the therapist at the end of 1 year of TFP. She did, however, show some resentment and conflict about her therapy. She described her therapist as reliable, dignified, important, mildly frustrating, and confusing. She could provide coherent examples of each of the adjectives describing the relationship with the therapist. She admitted feeling rejected and frustrated by the therapist but took ownership of these feelings without blaming him. She could discuss what to her were negative aspects of the relationship (e.g., she felt the therapist was cold and strict), but over time she began to feel a trusting connection to him.

From the therapist's point of view, after 1 year of TFP, he experienced Patient A as committed, stable, creative, interesting, and enjoyable. The positive aspects of the relationship with her were accompanied by feelings of intimidation by her dramatic episodes of self-destructive behavior in the early phase of TFP. The therapist was classified as secure/autonomous with respect to the patient on the PT-AAI. In fact, both patient and therapist were rated as secure/autonomous at the end of 1 year of TFP, suggesting that both of them had a clear conception of the difficulties in their relationship but with a rational, accepting, and even at times humorous view of their interaction.

CASE EXAMPLE: PATIENT B

Patient B, a 29-year-old single female, had an attachment state of mind that was in sharp contrast to that of Patient A. Patient B was referred to TFP by another therapist who terminated treatment with the patient following a near-lethal suicide attempt by Patient B that the therapist experienced as totally unexpected and "out of the blue."

On the initial AAI, Patient B received a primary classification of dismissing of attachment, with the subtype of devaluing of attachment. She could recall few memories from her childhood and described her parents as detached and derogatory. She described her mother as cold, sometimes warm, not very motherly, calm, and sparse. Following 1 year of TFP, Patient B was classified on a repeat AAI as having a secure state of mind, although she remained on the dismissing end of secure. There were indications in the material that she had consciously set aside early disappointing attachment relationships and redirected her attention to new relationships.

After 1 year of TFP, Patient B described her therapist on the PT-AAI as professional, controlled, understanding, concerned, and "not that personal." The memories that she produced to explicate these adjectives were quite vague and not totally convincing. She was classified with a dismissing state of mind with respect to the therapist, which was quite similar to her state of mind on the AAI prior to therapy. She minimized any feeling of loss during separations from the therapist. Likewise, she minimized the impact of the patient-therapist relationship on her functioning and did not have a clear idea of why the therapist behaved in certain ways during the treatment. She did offer that the therapy helped her realize more about herself, even though she struggled during the therapy to hide her feelings from the therapist.

The therapist was classified with a secure state of mind in his relationship with Patient B. He described their relationship during 1 year of TFP as distant, rigid, formal, cold, and superficial. With frustration, the therapist felt excluded from Patient B's inner life. He rarely thought about the patient outside of the therapy hours.

TREATMENT IMPLICATIONS

With these two patients, both having the clinical diagnosis of BPD but with contrasting attachment states of mind toward early caregivers, we can examine in microcosm each patient's attachment state of mind and the evolution of the attachment state of mind toward the therapist in TFP. Patient A manifested both symptom change and dramatic changes in her intimate relations and work life, although this eventual positive change was not without difficulties. Her early course of TFP was characterized by episodes of acting out in the first 3 months of therapy. The dominant object relations that arose in the therapeutic relationship were multiple and included 1) a neglected child in relation to a cold, uncaring parent; 2) a sadistic provocateur in relation to her victim; 3) a cared-for child in relation to a concerned parent; and 4) a sophisticated and seductive woman in relation to the object of her desire.

Patient A's aggressive self-destructive behavior in the form of suicide attempts ended during the first 6 months of treatment. She expanded her life experience by having and raising a child and by furthering her college education. Over time, the mistrust of others in her environment decreased as she became more aware of and tolerated her own aggressive impulses, understanding the role of projected aggression in her anxiety in relation to others. Her relationship with her therapist evolved from one of mistrust and distance to an acceptance of the treatment method and appreciation of the security that the relationship provided.

Patient B was characterized by a dismissing attachment state of mind, both toward early parental figures and toward her therapist. Her clinical course during 1 year of TFP was relatively uneventful: no suicidal behavior, quiet functioning at work, and a developing relationship with a new boyfriend. Her symptomatic states were decreased and functioning remained steady, but there was little in the way of significant change in her internal representations of self and others, which remained vague and impoverished as evidenced by her low reflective functioning score.

It is most informative to compare the attitude of the therapist toward the two patients. With Patient A, the therapist was curious, was very involved, and had a very positive attitude toward many of her qualities despite her serious pathology. The therapist became deeply involved in his own mind with the preoccupied patient. In contrast, the same therapist felt a distance from the dismissing Patient B. A clinical hypothesis would be that the treatment frame and consistency, as well as the therapist's focus on the patients' behavior and internal representations of self and others, assisted in symptom and behavioral change for both of the patients. However, in the case of Patient A, something more happened. The resolution of angry, aggressive acting out decreased, and the patient began to put more trust in the security of the therapeutic relationship and then gradually achieved more trusting relationships with those in her daily life. The latter is reflected in Patient A's improvement in the capacity for reflective functioning, which evolved over the course of 1 year of TFP from a truncated or impaired capacity to understand or elaborate the mental states of self and others to a more fully developed and clearly articulated capacity to think in terms of internal mental states.

EMPIRICALLY DERIVED TRAJECTORIES OF CHANGE

In the randomized controlled trial described above involving 56 borderline patients assigned to one of three treatments (TFP, dialectical behavioral therapy, or supportive treatment), we and our colleagues examined the domains of function as they changed across a treatment duration of 1 year (Lenzenweger et al. 2012a). Because there were few differences in behavioral and symptom change across the three treatments, we combined the patients across these treatments for this analysis.

One approach to examining change, whether across time or with treatment intervention, is to focus on end point/follow-up outcomes. These bivariate associations do not capture the dynamic process of change because they are derived from static cross-sectional assessments, usually made at baseline and end point. In our study (Lenzenweger et al. 2012a) we examined baseline psychological predictors as they related to rates of change (i.e., change in variables measured multiple times on each patient during the course of 1 year of treatment) across wide domains of functioning, such as suicidality, aggression, impulsivity, depression, and social adjustment.

We selected potential *predictors* of change on the basis of two models of severe personality pathology: a neurobehavioral model (e.g., agentic extroversion, affiliation, negative emotion, fear, nonaffective constraint) (Depue and Lenzenweger 2005) and an object relations model (e.g., identity diffusion, defenses, variable reality testing) (Kernberg and Caligor 2005).

A principal components analysis (PCA) on the rate of change for 11 different dimensional measures of domains of change yielded three factors of change: change in aggressive dyscontrol, change in psychosocial adjustment (global functioning and social adjustment), and change in conflict tolerance (anxiety/depression and impulsivity). This result indicates that different areas of functioning and symptomatology change at different rates and certain sets of variables change at the same rate—that is, as a domain.

In addition to identifying these three domains of change, we examined the relations between baseline characteristics (predictors) and scores for each of the three domains of change. Baseline negative affectivity and aggression predicted change in the aggressive dyscontrol domain. Lower pretreatment levels of negative affect and aggression were associated with more rapid clinical improvement in this domain. Baseline identity diffusion predicted the global social adjustment/self-acceptance domain of change. Higher pretreatment identity diffusion was associated with more rapid clinical improvement in the global functioning domain. Baseline social potency (persuasive, likes to influence others, decisive, takes charge, likes to be noticed) predicted the conflict tolerance change domain. Lower initial levels of social potency were associated with more rapid improvement in anxiety/depression and impulsivity.

TREATMENT IMPLICATIONS

The data from the study by Lenzenweger et al. (2012a) suggest that there are differentiable domains of change in the treatment of patients with BPD. Furthermore, change in each of these domains is predicted by relatively unique baseline personality and psychological variables. These predictors—negative affect and aggression, identity diffusion, and social potency—suggest a theoretical focus for the mechanisms of change in the treatment of borderline patients and suggest foci for clinical intervention.

CLINICAL INDICATORS OF CHANGE

The alert and sensitive TFP therapist will consistently monitor symptom, structural, and behavioral changes manifested in the patient-therapist interaction and reported in therapy sessions. The focus of attention in this therapist process is on both the process of the relationship between patient and therapist and the patient's current ongoing adjustment to the environment. Clinical indicators of structural change are listed in Table 11–1. There is a progression in the changes detailed in Table 11–1. For example, reduction in acting out is necessary for the major efforts to shift to understanding the intense underlying conflicted self-other representations that become salient in the therapeutic relationship. As described in the cases of Amy and Betty in Chapters 4 and 8–10, there was a growing recognition of each patient's aggressive affects, integration of these affects as perceptions of self and other changed, and a growing attempt to broaden investments in relationships and work as the interference of projections in interpersonal interactions diminished. The dual focus of TFP on both the internal representations of self and other and current functioning in relations and work is necessary for change in both realms. The usual progression of change that we have seen clinically is reduction of problem behaviors; modification in the representations of self and others, especially as manifested in the transference in the therapeutic relationship; and growing productive involvement in current functioning in work and relationships. The capacity for intimate relationships is often the last area of change.

TABLE 11–1.   Clinical indicators of structural change

Shift from antisocial and narcissistic transferences, if present, toward paranoid and ultimately depressive transferences

Reduction in acting out and somatization and increase in the ability to tolerate and reflect on internal conflict

Shift toward an integration of split-off positive and negative experiences; a growing capacity to become aware of one's own ambivalences and complicated affects (e.g., aggression, affectionate attachment)

Shift from primitive defenses toward more advanced defenses; capacity to utilize interpretation of defenses and incorporate an understanding (see Chapter 10, "Advanced Phase of Treatment and Termination," for a clinical illustration with quotes from a patient)

In patients with narcissistic features, resolution of conflicts involving envy with a growing capacity for gratitude and enjoyment

Increased triangulation of relationships (i.e., a growing capacity for the patient to be an objective observer of self in relating to others); more dominance of oedipal and sexual issues, in contrast to earlier dominance of dyadic pre-oedipal issues

Resolution of major symptom areas and growing productive involvement in work and professional life and in intimate love relations

SUMMARY

The successful treatment of borderline patients is much more complicated than the research literature suggests. The group of patients identified by the borderline diagnosis is a very heterogeneous group, with significant differences in severity of psychosocial adjustment, differences in attachment style that affect the therapeutic relationship, and differences in the severity of symptomatology. The treatment takes place over a long period of time in which the relationship between patient and therapist takes on a life of its own with its distinctive interaction. Treatment outcomes are not a simple matter of success versus failure but rather involve a number of domains of functioning, with the possibility of successful change in one domain and minimal change in another. Most importantly, change can occur in behavior with or without change in the powerful underlying organization of identity and moral values. We have organized TFP to try to maximize change in these latter categories as well as in the former ones.

We have presented a detailed investigation of the treatment of borderline patients that might contribute both to the sophisticated approach of clinicians to these complex patients and to the generation of hypotheses for future research. In our clinical work, we continue to explore new developments in our technical approach, with the basic goal of using TFP to achieve fundamental changes in the personality structure of these patients. Our goal is not only to bring about symptomatic improvement but also to influence the functioning of these patients by helping them to be able to increase their efficiency and satisfaction in their work and profession; to develop mature love relations in which eroticism, tenderness, and concern are integrated; and to enjoy a rich social life with friendship and creativity.

Key Clinical Concepts

- The heterogeneity of patients who meet the criteria for a diagnosis of borderline personality disorder results in a heterogeneity of trajectories of change in the psychotherapy process.

- Borderline patients begin treatment with very different levels of adjustment.

- Attachment states of mind between patient and therapist capture some of the individuality of the treatment process.

- The clinician must consider the individuality of the borderline patient because heterogeneity among borderline individuals is marked.

- Multiple patient factors (e.g., high- or low-level borderline status, attachment style), combined with the nature of the therapeutic relationship, lead to different pathways of change.

SELECTED READING

Lenzenweger MF, Clarkin JF, Levy KN, et al: Predicting domains and rates of change in borderline personality disorder. Personal Disord 3:185–195, 2012

REFERENCES

Ahadi SA, Rothbart MK: Temperament, development, and the big five, in The Developing Structure of Temperament and Personality From Infancy to Adulthood. Edited by Halverson CF, Kohnstamm GA. Hillsdale, NJ, Erlbaum, 1994, pp 189–207

American Psychiatric Association: Diagnostic and Statistical Manual of Mental Disorders, 3rd Edition. Washington, DC, American Psychiatric Association, 1980

American Psychiatric Association: Diagnostic and Statistical Manual of Mental Disorders, 3rd Edition Revised. Washington, DC, American Psychiatric Association, 1987

American Psychiatric Association: Diagnostic and Statistical Manual of Mental Disorders, 4th Edition. Washington, DC, American Psychiatric Association, 1994

American Psychiatric Association: Diagnostic and Statistical Manual of Mental Disorders, 5th Edition. Washington, DC, American Psychiatric Association, 2013

Auchincloss EL, Samberg E (eds): Psychoanalytic Terms and Concepts. New Haven, CT, Yale University Press, 2012

Ayduk O, Mendoza–Denton R, Mischel W, Downey G, Peake PK, Rodriguez Met al: Regulating the interpersonal self: strategic self-regulation for coping with rejection sensitivity. J Pers Soc Psychol 79:776-792, 2000

Ayduk O, Zayas V, Downey G, et al: Rejection sensitivity and executive control: joint predictors of borderline personality features. J Res Pers 42:151–168, 2008 18496604

Baker L, Silk KR, Westen D, Nigg JT, Lohr NE: Malevolence, splitting, and parental ratings by borderlines. J Nerv Ment Dis 180:258–264, 1992 1556566

Barnicot K, Katsakou C, Marougka S, Priebe S: Treatment completion in psychotherapy for borderline personality disorder: a systematic review and meta-analysis. Acta Psychiatr Scand 123(5):327–338, 2011 21166785

Barone L: Developmental protective and risk factors in borderline personality disorder: a study using the Adult Attachment Interview. Attach Hum Dev 5(1):64–77, 2003 12745829

Bartlett FC: Thinking: An Experimental and Social Study. New York, Basic Books, 1958

Bateman A, Fonagy P: Effectiveness of partial hospitalization in the treatment of borderline personality disorder: a randomized controlled trial. Am J Psychiatry 156(10):1563–1569, 1999 10518167

Bateman A, Fonagy P: Psychotherapy for Borderline Personality Disorder: Mentalization-Based Treatment. New York, Oxford University Press, 2004

Beck AT, Freeman A, Davis DD, et al: Cognitive Therapy of Personality Disorders, 2nd Edition. New York, Guilford, 2004

Bender DS, Skodol AE: Borderline personality as a self-other representational disturbance. J Pers Disord 21(5):500–517, 2007 17953503

Berenson KR, Gyurak A, Ayduk O, et al: Rejection sensitivity and disruption of attention by social threats cues. J Res Pers 43:1064–1072, 2009 20160869

Berenson,KR, Downey G, Rafaeli E, et al: The rejection-rage contingency in borderline personality disorder. J Abnorm Psychol 120:681–690, 2011 21500875

Bion WR: Learning From Experience. New York, Basic Books, 1962

Bion WR: Notes on memory and desire. Psychoanalytic Forum 2:271–280, 1967

Blum HP: The concept of erotized transference. J Am Psychoanal Assoc 21(1):61–76, 1973 4713717

Bowlby J: A Secure Base: Parent-Child Attachment and Healthy Human Development. New York, Basic Books, 1988

Britton R: Subjectivity, objectivity, and triangular space. Psychoanal Q 73(1):47–61, 2004 14750465

Calabrese ML, Farber BA, Westen D: The relationship of adult attachment constructs to object relational patterns of representing self and others. J Am Acad Psychoanal Dyn Psychiatry 33(3):513–530, 2005 16238476

Caligor E, Clarkin JF: An object relations model of personality and personality pathology, in Psychodynamic Psychotherapy for Personality Disorders: A Clinical Handbook. Edited by Clarkin JF, Fonagy P, Gabbard GO. Washington DC, American Psychiatric Publishing, 2010, pp 3–36

Caligor E, Kernberg OF, Clarkin JF: Handbook of Dynamic Psychotherapy for Higher Level Personality Disorder. Washington, DC, American Psychiatric Publishing, 2007

Caligor E, Diamond D, Yeomans FE, et al: The interpretive process in the psychoanalytic psychotherapy of borderline personality pathology. J Am Psychoanal Assoc 57: 271–301, 2009 19516053

Carlson EA, Egeland B, Sroufe LA: A prospective investigation of the development of borderline symproms. Dev Pychopathol 21:1311–1334, 2009

Carsky M, Yeomans F: Overwhelming patients and overwhelmed therapists. Psychodyn Psychiatry 40(1):75–90, 2012 23006030

Caspi A, Roberts BW, Shier R: Personality development. Annu Rev Psychol 56: 453–484, 2005

Cervone D: Personality architecture: within-person structures and processes. Annu Rev Psychol 56:423–452, 2005 15709942

Cicchetti D, Beeghly M, Carlson V, et al: The emergence of the self in atypical populations, in The Self in Transition: Infancy to Childhood. Edited by Cicchetti D, Beeghly M. Chicago, IL, University of Chicago Press, 1990, pp 309–344

Clark LA: Assessment and diagnosis of personality disorder: perennial issues and an emerging reconceptualization. Annu Rev Psychol 58:227–257, 2007

Clarkin JF, De Panfilis C: Developing conceptualization of borderline personality disorder. J Nerv Ment Dis 201(2):88–93, 2013 23364115

Clarkin JF, Posner M: Defining the mechanisms of borderline personality disorder. Psychopathology 38(2):56–63, 2005 15802943

Clarkin JF, Widiger TA, Frances A, et al: Prototypic typology and the borderline personality disorder. J Abnorm Psychol 92: 263-275, 1983 6619404

Clarkin JF, Hull JW, Hurt SW: Factor structure of borderline personality disorder criteria. J Pers Disord 7:137–143, 1993

Clarkin JF, Yeomans FE, Kernberg OF: Psychotherapy for Borderline Personality. New York, Wiley, 1999

Clarkin JF, Foelsch PA, Levy KN, et al: The development of a psychodynamic treatment for patients with borderline personality disorder: a preliminary study of behavioral change. J Pers Disord 15(6):487–495, 2001 11778390

Clarkin JF, Yeomans FE, Kernberg OF: Psychotherapy for Borderline Personality: Focusing on Object Relations. Washington, DC, American Psychiatric Publishing, 2006

Clarkin JF, Levy KN, Lenzenweger M-F, Kernberg OF: Evaluating three treatments for borderline personality disorder: a multiwave study. Am J Psychiatry 164(6):922–928, 2007 17541052

Clarkin JF, Fonagy P, Levy KN, et al: Borderline personality disorder, in Handbook of Contemporary Psychodynamic Approaches to Psychopathology. Edited by Luyten P, Mayes LC, Fonagy P, et al. New York, Guilford, in press

Coifman KG, Berenson KR, Rafaeli R, et al: From negative to positive and back again: polarized affective and relational experience in borderline personality disorder. J Abnorm Psychol 121:668–679, 2012 22686872

Connolly MB, Crits-Christoph P, Shappell Sandi, et al; The relation of transference interpretations to outcome in the early sessions of brief supportive-expressive psychotherapy. Psychotherapy Research 9(4):485–495,1999

Crits-Christoph P, Gibbons M, Murkherjee D: Psychotherapy process-outcome research, in Bergin and Garfield's Handbook of Psychotherapy and Behavior Change, 6th Edition. Edited by Lambert MJ. New York, Wiley, 2013, pp 298–340

Depue RA, Lenzenweger MF: A neurobehavioral dimensional model, in Handbook of Personality Disorders: Theory, Research and Treatment. Edited by Livesley WJ. New York, Guilford, 2001, pp 136–176

Depue RA, Lenzenweger MF: A neurobehavioral dimensional model of personality disturbance, in Major Theories of Personality Disorder, 2nd Edition. Edited by Lenzenweger MF, Clarkin JF. New York, Guilford, 2005, pp 391–454

Diamond D, Clarkin JF, Stovall-McClough KC, et al: Patient-therapist attachment: impact on therapeutic process and outcome, in Attachment Theory and the Psychoanalytic Process. Edited by Cortina M, Marrone M. London, Whurr, 2003, pp 179–203

Diamond D, Yeomans FE, Levy K: Psychodynamic psychotherapy for narcissistic personality disorder, in The Handbook of Narcissism and Narcissistic Personality Disorder: Theoretical Approaches, Empirical Findings, and Treatment. Edited by Campbell K, Miller J. New York, Wiley, 2011, pp 423–433

Distel MA, Willemsen G, Ligthart L, et al: Genetic covariance structure of the four main features of borderline personality disorder. J Pers Disord 24(4):427–444, 2010 20695804

Dixon-Gordon KL, Chapman AL, Lovasz N, et al: Too upset to think: the interplay of borderline personality features, negative emotions, and social problem solving in the laboratory. Personal Disord 2:243–260, 2011 22448801

Doering S, Hörz S, Rentrop M, et al: Transference-focused psychotherapy v. treatment by community psychotherapists for borderline personality disorder: randomised controlled trial. Br J Psychiatry 196(5):389–395, 2010 20435966

Downey G, Feldman SI: Implications of rejection sensitivity for intimate relationships. J Pers Soc Psychol 6:1327–1343, 1996 8667172

Dozier M, Cue K, Barnett L. Clinicians as caregivers: role of attachment organization in treatment. J Consult Clin Psychol 62:793–800 2003 7962883

Dziobek I, Preißler S, Grozdanovic Z, Heuser I, Heekeren HR, Roepke S: Neuronal correlates of altered empathy and social cognition in borderline personality disorder. Neuroimage 57:539-548, 2011

Eisenberg N, Smith CL, Sadovsky A, et al: Effortful control: relations with emotional regulation, adjustment, and socialization in childhood, in Handbook of Self-Regulation: Research, Theory, and Applications. Edited by Baumeister RF, Vohs KD. New York, Guilford, 2004, pp 259–282

Eisenberger NI, Lieberman MD, Williams KD: Does rejection hurt? An fMRI study of social exclusion. Science 302:290–292, 2003 14551424

Fairbairn WRD: An Object-Relations Theory of the Personality. New York, Basic Books, 1943

Fairbairn WRD: Psychoanalytic Studies of Personality. London, Tavistock, 1952

Fertuck EA, Lenzenweger MF, Clarkin JF, et al: Executive neurocognition, memory systems, and borderline personality disorder. Clin Psychol Rev 26(3):346–375, 2006 15992977

Fonagy P, Leigh T, Steele M, et al: The relation of attachment status, psychiatric classification, and response to psychotherapy. J Consult Clin Psychol 64(1):22–31, 1996 8907081

Fonagy P, Steele M, Steele H, et al: Reflective-function manual: version 5.0. For application to the Adult Attachment Interview. Unpublished manuscript, University College, London, 1998

Fonagy P, Gergely G, Target M: The parent-infant dyad and the construction of the subjective self. J Child Psychol Psychiatry 48(3-4):288–328, 2007 17355400

Freud S: Observations on transference-love (1915), in The Standard Edition of the Complete Psychological Works of Sigmund Freud, Vol 12. Translated and edited by Strachey J. London, Hogarth, 1958, pp 157–171

Freud S: Mourning and melancholia (1917), in The Standard Edition of the Complete Psychological Works of Sigmund Freud, Vol 14. Translated and edited by Strachey J. London, Hogarth, 1958, pp 237–258

Freud S: Beyond the pleasure principle (1920), in The Standard Edition of the Complete Psychological Works of Sigmund Freud, Vol 18. Translated and edited by Strachey J. London, Hogarth, 1958, pp 3–64

Frith CD, Frith U: Mechanisms of social cognition. Annu Rev Psychol 63:287–313, 2012 21838544

Gabbard GO: Technical approaches to transference hate in the analysis of borderline patients. Int J Psychoanal 72(4):625–637, 1991 1797717

Gergely G, Watson JS: The social biofeedback theory of parental affect-mirroring: the development of emotional self-awareness and self-control in infancy. Int J Psychoanal 77(Pt 6):1181–1212, 1996 9119582

Giesen-Bloo J, van Dyck R, Spinhoven P, et al: Outpatient psychotherapy for borderline personality disorder: randomized trial of schema-focused therapy vs transference-focused psychotherapy. Arch Gen Psychiatry 63(6):649–658, 2006 16754838

Gill M: The connection of all transference to the actual analytic situation, in Analysis of Transference, Vol 1: Theory and Technique. New York, International Universities Press, 1982, pp 96–106

Green A: Le Travail du Négatif. Paris, Editions de Minuit, 1993

Green A: La position phobique centrale, in La Pensée Clinique. Paris, Editions Odile Jacob, 2002 pp 149–186

Grinker R, Werble B, Drye R: The Borderline Syndrome. New York, Basic Books, 1968

Gross JJ, John OP: Individual differences in two emotion regulation processes: implications for affect, relationships, and well-being. J Pers Soc Psychol 85:348–362, 2003 12916575

Gross JJ, Thompson RA: Emotion regulation: conceptual foundations, in Handbook of Emotion Regulation. Edited by Gross JJ. New York, Guilford, 2007, pp 351–372

Gunderson JG, Kolb JE: Discriminating features of borderline patients. Am J Psychiatry 135(7):792–796, 1978 665789

Gunderson JC, Links P: Handbook of Good Psychiatric Management for Borderline Personality Disorder. Washington DC, American Psychiatric Publishing, 2014

Gunderson JG, Lyons-Ruth K: BPD's interpersonal hypersensitivity phenotype. J Pers Disord 22: 22-41, 2008 18312121

Hallquist MN, Pilkonis PA: Refining the phenotype of borderline personality disorder: diagnostic criteria and beyond. Pers Disord 3(3):228–246, 2012 22823231

Hampson SE: Personality processes: mechanisms by which personality traits "get outside the skin." Annu Rev Psychol 63:315–339, 2012 21740225

Harter S: The Construction of the Self: A Developmental Perspective. New York, Guilford, 1999

Heatherton TF, Wagner DD: Cognitive neuroscience of self-regulation failure. Trends Cogn Sci 15(3):132–139, 2011 21273114

Herpertz S: Self-injurious behavior: psychopathological and nosological characteristics in subtypes of self-injurers. Acta Psychiatr Scand 91: 57–68, 1995 7754789

Hesse E: The Adult Attachment Interview: protocol, method of analysis, and empirical studies, in Handbook of Attachment: Theory, Research, and Clinical Applications. Edited by Cassidy J, Shaver P. New York, Guilford, 2010, pp 552–598

Hill D: Special place of the erotic transference in psychoanalysis. Psychoanal Inq 14:483–498, 1994

Høglend P, Bøgwald KP, Amlo S, et al: Transference interpretations in dynamic psychotherapy: do they really yield sustained effects? Am J Psychiatry 165(6):763–771, 2008 18413707

Hooker CI, Gyurak A, Verosky SC, et al: Neural activity to a partner's facial expression predicts self-regulation after conflict. Biol Psychiatry 67:406–413, 2010 20004365

Horowitz LM: Interpersonal Foundations of Psychopathology. Washington, DC, American Psychological Association, 2004

Jacobson E: Contribution to the metapsychology of psychotic identifications. J Am Psychoanal Assoc 2:239–262, 1954 13151997

Jacobson E: Denial and repression. J Am Psychoanal Assoc 5: 61–92, 1957 13398327

Jacobson E: The Self and the Object World. New York, International Universities Press, 1964

Jacobson E: On the paranoid urge to betray, in Depression: Comparative Studies of Normal, Neurotic, and Psychotic Conditions. New York, International Universities Press, 1971, pp 302–318

Johansen M, Karterud S, Pedersen G, et al: An investigation of the prototype validity of the borderline DSM-IV construct. Acta Psychiatr Scand 109(4):289–298, 2004 15008803

Joseph B: Transference: the total situation. Int J Psychoanal 66:447–454, 1985

Jovev M, Jackson HJ: The relationship of borderline personality disorder, life events and functioning in an Australian psychiatric sample. J Pers Disord 20:205–217, 2006 16776551

Kazdin A: Psychotherapy for children and adolescents, in Bergin and Garfield's Handbook of Psychotherapy and Behavior Change, 5th Edition. Edited by Lambert MJ. New York, Wiley, 2004, pp 543–589

Kernberg OF: Borderline Conditions and Pathological Narcissism. New York, Aronson, 1975

Kernberg OF: Internal World and External Reality: Object Relations Theory Applied. New York, Jason Aronson, 1980

Kernberg OF: Severe Personality Disorders: Psychotherapeutic Strategies. New Haven, CT, Yale University Press, 1984

Kernberg OF: Aggression in Personality Disorders and Perversions. New Haven, CT, Yale University Press, 1992

Kernberg OF: Aggression, trauma, and hatred in the treatment of borderline patients. Psychiatr Clin North Am 17(4):701–714, 1994 7877899

Kernberg OF: Love Relations: Normality and Pathology. New Haven, CT, Yale University Press, 1995

Kernberg OF: Aggressivity, Narcissism, and Self-Destructiveness in the Psychotherapeutic Relationship: New Developments in the Psychopathology and Psychotherapy of Severe Personality Disorders. New Haven, CT, Yale University Press, 2004

Kernberg OF: New developments in transference-focused psychotherapy. Int J Psychoanal, in press

Kernberg OF, Caligor E: A psychoanalytic theory of personality disorders, in Major Theories of Personality Disorder, 2nd Edition. Edited by Lenzenweger ML, Clarkin JF. New York, Guilford, 2005, pp 114–156

Kernberg OF, Diamond D, Yeomans FE, et al: Mentalization and attachment in borderline patients in transference focused psychotherapy, in Mind to Mind: Infant Research, Neuroscience, and Psychoanalysis. Edited by Jurist EJ, Slade A, Bergner S. New York, Other Press, 2008, pp 167–201

King-Casas B, Sharp C, Lomax-Bream L, et al: The rupture and repair of cooperation in borderline personality disorder. Science 321(5890):806–810, 2008 18687957

Klein M: Notes on some schizoid mechanisms. Int J Psychoanal 27(Pt 3-4):99–110, 1946 20261821

Klein M: Mourning and its relation to manic-depressive states, in Contributions to Psychoanalysis. London, Hogarth Press, 1948, pp 311–338

Klein M: Envy and Gratitude, a Study of Unconscious Sources. New York, Basic Books, 1957

Knight RP: Borderline states, in Psychoanalytic Psychiatry and Psychology. Edited by Knight RP, Friedman CR. New York, International Universities Press, 1954, pp 97–109

Kochanska G: Emotional development in children with different attachment histories: the first three years. Child Dev 72(2):474–490, 2001 11333079

Kochanska G, Knaack A: Effortful control as a personality characteristic of young children: antecedents, correlates, and consequences. J Pers 71(6):1087–1112, 2003 14633059

Koenigsberg H, Kernberg OF, Stone MH, et al (eds): Borderline Personality Disorder: Extending the Limits of Treatability. Basic Books, New York, 2000a

Koenigsberg HW, Kernberg OF, Stone MH, et al: Transference-focused psychotherapy in sequence with other modalities, in Borderline Patients: Extending the Limits of Treatability. New York, Basic Books, 2000b, pp 247–266

Koenigsberg HW, Kernberg OF, Stone MH, et al: Using dream material, in Borderline Patients: Extending the Limits of Treatability. New York, Basic Books, 2000c, pp 207–228

Koenigsberg HW, Fan J, Ochsner KN, et al: Neural correlates of the use of psychological distancing to regulate responses to negative social cues: a study of patients with borderline personality disorder. Biol Psychiatry 66(9):854–863, 2009a 19651401

Koenigsberg HW, Siever LJ, Lee H, et al: Neural correlates of emotion processing in borderline personality disorder. Psychiatry Res 172(3):192–199, 2009b 19394205

Korfine L, Hooley JM: Directed forgetting of emotional stimuli in borderline personality disorder. J Abnorm Psychol 109(2):214–221, 2000 10895559

Korfmacher J, Adam E, Ogawa J, et al: Adult attachment: implications for the therapeutic process in a home visitation intervention. Appl Dev Sci 1:43–52, 1997

Krueger F, Mccabe K, Moll J, et al: Neural correlates of trust. Proc Natl Acad Sci 104:20084-9, 2007 18056800

Lenzenweger MF: Current status of the scientific study of the personality disorders: an overview of epidemiological, longitudinal, experimental psychopathology, and neurobehavioral perspectives. J Am Psychoanal Assoc 58(4):741–778, 2010 21115756

Lenzenweger MF, Cicchetti D: Toward a developmental psychopathology approach to borderline personality disorder. Dev Psychopathol 17(4):893–898, 2005 16613423

Lenzenweger MF, Clarkin JF: Major Theories of Personality Disorder, 2nd Edition. New York, Guilford, 2005

Lenzenweger MF, Clarkin JF, Kernberg OF, et al: The Inventory of Personality Organization: Psychometric properties, factorial composition, and criterion relations with affect, aggressive dyscontrol, psychosis proneness, and self-domains in a nonclinical sample. Psychol Assess 13:577–591, 2001 11793901

Lenzenweger MF, Johnson MD, Willett JB: Individual growth curve analysis illuminates stability and change in personality disorder features: the longitudinal study of personality disorders. Arch Gen Psychiatry 61(10):1015–1024, 2004 15466675

Lenzenweger MF, Clarkin JF, Yeomans FE, et al: Refining the borderline personality disorder phenotype through finite mixture modeling: implications for classification. J Pers Disord 22(4):313–331, 2008 18684047

Lenzenweger MF, Clarkin JF, Levy KN, et al: Predicting domains and rates of change in borderline personality disorder. Pers Disord 3(2):185–195, 2012a 22452776

Lenzenweger MF, McClough JF, Clarkin JF, Kernberg OF: Exploring the interface of neurobehaviorally linked personality dimensions and personality organization in borderline personality disorder: the Multidimensional Personality Questionnaire and Inventory of Personality Organization. J Pers Disord 26(6):902–918, 2012b 23281675

Levy KN, Meehan KB, Kelly KM, et al: Change in attachment patterns and reflective function in a randomized control trial of transference-focused psychotherapy for borderline personality disorder. J Consult Clin Psychol 74(6):1027–1040, 2006 17154733

Levy KN, Meehan KB, Beeney JE, et al: Mechanisms of change in the psychodynamic treatment of borderline personality disorder: findings from experimental psychopathology and psychotherapy process and outcome. Paper presented at the Annual Meeting of the Society for Psychotherapy Research, Bern, Switzerland, June 2011

Levy KN, Meehan KB, Yeomans FE: An update and overview of the empirical evidence for transference-focused psychotherapy and other psychotherapies for borderline personality disorder, in Psychodynamic Psychotherapy Research: Evidence-Based Practice and Practice-Based Evidence. Edited by Levy RA, Ablon JS, Kächele H. New York, Springer, 2012, pp 139–167

Lieberman MD: Social cognitive neuroscience: a review of core processes. Annu Rev Psychol 58:259–289, 2007 17002553

Linehan MM: Cognitive-Behavioral Treatment of Borderline Personality Disorder. New York, Guilford, 1993

Linehan MM, Armstrong HE, Suarez A, et al: Cognitive-behavioral treatment of chronically parasuicidal borderline patients. Arch Gen Psychiatry 48(12):1060–1064, 1991 1845222

Livesley WJ: Conceptual and taxonomic issues, in Handbook of Personality Disorders: Theory, Research, and Treatment. Edited by Livesley WJ. New York, Guilford, 2001, pp 3–38

Mahler MS: A study of the separation-individuation process and its possible application to borderline phenomena in the psychoanalytic situation. Psychoanal Study Child 26:403–424, 1971 5163236

McMain SF, Guimond T, Streiner DL, et al: Dialectical behavior therapy compared with general psychiatric management for borderline personality disorder: clinical outcomes and functioning over a 2-year follow-up. Am J Psychiatry 169(6):650–661, 2012 22581157

Meyer B, Pilkonis PA: An attachment model of personality disorders, in Major Theories of Personality Disorder, 2nd Edition. Edited by Lenzenweger MF, Clarkin JF. New York, Guilford, 2005, pp 231–281

Miano A, Fertuck EA, Arntz A, Stanley B: Rejection sensitivity is a mediator between borderline personality disorder features and facial trust appraisal. J Pers Disord 27(4):442–456, 2013 23586933

Mischel W, Shoda Y: Toward a unified theory of personality: integrating dispositions and processing dynamics within the cognitive-affective processing system, in Handbook of Personality: Theory and Research, 3rd Edition. Edited by John OP, Robins RW, Pervin LA. New York, Guilford, 2008, pp 208–241

Mitchell S, Aron L (eds): Relational Psychoanalysis: The Emergence of a Tradition. Relational Perspectives Book Series, Vol 14. Hillsdale, NJ, Analytic Press, 1999

Nelson K, Fivush R: The emergence of autobiographical memory: a social cultural developmental theory. Psychol Rev 111(2):486–511, 2004 15065919

Ochsner KN, Gross JJ: Cognitive emotion regulation: insights from social cognitive and affective neuroscience. Curr Dir Psychol Sci 17:153–158, 2008

Paris J: Borderline Personality Disorder: A Multidimensional Approach. Washington DC, American Psychiatric Press, 1994

Patrick M, Hobson RP, Castle D, et al: Personality disorder and the mental representation of early social experience. Dev Psychopathol 6:375–388, 1994

Perry JC, Herman JL: Trauma and defense in the etiology of borderline personality disorder, in Borderline Personality Disorder: Etiology and Treatment. Edited by Paris J. Washington DC, American Psychiatric Press, 1993, pp 123–139

Pincus AL: A contemporary integrative interpersonal theory of personality disorders, in Major theories of personality disorder, 2nd Edition. Edited by Lenzenweger M, Clarkin J. New York, Guilford, 2005, pp 282–331

Piper WE, Duncan SC: Object relations theory and short-term dynamic psychotherapy: findings from the Quality of Object Relations Scale. Clin Psychol Rev 19(6):669–685, 1999 10421951

Piper WE, Azim HFA, Joyce AS, McCallum M: Transference interpretations, therapeutic alliance, and outcome in short-term individual psychotherapy. Arch Gen Psychiatry 48(10):946–953, 1991 1929765

Posner MI, Rothbart MK: Developing mechanisms of self-regulation. Dev Psychopathol 12(3):427–441, 2000 11014746

Posner MI, Rothbart MK, Vizueta N, et al: Attentional mechanisms of borderline personality disorder. Proc Natl Acad Sci 99:16366–16370, 2002

Racker H: The meanings and uses of countertransference. Psychoanal Q 26(3):303–357, 1957 13465913

Reich W: Character Analysis. New York, Farrar, Straus, and Giroux, 1972

Renneberg B, Herm K, Hahn A, et al: Perception of social participation in borderline personality disorder. Clin Psychol Psychother 19(6):473–480, 2012 22076727

Rockland LH: Supportive Therapy for Borderline Patients: A Psychodynamic Approach. New York, Guilford, 1992

Rothbart MK, Bates JE: Temperament, in Handbook of Child Psychology, Vol 3, 5th Edition. Edited by Damon W, Eisenberg N. New York, Wiley, 1998, pp 105–176

Russell JJ, Moskowitz DS, Zuroff DC, et al: Stability and variability of affective experience and interpersonal behavior in borderline personality disorder. J Abnorm Psychol 116(3):578–588, 2007 17696713

Sadikaj G, Russell JJ, Moskowitz DS, Paris J: Affect dysregulation in individuals with borderline personality disorder: persistence and interpersonal triggers. J Pers Assess 92(6):490–500, 2010 20954051

Sanderson C, Clarkin JF: Further use of the NEO-PI-R personality dimensions in differential treatment planning, in Personality Disorders and the Five-Factor Model of Personality, 3rd Edition. Edited by Widiger TA, Costa Jr PT. Washington, D.C., American Psychological Association, 2013, pp 325–348

Sanislow CA, Grilo CM, McGlashan TH: Factor analysis of the DSM-III-R borderline personality disorder criteria in psychiatric inpatients. Am J Psychiatry 157(10):1629–1633, 2000 11007717

Selby EA, Ward AC, Joiner TE Jr: Dysregulated eating behaviors in borderline personality disorder: are rejection sensitivity and emotion dysregulation linking mechanisms? Int J Eat Disord 43(7):667–670, 2010 19806606

Shea M, Stout R, Gunderson J, et al: Short-term diagnostic stability of schizotypal, borderline, avoidant, and obsessive-compulsive personality disorders. Am J Psychiatry 159:2036–2041, 2002 12450953

Shedler J, Westen D: The Shedler-Westen assessment procedure: making personality diagnosis clinically meaningful, in Psychodynamic Psychotherapy for Personality Disorders: A Clinical Handbook. Edited by Clarkin JF, Fonagy P, Gabbard GO. Washington, DC, American Psychiatric Publishing, 2010, pp 125–161

Silbersweig D, Clarkin JF, Goldstein M, et al: Failure of frontolimbic inhibitory function in the context of negative emotion in borderline personality disorder. Am J Psychiatry 164(12):1832–1841, 2007 18056238

Silk KR, Friedel RO: Psychopharmacological and neurobiological considerations, in The Integrated Treatment of Borderline Personality Disorder. Edited by Livesley WJ, Dimaggio G, Clarkin JF. New York, Guilford, in press

Skodol AE, Pagano ME, Bender DS, et al: Stability of functional impairment in patients with schizotypal, borderline, avoidant, or obsessive-compulsive personality disorder over two years. Psychol Med 35:443–451, 2005 15841879

Staebler K, Helbing E, Rosenbach C, Renneberg B: Rejection sensitivity and borderline personality disorder. Clin Psychol Psychother 18(4):275–283, 2011a 21110407

Staebler K, Renneberg B, Stopsack M, et al: Facial emotional expression in reaction to social exclusion in borderline personality disorder. Psychol Med 41(9):1929–1938, 2011b 21306661

Steiner J: Psychic Retreats: Pathological Organization of the Personality in Psychotic, Neurotic and Borderline Patients. London, Routledge and The Institute of Psychoanalysis, 1993

Stepp SD, Pilkonis PA, Yaggi KE, et al: Interpersonal and emotional experiences of social interactions in borderline personality disorder. J Nerv Ment Dis 197(7):484–491, 2009 19597355

Stern BL, Yeomans FE, Diamond D, et al: Transference-focused psychotherapy for narcissistic personality disorder, in Treating Pathological Narcissism. Edited by Ogrodniczuk J. Washington, DC, American Psychological Association, 2013

Stiglmayr CE, Ebner-Priemer UW, Bretz J, et al: Dissociative symptoms are positively related to stress in borderline personality disorder. Acta Psychiatr Scand 117:139-147, 2008 18028248

Stoffers J, Völlm BA, Rücker G, et al: Pharmacological interventions for borderline personality disorder. Cochrane Database Syst Rev (6):CD005653, 2010 20556762

Stone MH: Personality Disordered Patients: Treatable and Untreatable. Washington, DC, American Psychiatric Publishing, 2006

Trull TJ, Ebner-Priemer UW: Using experience sampling methods/ecological momentary assessment (ESM/EMA) in clinical assessment and clinical research: introduction to the special section. Psychol Assess 21(4):457–462, 2009 19947780

Westen D: The impact of sexual abuse on self structure, in Disorders and Dysfunctions of the Self (5th Rochester Symposium on Developmental Psychopathology, 1991). Edited by Cicchetti D, Toth SL. Rochester, NY, University of Rochester Press, 1993, pp 223–250

Widiger TA, Simonsen E: Alternative dimensional models of personality disorder: finding a common ground, in Dimensional Models of Personality Disorders: Refining the Research Agenda for DSM-V. Edited by Widiger TA, Simonsen E, Sirovatka P, et al. Washington, DC, American Psychiatric Association, 2006, pp 1–21

Winnicott DW: Hate in the counter-transference. Int J Psychoanal 30:69–74, 1949

Wnuk S, McMain S, Links PS, et al: Factors related to dropout from treatment in two outpatient treatments for borderline personality disorder. J Pers Disord 27(6):716–726, 2013 23718760

Yeomans FE, Selzer MA, Clarkin JF: Treating the Borderline Patient: A Contract-Based Approach. New York, Basic Books, 1992

Yeomans FE, Gutfreund J, Selzer MA, et al: Factors related to drop-outs by borderline patients. J Psychother Pract Res 3(1):16–24, 1994 22700170

Yeomans FE, Clarkin JF, Kernberg OF: A Primer of Transference-Focused Psychotherapy for the Borderline Patient. Northvale, NJ, Jason Aronson, 2002

Yun RJ, Stern BL, Lenzenweger MF, et al: Refining personality disorder subtypes and classification using finite mixture modeling. Pers Disord 4(2):121–128, 2013 23046042

Zanarini MC, Williams AA, Lewis RE, et al: Reported pathological childhood experiences associated with the development of borderline personality disorder. Am J Psychiatry 154(8):1101–1106, 1997 9247396

Zanarini MC, Frankenburg FR, Hennen J, et al: The longitudinal course of borderline psychopathology: 6-year prospective follow-up of the phenomenology of borderline personality disorder. Am J Psychiatry 160:274–283, 2003 12562573

Zanarini MC, Frankenburg FR, Reich DB, Fitzmaurice G: Attainment and stability of sustained symptomatic remission and recovery among patients with borderline personality disorder and axis II comparison subjects: a 16-year prospective follow-up study. Am J Psychiatry 169(5):476–483, 2012 22737693

INDEX

Page numbers printed in **boldface** refer to tables or figures. Page numbers followed by *n* indicate note numbers.